Religion as a Social Determinant of Public Health

Religion as a Social Determinant of Public Health

Edited by **ELLEN L. IDLER**

OXFORD
UNIVERSITY PRESS

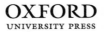

OXFORD
UNIVERSITY PRESS

Oxford University Press is a department of the University of Oxford.
It furthers the University's objective of excellence in research, scholarship,
and education by publishing worldwide.

Oxford   New York
Auckland   Cape Town   Dar es Salaam   Hong Kong   Karachi
Kuala Lumpur   Madrid   Melbourne   Mexico City   Nairobi
New Delhi   Shanghai   Taipei   Toronto

With offices in
Argentina   Austria   Brazil   Chile   Czech Republic   France   Greece
Guatemala   Hungary   Italy   Japan   Poland   Portugal   Singapore
South Korea   Switzerland   Thailand   Turkey   Ukraine   Vietnam

Oxford is a registered trade mark of Oxford University Press
in the UK and certain other countries.

Published in the United States of America by
Oxford University Press
198 Madison Avenue, New York, NY 10016

© Oxford University Press 2014

Cataloging-in-Publication data is on file with the Library of Congress

9780199362202 (hbk.)
9780199362219 (pbk.)

1   3   5   7   9   8   6   4   2

Printed in the United States of America on acid-free paper

CONTENTS

FOREWORD

I n 2005, Emory University embarked on a set of strategic initiatives, among them, one on religion and the human spirit; the Religion and Public Health Collaborative, created as part of that initiative, built on the intellectual traditions of the Interfaith Health Program and the Carter Center. Ellen Idler was hired as part of that effort; her joint appointments in sociology and public health sparked conversations about the relationship between religion and public health across campus and among colleagues worldwide. This work of scholarship has sprung from this committed conversation, across unusually distant disciplinary boundaries.

Is religion a social determinant of health? Does affiliation with a congregation or attendance at religious functions contribute to social capital? What impact does religious practice and observance have on the health of individuals and the larger communities? These and other questions are explored throughout this volume.

In a 1988 report on the future of public health, the Institute of Medicine of the National Academies of Science defined the mission of public health as "fulfilling society's interest in assuring conditions in which people can be healthy."[1] The focus of public health is often on the prevention of disease or disability, and the frame of reference is on populations rather than individuals. The first function of public health is to assess the health problems or threats and risk factors in a population. Next, public health should set policies to improve or protect the health of the populations. The final public health function has been termed "assurance"—making sure that resources are adequate to meet identified public health needs. These resources could include specialized programs to improve health literacy, provide immunizations or reproductive health services, or expand health insurance.

It has long been recognized that individual health is influenced not only by genetics, biologic exposures, individual behaviors, and access to quality health services but also by the social and cultural environment. The World Health Organization's recently formed Commission on the Social Determinants of Health noted, "Together, the structured determinants and conditions of daily life constitute the social determinants of health and are responsible for a major part of the health inequities between and within countries."[2] It would seem that religious institutions clearly qualify as "determinants and conditions of daily life" but in what way might they influence health? Furthermore, religious beliefs often unite people within and between communities, sometimes to the exclusion of nonbelievers. In that regard, religious communities influence "social capital," which is seen as "cooperation and trust at the level of societies."[3]

So, even if religion influences social capital and religious practices and beliefs are themselves social determinants of health, why does it matter to public health? First, improvement in the health of populations depends upon a strong assessment of all factors affecting health, including the knowledge and beliefs of constituents. Policies to improve health must take into account this assessment. In many situations, in fulfillment of their social mission, religious communities can provide substantial and sustained resources to address health inequities to improve the public health.

This volume provides many detailed examples of religion as a health determinant and is a rich source for those involved in both religion and public health.

James W. Curran, MD, MPH
Rollins School of Public Health
Emory University
2013

PREFACE | *Religious Literacy Is a Twenty-First-Century Skill*

ELLEN IDLER AND LAURIE PATTON

This volume presents original scholarship at the intersection of religion and public health, two disciplines not often thought of together. Although it is now commonplace thinking in the world of public health that the social conditions in which people grow and live are primary determinants of population health, these determinants are usually framed in terms of economic and political conditions. Religion is rarely if ever mentioned in treatments of the subject. The authors of this volume all share the view that we ignore the role of religion in public health—particularly global public health—to our own disadvantage.

In the study of religion, there is a growing interest in health as it affects and is affected by religious behavior. This interest is part of a larger pattern: gone are the days when religion was understood as a separate sphere of human activity. Scholars have increasingly focused on the connections between religious activity and other modes of activity (economic, political, cultural, psychological, and so on). The increased interest in health among religion scholars is thus part of a larger phenomenon, one that requires deeper description and analysis of religious practices and institutions, both historically and in the present day.

Health literacy is a key concern of global health; religious literacy should also be a focus for scholars of both religion and public health. Many recent studies show a profound ignorance in many quarters about other people's religions, but knowledge about religious practices, particularly as they affect health, is essential for human flourishing in this increasingly multireligious world. Religious literacy is a twenty-first-century skill in many fields but especially in public health.

Under the umbrella of scholarship in religion and health, much of the space and almost all of the popular perception is taken up by work on religion and *medicine*. Does prayer heal? Should spiritual needs be assessed in physician visits? Can traditional or alternative healing practices be integrated into Western medical care systems? Can spirituality help one cope with illness? There is a tendency to want a single answer to these questions—a resounding "yes" for those who would like religion to be better integrated into health systems and a "no" or at the very most a "maybe" for those who are more skeptical. In this volume, we take a more complex approach. We begin with the assumption that the intersections of health and religion have barely been described, much less analyzed, and that "thick description" is the first order of business. New religious practices and communities and new health practices and communities are coming into being and interacting in new ways every day, and there is every reason to assume that such dynamic interactions also took place in history. Such dynamism is at the heart of our work.

Moving beyond medicine and the health of individual patients, we are concerned with the health of populations and communities. We pair that concern with a focus on religion—*religions*—as shared practices, beliefs, and institutions, distinct from the subjective and potentially idiosyncratic spirituality of individuals. We are interested in exploring the complex, multifaceted role that faith traditions play in determining indicators of public health such as infant mortality, life expectancy, and cause-specific deaths. Some of that health-determining influence flows through people's participation in religious practices and affiliation with mosques, synagogues, and churches. Some of it flows through lifestyle factors associated with religious observance. Some comes from relationships between religious institutions and institutions of public health and medical care. Some comes from the role that religious institutions play in their communities, in providing help for those in need and leveraging social capital.

We argue that the influence of religion on public health is ubiquitous in most societies, but we emphatically do *not* argue that this influence is always benign. Sometimes social determinants are beneficial for health, but sometimes they are not. Sometimes the interests of public health institutions and religious institutions are aligned, and sometimes they are at odds. Only rarely are they not related to each other at all.

The chapters in this work are written by distinguished scholars at Emory University's Schools of Public Health, Theology, Nursing, Medicine, Law, its Center for Ethics, and the Arts and Sciences departments of anthropology, religion, and sociology. They have a variety of scholarly, scientific, professional, and clinical backgrounds, but they share a commitment to interdisciplinary inquiry. As a result, while individual articles may have particular emphases, the volume as a whole weaves together social scientific, humanistic, and scientific inquiry in a subtle interdisciplinary texture.

The volume is the result of a faculty seminar that ran at Emory from 2010 to 2013. Almost all of the participants were present or former faculty members at Emory University, with the exception of two of the founding members of the African (now International) Religious Health Assets Programme, an international collaborative with close ties to Emory. The group met monthly to discuss outlines and chapters (including overseas participants via Skype). Manuscripts were posted on a secure website, allowing members to share resources and comment on each other's work. The process of producing this work was an exemplar of contemporary interdisciplinary scholarship facilitated by technology. Sustaining it over a period of years was only possible because of the dedicated commitment of members, with some occasional extra doses of enthusiasm from the editor. We believe the coherence of the intellectual exchange of this interdisciplinary faculty seminar will carry over to practitioners, students, and researchers in public health and faith institutions and that it will play a role in initiating dialogue between them.

The overall argument of the book is laid out in chapter 1, "Religion: The Invisible Social Determinant." This chapter, written by Ellen Idler, reviews the logic of the social determinants of health approach and explains why religion belongs among the social determinants. Briefly, the answer is twofold: religious practices and institutions have both a direct impact on health through a variety of pathways and an indirect impact through their articulation with economic and political determinants.

Following chapter 1, the work is divided into five parts, each containing several chapters written by experts in many fields. Part I engages in the kind of "thick description" of religious practice that establishes the foundation for exploring the dynamic connections between religion and public health. Each description in this section is written by a scholar of the religious tradition described, one who in many cases is also an active, observant member of the faith. Our description of these practices is organized by their cycles of repetition. Geshe Lobsang Tenzin Negi and Brendan Ozawa-de Silva ("Refuge Meditation in Tibetan Buddhism"), Eric Reinders ("Taiji in Taoism"), Kathryn Yount ("Hijab in Islam"), and George Grant and Jose Montenegro ("Vegetarianism in Seventh-day Adventism"), describe practices engaged in on a daily basis. Descriptions of weekly practices include Phillip Thompson's "The Eucharist in Roman Catholicism" and Don

Saliers's "Congregational Song and Health," in mainline Protestantism. Religious practices engaged in just once per year are represented by Chikako Ozawa-de Silva's look at the New Year's visitation of Shinto shrines and Abdullahi An-Na'im's description of Ramadan fasting. Finally, we take one-time rituals in order of their occurrence in the life course: Don Seeman writes about circumcision in Judaism, Emmanuel Lartey describes girls' puberty rituals in African religious traditions, Wesley de Souza discusses adult baptism by immersion in Latin American Pentecostalism, and Bhagirath Majmudar writes about funeral and cremation rites in Hinduism. Each of these pieces is followed by resources for further reading on the practice and a note from the editor outlining the state of health research on it.

Part II takes a historical perspective on the understudied, underappreciated relationship between religion and public health in England and the United States. In the eighteenth and nineteenth centuries, as public health institutions were being created, religious institutions were already powerful and well established. Religious leaders were frequently in the forefront of public health reform movements, often bringing to the effort a strong social justice orientation that linked economic and living conditions to health. Karen Scheib writes about the contributions of John Wesley, the founder of Methodism, to increasing lay health knowledge and access to affordable care in eighteenth-century England. John Blevins focuses on the quite different situation in the United States in the nineteenth century, with its sanitary reform movement, temperance movement, and the important role of the Social Gospel tradition in influencing the shape of public health institutions. The two institutions have not always been cooperative partners, however, and we also take a look at a period in US history when religious motivations dictated reproductive health policy in a way that did not improve the public's health. Carol Hogue and Lynn Hogue detail the sweeping effects of nineteenth-century Comstock laws, which severely limited sex education and access to information about contraceptive practice, abortion, and, by extension, women's reproductive health. This section exclusively focuses on the United States and England because the little research that exists comes from these two countries. However, we view this work as critical background. For example, the effects of religious commitment on AIDS education and public discourse in developing countries might be informed by consideration of the debate over the Comstock laws. The roles of charismatic religious reformers in Eastern Europe or the former Soviet states might be informed by the study of John Wesley's role in ensuring public health.

In Part III, we examine the life course consequences of religious practices and their relationship to the social support, social constraints, and social capital provided by religious institutions. Just as the health effects of early childhood economic adversity play out over time, we see the public health implications of cyclical religious practices, and the institutions in which they take place, as having an accumulating effect on physical and mental health as people grow up, mature, and grow old. Laura Gaydos and Patricia Page begin at the beginning with religious influences on reproductive health. Ellen Idler reviews the research on religion and health through the life course with an emphasis on mortality outcomes, summarizing the research from studies of specific religious groups and individuals in population-based studies. Brendan Ozawa-de Silva completes this section with a chapter on religion and mental health problems and well-being, focusing especially on the development of meditation practices derived from contemplative Buddhism.

Part IV takes the global perspective. Religious institutions have long had an impact on the health of communities around the world through the direct provision of health services and through relief and development efforts. Peter Brown discusses the historical and contemporary role of religious institutions in the burgeoning field of global health and the need for religious literacy to move the field forward. Matthew Bersagel Braley tells the surprising story of the World Council of Churches' Christian Medical Commission and its influence on its neighbor in Geneva, the World Health Organization, while laying out the changes in theological thinking that drove the changes in both institutions. Ellen Idler writes about the religious origins of some well-known social institutions, such as the La Leche League, that have addressed community health problems with entirely novel, religiously inspired solutions. James Cochrane, Gary Gunderson, and Deborah McFarland, founders of the African Religious Health Assets Programme, write about the origins and mission of that innovative institution. Each of these cases has a kind of bidirectionality: while religious groups are a social determinant of health, so, too, health considerations may influence theological thinking and the shape of religious institutions and practices.

In Part V, we examine three worldwide epidemics and take a look at the role that religion is playing or could play in finding solutions. Safiya George Dalmida and Sandra Thurman write about the complex role of religion in the progression of the HIV/AIDS epidemic in the United States and abroad. Mimi Kiser and Scott Santibañez discuss the serious potential for a global influenza pandemic and explore the role local faith communities have played as partners with public health officials in education and immunization efforts. Kenneth Hepburn and Theodore Johnson examine the role of religious institutions in providing long-term care for Alzheimer's patients, as that disease reaches epidemic proportions in developed countries.

We close the book by looking to the future to imagine religion's role as a social determinant of twenty-first-century health and to see what productive partnerships can be constructed to face emerging challenges to public health. In keeping with the interdisciplinary approach of the book, we have perspectives from ethicist Paul Root Wolpe, health policy expert Walter Burnett, and sociologist Ellen Idler.

A full understanding of the social determinants of global public health—a field growing in importance for public health scholars and practitioners as well as religious bodies and leaders—cannot be reached without including religious practices and religious institutions. Conversely, religious institutions cannot help but be shaped by global health and public health concerns. Our hope is that this volume will begin to end the exclusion of this essential sector from paradigms in the study of both health and religion.

ACKNOWLEDGMENTS

The long undertaking of developing these ideas has been supported by many organizations and individuals within Emory University. Initial financial support for the seminar came from the University Strategic Initiative's funding for the Religion and Public Health Collaborative (Ellen Idler, Director) and from the Center for Faculty Development and Excellence (Laurie Patton, Director until 2011). Many of the ideas for the volume were developed in a cross-listed interdisciplinary graduate seminar on Religion and Public Health taught by Ellen Idler in 2010 and 2011; she would like to thank the wonderful students from the Rollins School of Public Health, the Candler School of Theology, and the departments of sociology, anthropology, and religion for their willingness to register for such an unconventional course and their openness in engaging with each other across disciplinary lines. Specific graduate students who contributed many hours of research assistance and who deserve special thanks include Kate Cartwright, Jill Daugherty, and Patrick McLaughlin. Susan Landskroener provided indefatigable staff support.

Normally one would thank those colleagues who provided comments on the manuscript along the way and offered insights, pushback, or connections to readings one didn't know about. But in this volume those people already have their names in the table of contents. The production of this volume has been a remarkable group effort that was not without arguments or strongly stated positions but was sustained by a shared commitment to the importance of the ideas and the need to bring them forward. Many of us will find a sad gap on our calendars on the third Wednesday of each month.

The editor wishes to thank her mentors, Stanislav Kasl and Peter Berger, for cultivating her intellectual interest in religion, and her father for her exposure to its practice. Finally, long-suffering spouses come in for thanks for their forbearance; the editor's, however, sacrificed far more than she had any right to expect, and it is not even a slight exaggeration to say that this volume would not have existed without him.

Notes

1. National Research Council, *The Future of Public Health* (Washington, DC: National Academies Press, 1988).
2. World Health Organization, *Closing the Gap in a Generation: Health Equity Through Action on the Social Determinants of Health—Final Report of the Commission on Social Determinants of Health* (Geneva, Switzerland, 2008).
3. Robert Putnam, *Bowling Alone: The Collapse and Revival of American Community* (New York: Simon and Schuster, 2000).

1 | Religion: The Invisible Social Determinant

ELLEN IDLER

T HE CUMBERLAND VALLEY IN SOUTH-CENTRAL Pennsylvania is beautiful country, with expansive, well-kept farms and fields and orchards in every shade of green and gold. Some of the country's earliest settlers came here from the British Isles to find religious freedom, building their barns and houses from gray stone and raising herds of black-and-white dairy cows. The Cumberland county seat, Carlisle, Pennsylvania, located just north of the Gettysburg battlefield, was first settled by Scots-Irish immigrants who founded the First Presbyterian Church there in 1734. Carlisle's Second Presbyterian Church split off from that congregation a hundred years later, in 1833.

Jennifer McKenna grew up in this valley in the 1960s. When she returned as an adult to become associate pastor of the Second Presbyterian Church in 2004, she was struck by something that had changed dramatically since her childhood: the quality of the air. Although one would not expect a small town in an agricultural valley to have a serious problem with air pollution, the American Lung Association had listed Cumberland County as the fourteenth most polluted county in the United States. Rates of asthma, emphysema, and bronchitis had climbed, especially in children. School nurses were reporting a dramatic increase in inhaler use, and physicians noted that they were prescribing stronger and stronger medications for their patients with respiratory ailments.

The source of the poor air quality, especially the high levels of particulate matter in the air, was the three thousand diesel trucks that drove through the area each day and often made rest stops along a short highway that connects US 81 to the Pennsylvania Turnpike; local residents call it the "Miracle Mile." The problem wasn't just the sheer volume of trucks; it was the fact that truckers would take their mandated ten-hour rest periods in one of the many truck service areas *without ever turning off their motors.* Although some service areas had hook-up facilities to provide power to the trucks, many drivers preferred to keep their trucks running.

In 2004, a group of physicians concerned that the air quality was compromising the health of the community ran an ad in the local paper calling attention to the problem. Reverend McKenna responded by putting a notice in her church bulletin asking, "Anybody interested in trying to figure out what we can do about the air?" Twenty people showed up for a meeting to discuss possible solutions. This group and those who joined them from other religious congregations and community groups formed the Clean Air Board of Central Pennsylvania in 2005. The members of the Clean Air Board quickly went to work. They went to truck stops, diners, schools, and government offices to share information about the problem; they circulated petitions and conducted workshops. In 2008, they succeeded in getting the Pennsylvania Department of Environmental Protection to consider an anti-idling regulation that required trucks to use external power sources when they are parked and running. Eventually, the legislature took action to enshrine the requirement in law; the Diesel-Powered Motor Vehicle Idling Act was signed by Governor Ed Rendell in October 2008 went into effect in February 2009.

When asked by the head of the Pennsylvania Department of Environmental Protection why she was interested in this effort, Reverend McKenna replied, "We are a faith-based organization of citizens because I believe that we are supposed to be good stewards of the earth and take care of it."[1] She might well have added, "We take care of the earth for everyone who lives on it." After all, the air of the Cumberland Valley and the state of Pennsylvania is breathed by everyone—not only Presbyterians but also members of other religious congregations as well as those who have never set foot in a church, synagogue, or mosque.

Reverend McKenna was suggesting a role for religious institutions in ensuring public health. Reverend McKenna and her colleagues acted manifestly on behalf of the public's health to prevent disease by controlling the conditions of the environment, to educate key players, and to organize a community response when the health of the community was threatened. Community members came together to create a new social institution—the Clean Air Board—with a mission to change, through legal regulation, behaviors that were harming the health of all. It was a mission motivated at least in part by religious teachings.

It is public health and the role that religious institutions have played in shaping it that we take as the subject of this book. Public health is concerned with the health of populations—something more than the sum of the health of the individuals within them. It is, to paraphrase Charles-Edward Amory Winslow, one of the founders of the American Public Health Association: the science and practice of preventing disease and promoting health through sanitation, infection control, education, organized health services, and the provision of adequate standards of living for the maintenance of health to protect the ability of individuals to realize their birthright of health and longevity.[2] A population's health is measured by indicators such as life expectancy, infant mortality, and the distribution of disease and disability—a population is a living thing and these are its vital signs.

Our perspective on religion in this book corresponds to our view of health: religion, like public health, has an essentially social character and cannot be understood apart from the groups of people who form themselves into groups for the purpose of practicing their faith. Scholars disagree about the etymology, but one traditional derivation of the word "religion" is from the Latin *religio*, meaning the practice of rites, ceremonies, or a way of life that recognizes a divine higher power.[3] It probably evolved from the word *lego*, meaning to choose or take hold of something.[4] Together these derivations imply both a ritual-practicing social group and the force of belief that holds it together. But, importantly, religion is not one abstract thing; it is many specific, different, contrasting, and even conflicting things. Religious beliefs that bind people together in social groups are particular to those groups: A set of beliefs that binds like-minded believers together simultaneously marks them off from other sets of believers, and both of these sets are marked off from others who are not affiliated with any religious group. Taken together, these groups form populations, whose health may be influenced in various ways by their religious beliefs and practices.

For Good and Ill: The Health Effects of Religion

Researchers have long recognized the role of religious institutions in the health of populations. Sociologist Emile Durkheim was the first to use statistical data to link mortality by suicide to a range of social influences, including religion.[5] The son of a French rabbi, Durkheim was concerned with the rising suicide rates in Europe at the turn of the twentieth century. His research showed that suicides were distributed quite unequally within and between countries; he found higher rates for widowed and divorced individuals compared with those who were married, for men compared with women, and for Protestants compared with Roman Catholics and Jews.

Religion as Social Support

One of the forces that Durkheim saw causing the increased rate of suicide was alienation, that is, the loss of close relationships and all of the benefits that they provide. This critical support and nurturance may be provided by any of a number of social groups, including families, friends, neighbors, voluntary organizations, and religious groups. Ties to social groups give an individual multiple roles to play—as spouse, parent, sibling, worker, active citizen, or fellow congregant. These roles provide feedback, self-esteem, and social recognition, all of which provide a sense of well-being as well as material and emotional support when they are needed. An impressive amount of research on the importance of social connectedness is summarized in a recent meta-analysis of 148 studies from around the world;[6] this analysis shows that social involvement is unquestionably associated with better health and longer lives.

Religious group membership or participation in religious services is frequently included among the types of social ties in this research, as they were in Durkheim's work and in the Alameda County Study, the first of the modern epidemiological studies to link social networks to mortality from all causes.[7] A subgroup of these studies has focused specifically on religious ties; one recent example is an analysis of data from the US National Health Interview Survey.[8] In this study of twenty-two thousand adults, those who never attended religious services were almost 50 percent more likely to die from any cause over the fifteen years of the study than those who attended services more often than once per week. Other social ties were also important in this study—those who were married and socially active were also at less risk of dying—but the effect of religious attendance was independently significant.

We examine the research literature on religion and mortality in much more detail in chapter 18. For now, the important thing to note is that, in addition to whatever changes the Second Presbyterian Church and the Clean Air Board have brought about in Pennsylvania's air quality, they also represent social and community institutions that, like any other group, provide health-protective social ties in the lives of their members. They may represent extraordinary examples of religion and public health activism on one level, but, on another level, they are also perfectly ordinary contributors to public health.

Religion as Social Control

Social groups—including religious groups—may also contribute to the health of their members in other ways by helping to regulate behavior. Durkheim thought that at the same time that membership in groups prevented alienation—by providing the "carrots" of warmth and friendship—social ties also came with "sticks"—by providing pressure to regulate behavior. He saw the normal human condition as one in which people have insatiable desires for material things: the more we have, the more we want. One of the major functions of society, he thought, was to rein in those desires and control unbridled appetites to allow people to live together harmoniously by encouraging (or demanding) the sacrifice of some self-interest for the good of the whole. But Durkheim saw these curbs becoming less effective in the modern world, and this was another cause of the increasing suicide rates—he called it *anomie*, a state of being without social norms or rules.

Religious groups are excellent examples of social organizations that impose rules on members to control behavior. They expect sacrifices of time and money; they regulate sexual, marital, and family relationships; and they may impose restrictions on dress, days of rest, or other routines. Importantly, given our concern with health, they may require adherents to maintain strict dietary practices or to abstain from alcohol or cigarette smoking. Of course, some faith traditions, such as Seventh-Day Adventists, Orthodox Jews, or Muslims, regulate such personal behaviors much more strictly than others do. But research shows that even among members of mainstream Protestant churches in the United States (like Carlisle's Second Presbyterian), rates of smoking and alcohol use are significantly lower than they are for the nonreligious.[9]

Up to this point, we have been focusing on the health-protective side of social ties in general and religion in particular. Whether they are wielding carrots or sticks, the impact of belonging to social groups was shown to result in a lower risk of suicide in Durkheim's research over a century ago and has been shown to result in lower mortality from all causes wherever more modern studies have been done. The research shows a net benefit of social ties, religious or otherwise, for health.

However, Durkheim also saw the potential for harm from these same sources. Because the conditions of the modern world or at least modern Europe were turning toward isolated individualism, the effects of social integration and regulation were protective with respect to suicides. But Durkheim explicitly allowed that too intense a level of these influences could clearly be harmful to individuals and that people could also be driven to suicide by living in societies that were too restrictive, controlling, and punishing. The misuse of power by individuals within a religious institution can have devastating consequences; sexual abuse of children by Roman Catholic priests is a painful example of the potential for harm that can be inflicted by a trusted institution.

Religion can act in other ways that are directly or indirectly damaging to public health. In many places, religion acts particularly to restrict women's rights, justifying the unequal, even violent treatment of women and limiting women's ability to access education and reproductive health services. Religious beliefs may motivate anti-LGBT attitudes, greatly complicating public health efforts to control the HIV/AIDS epidemic. Through their power to enforce norms, religious groups may even compel their members to forgo practices that have clear public health benefits, such as immunizations, contraception, or condom use to prevent sexually transmitted diseases. Some religious beliefs forbid certain medical treatments, such as blood transfusions or organ donation. More benignly, some religious practices carry the potential for inadvertently spreading disease or injury. Nineteenth-century Christian missionaries inadvertently introduced deadly infections to indigenous populations at the same time that they brought modern medical treatments. Today, congregations meeting for services could allow the flu to spread through the air by handshakes or via the sharing of food and drink, sacramental or otherwise. In mass gatherings such as the Hajj or other pilgrimages, public water and sanitation systems may be overwhelmed, or crowds may stampede.

Some religious practices such as handling poisonous snakes, ingesting hallucinogenic drugs, or spending hours in sweat lodges are themselves inherently dangerous, even deadly. We can easily bring to mind places and incidents in which religion has served as a source of social strife and violent conflict that kills through war, terrorism, or mass suicide. The same ties that bind individuals together in supportive in-groups may blind them to the humanity of outsiders, justifying violence and cruelty.

There are other, less direct negative impacts of religion. Religious groups with high intermarriage rates can and do transmit serious genetic disorders to their children; well-known examples include the Amish and

Ashkenazi Jews. At the same time that some denominations refuse modern medical care, patients who say they use religion to cope with their serious illness are more likely to seek excessive expensive and fruitless intensive medical care at the end of life. Clearly, the potential for religion to have widespread negative effects on the physical and mental health of believers and nonbelievers alike is real and considerable, and we return to these themes in a number of chapters. We want to sketch out a role for religion as a social force in the same way that Durkheim saw it—a force that can harm both by its absence and by too overbearing a presence. Religion's role in public health is complicated and multifaceted, and in laying this picture out for the first time, we acknowledge that there are extremes in every direction.

Religion as Social Capital

There is yet a third way in which religion can directly influence population health in communities—by the creation of social capital. The health of populations is strongly affected by the physical capital of the places in which they live: their air, water, land, and infrastructure and their buildings, sidewalks, and streets. But communities are also composed of political, economic, educational, religious, and social institutions, resources collectively referred to as *social capital*.[10] Healthy societies are full of middle-level institutions, the civil society that exists in the space between individuals and the large-scale structures of the state. In their review of studies of the impact of social capital on population health, Kim, Subramanian, and Kawachi find that higher levels of social capital in communities are significantly associated with lower mortality rates and better self-ratings of health.[11]

Some of these middle-level institutions, like the First Presbyterian Church of Carlisle, have very long histories, with origins that predate the memories of those alive in the community today. Others, like the Clean Air Board, were created de novo by human beings seeking social solutions to problems. Religious institutions have a long history of creating social capital in their communities, by establishing schools, hospitals, and clinics and providing health and social services, often to the neediest members of their communities. Thus they exist not only as middle-level institutions themselves but also as points of contact for motivated individuals to create new institutions and new social capital.

Their capacity for such undertakings is enhanced by, on the one hand, ethical teachings that motivate concern for the wider community and, on the other hand, access to many parts of the community through the social ties of congregation members. Reverend McKenna's deep, lifelong knowledge of her community; her social networks, which included members of the medical and legal professions; her church-based communication channels, which brought interested individuals together; the legitimacy and authority of her role as pastor; and her concern for the community as a whole exemplify the kind of social capital that congregations can provide for their communities. Like the Reverend Henry Whitehead, whose critical role in uncovering the cause of London's 1854 cholera epidemic is recounted in Steven Johnson's *The Ghost Map*,[12] Reverend McKenna was already "on the ground" before the health threat arose, with invaluable local knowledge and strong ties to her neighbors and friends. This is a key to understanding social capital: in daily life it may be taken for granted, but in a crisis it takes on form and effectiveness.

Religion as a Social Determinant of Health

In 2008, the same year that the Diesel-Powered Motor Vehicle Idling Act was being written into law in the state of Pennsylvania, the World Health Organization (WHO) published the report of its Commission on the Social Determinants of Health (CSDH). The commission was made up of distinguished global health leaders, including WHO Secretary General Margaret Chen, Nobel laureate Amartya Sen, former US Surgeon General David Satcher, former director of the Centers for Disease Control William Foege, and the commission's leader, Sir Michael Marmot, epidemiologist at University College London. From 2005 to 2008, the commission engaged in a global process of collaboration with researchers from around the world and mobilized knowledge networks and evidence-gathering partnerships with health workers and community representatives with expertise at the local level. The goal of the commission's work is nicely expressed in the title of its report: *Closing the Gap in a Generation: Health Equity through Action on the Social Determinants of Health*. By "social determinants," the Commission means "the circumstances in which people are born, grow up, live, work, and age, and the systems put in place to deal with illness. These circumstances are in turn shaped by a wider set of forces: economics, social policies, and politics."[13] Notably, religious institutions are not mentioned among the "wider set of forces," nor were representatives of local, national, or international religious organizations mentioned as participants in the CSDH report, even in the description of the civil society sector's partnership with the commission. Nor is religion mentioned among the thematic areas on which evidence was gathered, including aging, indigenous peoples, food and nutrition, violence and conflict, and the environment.

The commission's activities and its report are the most recent and visible expression of the growing recognition on the part of researchers and policymakers of the importance of social factors as determinants of public health. The critical insight is that the primary determinants of health around the world are *not* health services and medical care, but the conditions in which people live their daily lives. Social, political, and economic determinants of health lie outside of what is thought of as the health sector, and yet they profoundly affect the public's health. The social determinants perspective is today the dominant research and policy paradigm in public health.

However, it is, in one respect, incomplete. Our purpose is not to single out the commission for criticism or to in any way diminish its achievement in calling attention to health inequalities in societies throughout the world. Its social justice orientation and concern for the health and living conditions of the most vulnerable members of society are in fact indistinguishable from the perspectives of many faith-based relief and development organizations.

But the commission's failure to include religion in its list of determinants reflects a blind spot in nearly all of the current work on social determinants. Although the term "social determinants" suggests a wide and inclusive set of determinants, it is specifically the political and economic conditions of life that have been seen as most central. We contend that religion belongs among the set of social determinants and should be considered not only as an independent determinant of health but also for the numerous ways in which it may interplay with economic determinants.

The Social Gradient

Research on economic determinants of mortality in the United States may be traced to the early 1970s, with the publication of Kitagawa and Hauser's *Differential Mortality in the United States*, which sought to explain why the United States—the most affluent country in the world—ranked sixteenth in the world in life expectancy.[14] They concluded that this poor showing was largely due to significant differences in life expectancy by race and socioeconomic status (which they equated with years of education). In the following decades, two studies in the United Kingdom, the Black Report[15] and the Acheson Report,[16] also found mortality differentials, this time by social class as determined by the British system of classifying occupations. The Acheson Report pointed out that, while mortality rates were declining for the population as a whole, the declines had been more rapid for those in the upper social classes, and therefore the gap in longevity between the rich and the poor was growing. Twin follow-on studies, the Whitehall Studies I and II (the latter of which is still ongoing), have provided perhaps the deepest understanding of the pervasive influence of social class on health.[17] Named for the street where the British Civil Service is located, the Whitehall Studies together have examined nearly thirty thousand civil servants (mostly male) in occupations ranging from janitors and messengers to top-level administrators. The studies' early findings were that those at the bottom of the civil service hierarchy had mortality rates three times as high as those in the highest positions. This was somewhat surprising since none of the jobs required extensive exposure to hazardous or dangerous environments. The civil service hierarchy simply served as an effective proxy for social class, arraying employees by both education and income.

Marmot's[18] work showed that differences in mortality rates existed not only between the top and bottom of the hierarchy but at every step in between; he called this the *social gradient*. Further, Marmot found, Whitehall civil servants were subject to a gradient not only for mortality but also for a wide range of physical and mental health problems, including cardiovascular disease, some cancers, gastrointestinal disease, depression, and suicide. Some mechanisms for these differences have been identified: employees in the lower grades were more likely to be smokers, to be overweight, and to exercise less often. Adjusting for these and other individual-level risk factors reduced but did not eliminate the effect of position in the employment hierarchy.

A second important explanation for the relationship between employment level and health is the actual conditions of work. Researchers have identified health-relevant features of the work environment, such as the balance between the demands of the job and the amount of control the worker has over how tasks are performed or between the effort put forth and the rewards received.[19] Menial, routine jobs may be difficult and time-pressured but bring little reward, either in the form of compensation or as recognition, and offer few opportunities for even the self-satisfaction that creative problem solving or innovation can bring.

A third explanation for the graded, step-by-step effect of social position on health relies on the concept of status. Inequalities in health may not be due simply to absolute differences in income and education but to the tendency of people to express their feelings of superiority over those who are lower in the hierarchy. Social distinctions exist in all social hierarchies, not only in employment. They are manifested in a myriad of ways, including dress, manners, ways of speaking, preferences in music and film, diet, and choice of friends. People who consider themselves more refined and sophisticated cultivate their tastes for more expensive and less accessible cultural goods and may display their disregard for what is "popular" with an air of snobbery. Thus, the social gradient is created and maintained by a number of possible mechanisms that appear—given the increasing mortality differentials—to be increasing in strength.

This idea of the social gradient in health, developed initially from research in a single sphere of a single society, has been extended since then to studies of income inequality between countries. Richard Wilkinson, a British epidemiologist and a colleague of Michael Marmot, has addressed the question of whether it is the absolute (or average) level of income of a country or its level of income inequality (the size of the difference between the richest and the poorest citizens) that produces the biggest difference in health.[20] Wilkinson ranked countries by comparing the bottom percentiles of their income distribution to the top percentiles; a country in which there are many people with relatively low incomes and a small number taking a large proportion of the total wealth would have a high level of income inequality (the United States would be an example). Japan would be an example of a country in which the differences between the poor and the wealthy are not as great, and Japan, with its more equal distribution of income, has a significantly higher life expectancy than the United States.

Another way to put this question is to ask whether more equal societies are healthier simply because they have fewer poor people, or if there is an effect of the inequality itself over and above the obvious effect of poverty on health. A recent meta-analysis of studies of income inequality, mortality, and self-reports of health suggests that there is an effect of inequality; data from industrialized countries around the world showed relatively small but significantly increased risks of mortality and poor self-rated health for individuals in countries with more income inequality.[21]

The Cumulative Effect of Social Determinants

The outcome of these four decades of research on the effects of income, education, and work on life expectancy has been a growing consensus that social factors play a determining role in the health of populations and that reducing poverty and income inequality would be the most effective way to promote population health. This was the intellectual and moral background for the formation of the CSDH. As Michael Marmot put it in announcing the formation of the commission, "The gross inequalities in health that we see within and between countries present a challenge to the world. That there should be a spread of life expectancy of 48 years among countries and 20 years or more within countries is not inevitable."[22]

The CSDH work is an attempt to address those gross inequalities by looking at social determinants of health on a global scale. The term "social determinant" is a good one because it has a neutral valence; it implies that social, political, and economic forces may have either negative or positive effects—or both—on health. The benefits to some of higher levels of education, income, and wealth may prove to cause harm to those with less, not only absolutely—because of material deprivation— but also relatively by comparison with those who have even a little bit more. An analogy could be made to a field of wheat. If the fertilizer needed to grow the crop to its full potential is spread unevenly, some of the wheat will shoot up and thrive, while the rest will grow more slowly and weakly. So there is a direct effect of the advantage or disadvantage of some wheat seedlings compared with others. But there is an added effect of the fertilizer that is manifested over time and mediated through other resources. The wheat seedlings that grow the fastest also absorb the most water from the soil, and because they rise more quickly, they shade the lower, smaller plants, gaining an advantage in sunlight as well.[23] So early advantages beget later ones.

The analogy of the wheat field illustrates another development in this area of research, and that is the growing appreciation of the importance of the impact of social determinants on health over time. For wheat, the effects of an advantage would be realized in a single season, but for human beings, the conditions of early life can have effects that play out over decades, from adolescence into adulthood and old age. It seems obvious that poverty and social inequality would adversely affect a child's health and development, and it is also obvious that we do not choose the time and place of our origins. The early social determinants research, however, focused on working people, hence adults already in midlife. More recent research programs, such as the British Birth Cohort studies, have looked at people enrolled from birth, which has allowed some estimation of the considerable impact of childhood social conditions on later life.[24]

That impact begins even before birth. In utero, the physical environment and nutrition of the mother will have a profound effect on the embryo's growth and development. After birth, infant and child growth patterns have been linked to a number of factors in adult health, specifically coronary heart disease, obesity, binge drinking, diabetes, and hypertension; adult respiratory disease is associated with poor growth in utero, early infection and chest illness, poor childhood growth, and short attained height.[25] Adverse circumstances in early life may affect adult health because they make children vulnerable to later insults: a child who has grown up in a household of smokers has already inhaled a significant amount of cigarette smoke before he sneaks his first cigarette. He is also more likely to try that first cigarette because it is obtainable in the household and because the behavioral norms that he has grown up with are different than they would be in a household of nonsmokers.

As a child grows, income inequality reproduces itself through the education system he or she is exposed to and the value placed on education by his or her parents. In fact, educational attainment is a strong determinant of adult economic success, independent of parents' social class,[26] and both educational attainment and parents' social class are factors that remain unchanged through adult life and old age. Just as important is the emotional and social support (or the absence of it), offered by parents, teachers, and other significant adults, which can inhibit children's growth and development or allow them to reach their full physical, social, and cognitive potential.[27] There can be upward (and downward) social mobility, to be sure. Children frequently grow up to achieve much more than their parents did. But we carry our childhoods with us: early-life circumstances can still have an impact on adult health. This complex set of determinants, some playing out slowly over time, underlies the social gradient of adult health.

The Role of Religion

Where is religion in all of this? A consideration of the effects on health of the social conditions of childhood and family life might suggest the presence or absence of religion as one of those conditions, but in fact religion is almost never mentioned in this literature. When there are brief references, religion is linked to ethnicity and understood as a cause of discrimination or violence against minority groups;[28] religious differences, along with language, race, and ethnic origin are "seen as markers of low social status and attract various downward prejudices."[29] There are also passing references to religion as antiquated or primitive, as in "Christians, Jews, Hottentots, and Eskimos,"[30] or as exceptional and out of the mainstream, as in studies finding low blood pressure in "pre-agricultural societies as well as some modern closed monastic communities."[31] The strongest proponents of income inequality as the primary social determinant of health, in fact, find all other social determinants subsidiary to that force, contending that ethnic, racial, religious, or language differences are magnified under conditions of high income inequality and are less likely to cause friction when material inequalities are smaller.[32] So, according to the leading expositions of the social determinants approach to understanding population health, economic factors are of the greatest importance, and religion, if it plays any role at all, is a minor factor whose primary importance is in the ways that it may lead to discrimination, thereby harming health.

We wish to put forward a broader vision of religion as a primarily important determinant, both positive and negative, of population health alongside economic inequality. We have already outlined some ways in which religion may act directly on population health, by integrating individuals in social networks that both care for them and regulate their behavior and by providing institutional actors and social capital to communities. But religious groups are not independent of the economic and political systems they live in and under, and religion has a relationship to income inequality that is extremely complex. The effects of religion and income inequality on health have been studied separately but not, to date, jointly; we see this as a shortcoming of both fields of study.

Let us briefly consider three ways in which religion and economic inequality may interact and affect each other. First, religion may reduce economic inequality by evoking charitable impulses and compassionate responses to the less fortunate. Focusing on inequality is all about paying attention to the differences between individuals and between groups. Wilkinson depicts the social impact of income inequality by connecting it to more authoritarianism in personal interactions, deteriorating family relations, lowered trust in neighbors, and less involvement in the community. As he writes, "Inequality promotes strategies that are more self-interested, less affiliative, often highly antisocial, more stressful, and likely to give rise to higher levels of violence, poorer community relations, and worse health."[33] Income inequality promotes increased social distance between individuals and between social groups. This distance is not lateral but vertical; relations are perceived in terms of hierarchy, dominance/subordination, and insider/outsider status. To cope, individuals become more competitive, more aware of and protective of status and material reward, and less generous toward and trusting of others. So on top of the material deprivation that has a direct effect on health, income inequality creates a host of social sequelae that have their own adverse effects on individual and community health alike; we see this in the social gradient.

Religion, too, is sometimes about drawing attention to differences. Insider/outsider status is to some extent an unavoidable feature of belonging in social groups—those into which one is born and those with which one affiliates by choice. Religions also contain socially stratified hierarchies within them, be they the Hindu caste system or the governance structure of the Presbyterian church. But religions, unlike other social structures, also offer belief systems that encourage us to pay attention to human commonalities and to work to reduce differences through charitable acts. The early twentieth-century sociologist of religion Max Weber noted that "the giving of alms is a universal and primary component of every ethical religion."[34] More recently, the religion scholar Karen Armstrong has argued that compassion, "the ability to *feel with* the other,"[35] is the central practice of all of the world's religions. The Buddhist doctrine of *anatta* ("no self") is the requirement to live without self-interest of any kind, to put away "me" and "mine." What is known in Western societies as the Golden Rule—"Do unto others as you would have them do unto you"—is taught almost identically in Confucianism, in which *Jen*—the capacity to *"measure the feelings of others by one's own"*[36]—is the "virtue of virtues." Ancient Judaism offers a similar admonition: "You shall not take vengeance or bear any grudge against the sons of your own people, but you shall love your neighbor as yourself: I am the LORD" (Leviticus 19:18).[37] Motivated concern for the disadvantaged, "the least of these my brethren" in the words of Jesus, puts members of religious groups into contact with the neediest and most vulnerable in their communities.

At the same time, religious narratives about overcoming slavery and injustice, as in the exodus of the people of Israel from Egypt or the cries of the Old Testament prophets for social reform, provide models for a moral response to power and hope for peace and justice in the future for those who are oppressed in the present. Regular attendance at religious services makes members aware of these faith contexts for the needs within and outside of the congregation and gives them invitations as well as motivation to serve others.

Moreover, religious groups have the social and physical capital to make these efforts effective. Congregations maintain presences in their communities. They have physical spaces and warmth and light—shelter—to offer midnight basketball for adolescents, housing for the homeless, or soup kitchens for the hungry. They have paper and copiers and phones and phone lists, and they offer members opportunities to develop leadership skills—public speaking, budgeting, organizing, decision-making, policy-making, problem solving. Sociologist Nancy Ammerman calls these "civic skills"; she observes that throughout American history, congregations have had a "meetinghouse" role and that they serve this purpose especially well for the least advantaged, who have fewer opportunities to develop these skills in their places of work.[38]

Much of this activity is on behalf of those who have even fewer advantages. In the 1998 National Congregation Survey, Mark Chaves finds that 57 percent of US congregations participated in social service activities, most frequently food, housing, or children's programs, and that, on average, congregations participated in more than three programs.[39] The Second Presbyterian Church of Carlisle is no exception. Members there participate regularly, along with those of other congregations in the area, in the programs of Habitat for Humanity, Heifer International, and the Interfaith Housing Network, and they make an annual trip to Honduras with the Presbyterian Church (USA) to build and improve housing in an isolated rural village.[40] In these activities, congregation members come into contact with the less fortunate and are forced to confront economic inequality; at the same time, by giving of their resources of money and time, they are alleviating some of that inequality, increasing the material resources of the less advantaged, and working to change the conditions that produce inequality.

There is a second way in which religion may moderate the health consequences of income inequality, and that is by alleviating its psychological effect. Wilkinson[41] depicts the psychological impact of income inequality in the form of higher levels of stress, depression, insecurity, shame, aggression, and social anxiety; these can lead to health-harming behaviors of violence, drug and alcohol use, and antisocial behavior. Religion offers an alternative status system that may subvert the materialist values that are the basis for the invidious comparisons of "the status syndrome." By placing ultimate value on the spiritual and ethical dimensions of other human beings instead of on their net worth, religions provide a different basis for comparison and different structures for developing both self-esteem and respect for others. Wealth and material goods are things of this world, and religion puts them into context with an emphasis on a higher spiritual plane, whether in this life or the next. Moreover, coming to know and experience the lives of those who are less fortunate can give one a sense of humility and gratitude for what one does have, however little—in stark contrast to the feelings of relative deprivation engendered by comparisons to those higher on the social status ladder.

This reduction of the psychological effect of income inequality would be especially marked in congregations in disadvantaged communities. Congregants whose daily life in the workplace is characterized by little control over the pace of work, who have few opportunities to make decisions about what is done or when or how, and who receive correspondingly little compensation or recognition may especially benefit from the opportunities to develop civic skills offered by a religious affiliation. Others with gifts of the spirit or the ability to sing, pray, or tell stories may find that their congregation affords them respect and dignity in ways that their work or school environment does not.

This perspective, in which religion substitutes spiritual values for earthly, material ones, can certainly also be cast as a pacifier, a tool for suppression, an opiate. Religion and religious institutions may indeed serve the purposes of a ruling class, allowing it to maintain civil order based on injustice and inequality in the present by offering the promise of reward in another life. These complex dynamics would be especially pronounced for racial and ethnic minority groups who experience both economic disadvantage and racial discrimination. African Americans in particular are often noted as a group for whom religion is especially important. Compared to whites, African Americans are more religiously observant by every measure, reporting higher rates of attendance at services, daily devotions, and stronger religious identity.[42] Yet, far from having a pacifying effect, the black church has played an extremely important role in the arc of African American history, from slavery to reconstruction, to Jim Crow, to the civil rights period, and on into the present.

The health inequalities of African Americans, often referred to as health disparities, are also well documented. African Americans have higher mortality rates at every age, with especially high rates in infancy and adolescence, compared with all other racial and ethnic groups in the United States. Some but certainly not all of the health differences are due to lower levels of education and income, and most analysts see an independent effect of racial discrimination.[43] As Nancy Krieger puts it, "Inequality hurts."[44] The particularly high level of religiousness among African Americans and their economic disadvantage make the relationship between religion and health especially complex and paradoxical. Analyses of US national data show that religious attendance does in fact offer a strongly significant protective effect, resulting in lower mortality rates among African American adults; this effect was especially pronounced for women and those living in the South.[45] One can only conclude that higher overall rates of religiousness protect the African American community from what would be even more dramatically elevated mortality rates than already exist.

Finally, in addition to reducing inequality or reducing the perception of inequality, there is a third way that we should consider religion to have a relationship with economic inequality, and that is a way in which it may be harmful to health. At the same time that it may alleviate or blunt the effects of economic inequality, religion may also act to reinforce or increase that inequality. Max Weber first linked Protestant concern with salvation to economic behaviors that gave rise to capitalism,[46] and he describes the economic behavior of the other world's religions in other work;[47] those behaviors, conditioned by religious beliefs, lead to marketplace advantages for some but disadvantages for others. Recent research by the Pew Foundation bears out the consequences of these differences: in surveys done in 2007 and 2010, the Foundation finds dramatic differences in US household income by religious affiliation. Hindus and Jews rank at the top, with 65 percent and 57 percent, respectively, of US households with those affiliations reporting income of $75,000 or more, and Jehovah's Witnesses and historically black Protestant churches rank at the bottom, with fewer than 20 percent of US households with these affiliations in the top income category.[48] Roman Catholics, Mormons, and Lutherans rank very near the national average, with 30 percent of households with these affiliations making $75,000 or more; Methodists and secular households are a little higher, Muslims and Baptists a little lower than the national average.[49] Dramatic differences in economic status by religion are seen in another recent study that focuses not on household *income* (the basis for the social determinants literature) but on household *wealth* and *assets*, which are even more important in many ways. Using data from the US National Longitudinal Survey of Youth, sociologist Lisa Keister finds an overall median net worth of $58,000 (assets such as stocks and bonds, trust accounts, and real estate minus debt) for this young adult sample by the time they reached their thirties and early forties. However, young adults raised as Jewish had a median net worth of $221,000 while young adults raised as Baptists had a median net worth of just $26,000, little more than a tenth as much.[50] Other groups in the survey, in descending order of net worth, included Episcopalians, Presbyterians, Lutherans, Methodists, Catholics, other Protestants, no religion, other religion, and Baptists.

The reasons different religions should produce such disparities in wealth and income are complex. Keister argues that participation in particular religious ceremonies and rituals inculcates skills, knowledge, and values that may apply directly to decisions about consumption, saving, and investment.[51] Others have stressed childrearing practices that are reinforced by religion; these may tend to inculcate obedience to authority or autonomy and independent thinking. Regardless of affiliation, respondents who attend services more frequently value obedience in parent–child relations over autonomy.[52] Other pathways may be traced even further back to childbearing. Avoiding early, premarital pregnancy is one factor in helping young people stay in school, another route to higher levels of wealth and income. Data from women in the US National Survey of Family Growth show that higher levels of religious participation are associated positively with both educational attainment and higher wages.[53] There is a consistent finding in the literature on religion and family life that more frequent attendance at services is associated with earlier childbearing if the mother is married, and with later childbearing if she is single.[54] Taking it back even a step further, other research shows that adolescents who say that religion is important to them and those who live in households with religiously observant parents are less likely to engage in sexual activity in the first place.[55]

These data are limited to the United States, with its unusual combination of extremes of income and income inequality, high levels of religious observance, and relatively poor population health indicators. By contrast, most of the world's wealthiest countries, particularly those in Europe, are largely secular. At the same time, the great majority of the world's population lives in countries with very low per capita GDP but with high levels reporting that religion is very important in their daily lives.[56] The poorest countries in the world are also most likely to be majority Muslim. Thus, on a country-by-country level, high levels of religiousness are strongly correlated with income inequality and poverty and, correspondingly, with poor health. The large amount of research finding a positive correlation between religion and health using data from the United States has probably obscured this important association at the global level.

As we said, it is a complicated topic. But the preeminent importance of religiousness in the world's poorest countries surely strengthens our central point—that religion needs to be considered among the social determinants of health if any progress is to be made in reducing health inequalities. We do not mean to convey the impression that we see religion as the answer to the problem of health inequalities. Indeed, in many cases it is surely part of the problem.

* * *

This is the rationale for this work, which has the goal of sketching out religion's relationship to public health and underpinning our claim that religion belongs among the social determinants of health. Where, when, and how do we see religion acting as a social determinant? This is unquestionably a broad agenda, perhaps broad beyond reason. But the topic is so important and so unexamined that we feel compelled to make the big case. The social determinants perspective is today the dominant research and policy paradigm in public health, but in its formal articulations, including the CSDH report, a critical piece of the puzzle has been missing. There are few if any communities in the world where there is no religious institution at all, and in many communities, particularly the most vulnerable, religious institutions may be the most important, vital, and functional social institutions in the lives of community members. Effective action on the social determinants of health at the local or global level cannot ignore these important social actors. In this book, we make the argument for how and why they must be included.

Notes

1. Ellen Simon, "Interview with Reverend Jennifer McKenna," October 26, 2007, http://carlislehistory.dickinson.edu/?page_id=154. For the enactment of the Diesel-Powered Motor Vehicle Idling Act, see Pennsylvania Business Association, "Act 124 (Idling Restrictions) and Motorcoaches," *PBA Reporter*, November 2008, http://www.pabus.org/documents/Bulletins/2008%20November%20%20Reporter%20 Idling%20ACT%20124.pdf.
2. Charles-Edward Amory Winslow, "The Untilled Fields of Public Health," *Science* 9, no. 51 (1920): 23–33. In the article, Winslow describes public health as "the science and the art of preventing disease, prolonging life, and promoting physical health" (p. 30).
3. C. T. Onions, ed., *The Shorter Oxford English Dictionary* (Oxford: Clarendon Press, 1933), 1697.
4. P. G. W. Glare, ed., *Oxford Latin Dictionary* (Oxford: Clarendon Press, 1976), 1605.
5. Emile Durkheim, *Suicide: A Study in Sociology*, trans. Joseph Swain (1897; repr, New York: Free Press, 1951).
6. Julianne Holt-Lunstad, Timothy B. Smith, and J. Bradley Layton, "Social Relationships and Mortality Risk: A Meta-Analytic Review," *PLoS Medicine* 7, no. 7 (2010), DOI: 10.1371/journal.pmed.1000316.
7. Lisa F. Berkman and S. Leonard Syme, "Social Networks, Host Resistance, and Mortality: A Nine-Year Follow-up Study of Alameda County Residents," *American Journal of Epidemiology* 109, no. 2 (1979): 186–204.
8. Richard G. Rogers, Patrick M. Krueger, and Robert A. Hummer, "Religious Attendance and Cause-Specific Mortality in the United States," in *Religion, Families, and Health: Population-Based Research in the United States*, ed. Christopher G. Ellison

and Robert A. Hummer (New Brunswick, NJ: Rutgers University Press, 2010), 292–320.

9. Mary A. Whooley, A. L. Boyd, J. M. Gardin, and David R. Williams, "Religious Involvement and Cigarette Smoking in Young Adults: The Cardia Study," *Archives of Internal Medicine* 162, no. 14 (2002): 1604–1610.

10. Robert Putnam, *Bowling Alone: The Collapse and Revival of American Community* (New York: Simon and Schuster, 2000).

11. Daniel Kim, S. V. Subramanian, and Ichiro Kawachi, "Social Capital and Physical Health: A Systematic Review of the Literature," in *Social Capital and Health*, ed. Ichiro Kawachi, S.V. Subramanian, and Daniel Kim (New York: Springer, 2008), 139–190.

12. Steven Johnson, *The Ghost Map: The Story of London's Most Terrifying Epidemic— and How It Changed Science, Cities, and the Modern World* (New York: Riverhead Books, 2006).

13. Commission on the Social Determinants of Health, *Closing the Gap: Health Equity through Action on the Social Determinants of Health. Final Report of the Commission on Social Determinants of Health* (Geneva: World Health Organization, 2008), i.

14. Evelyn M. Kitagawa and Philip M. Hauser, *Differential Mortality in the United States: A Study in Socioeconomic Epidemiology* (Cambridge, MA: Harvard University Press, 1973).

15. Douglas Black, *Inequalities in Health: The Black Report* (London: Pelican, 1982).

16. Donald Acheson, *Independent Inquiry in Inequalities in Health Report* (London: Stationary Office, 1998).

17. Michael G. Marmot and Martin J. Shipley, "Do Socioeconomic Differences in Mortality Persist after Retirement? 25 Year Follow up of Civil Servants from the First Whitehall Study," *British Medical Journal* 313, no. 7066 (1996): 1177–1180.

18. Michael G. Marmot, *The Status Syndrome: How Social Standing Affects Our Health and Longevity* (New York: Henry Holt, 2004).

19. Johannes Siegrist and Töres Theorell, "Socio-Economic Position and Health: The Role of Work and Employment," in *Social Inequalities in Health: New Evidence and Policy Implications*, ed. Johannes Siegrist and Michael Marmot (Oxford: Oxford University Press, 2006), 73–100.

20. Richard Wilkinson, *The Impact of Inequality: How to Make Sick Societies Healthier* (New York: New Press, 2005).

21. Naoki Kondo, Grace Sembajwe, Ichiro Kawachi, Rob M. van Dam, S. V. Subramanian, and Zentaro Yamagata, "Income Inequality, Mortality, and Self-Rated Health: Meta-Analysis of Multilevel Studies," *British Medical Journal* 339, no. 7731 (2009): 1178–1181.

22. M. Marmot, "Social Determinants of Health Inequalities," *Lancet* 365, no. 9464 (2005): 1099.

23. Stephen Senn, "Mortality and Distribution of Income: Societies with Narrower Income Distributions Are Healthier," *British Medical Journal* 316, no. 7144 (1998): 1611–1612.

24. Diana Kuh and Yoav Ben-Shlomo, *A Life Course Approach to Chronic Disease Epidemiology*, 2d ed. (Oxford: Oxford University Press, 2004).

25. Chris Power and Diana Kuh, "The Life Course Development of Unequal Health," in *Social Inequalities in Health: New Evidence and Policy Implications*, ed. Johannes Siegrist and Michael Marmot (Oxford: Oxford University Press, 2006), 27–53.

26. George Davey Smith, Carole Hart, David Hole, Pauline MacKinnon, Charles Gillis, Graham Watt, David Blane, and Victor Hawthorne, "Education and Occupational Social Class: Which Is the More Important Indicator of Mortality Risk?" in *Health Inequalities: Lifecourse Approaches*, ed. George Davey Smith (Bristol, UK: Policy Press, 2003), 171–189.

27. Michael Wadsworth and Suzie Butterworth, "Early Life," in *Social Determinants of Health*, 2d ed., ed. Michael Marmot and Richard Wilkinson (Oxford: Oxford University Press, 2006), 31–53.

28. Mel Bartley, *Health Inequality: An Introduction to Theories, Concepts and Methods* (Cambridge, UK: Polity Press, 2004), 151; Nancy Krieger, "Discrimination and Health," in *Social Epidemiology*, ed. Lisa Berkman and Ichiro Kawachi (Oxford: Oxford University Press, 2000), 36–75.

29. Richard Wilkinson and Kate Pickett, *The Spirit Level: Why Greater Equality Makes Societies Stronger* (New York: Bloomsbury Press, 2009), 185.

30. Marmot, *The Status Syndrome*, 89.

31. Wilkinson, *The Impact of Inequality*, 277.

32. Wilkinson, *The Impact of Inequality*, 228.

33. Wilkinson, *The Impact of Inequality*, 23.

34. Max Weber, *The Sociology of Religion* (1922; repr. Boston: Beacon Press, 1964), 212.

35. Karen Armstrong, *The Case for God* (New York: Knopf, 2009), 24; emphasis in the original.

36. Huston Smith, *The Illustrated World's Religions: A Guide to Our Wisdom Traditions* (New York: Harper Collins, 1994), 110; emphasis in the original.

37. All biblical quotations are taken from the Revised Standard Version.

38. Nancy Ammerman, *Congregation and Community* (New Brunswick, NJ: Rutgers University Press, 2001), 364.

39. Mark Chaves, *Congregations in America* (Cambridge, MA: Harvard University Press, 2004). Although in this survey health programs did not figure prominently among the types of social services congregations are involved in, they are certainly of vital importance to particular religious groups; genetic screening for Tay-Sachs disease in Ashkenazi Jewish congregations and clinics for hypertension in African American churches in the "stroke belt" are common examples of action by religious congregations to respond to specific health threats.

40. Jennifer McKenna, telephone interview, July 13, 2011.

41. Wilkinson, *The Impact of Inequality*.

42. Christopher G. Ellison, Robert A. Hummer, Amy M. Burdette, and Maureen Benjamins, "Race, Religious Involvement, and Health: The Case of African Americans," in Rogers, Krueger, and Hummer, *Religion, Families, and Health*, 321–348.

43. Gary King and David Williams, "Race and Health: A Multidimensional Approach to African-American Health," in *Society and Health*, ed. Benjamin Amick, Sol Levine, Alvin R. Tarlov, and Diana Chapman Walsh (New York: Oxford University Press, 1995), 93–132.

44. Krieger, "Discrimination and Health," 36.

45. Ellison et al., "Race, Religious Involvement, and Health."
46. Max Weber, *The Protestant Ethic and the Spirit of Capitalism* (1904/1905; repr. New York: Scribner, 1958).
47. Weber, *The Sociology of Religion.*
48. The Pew Forum on Religion and Public Life, "Income Distribution within U.S. Religious Groups," January 30, 2009, http://www.pewforum.org/Income-Distribution-Within-US-Religious-Groups.aspx.
49. David Leonhardt, "Is Your Religion Your Financial Destiny?," *New York Times Sunday Magazine*, May 11, 2011.
50. Lisa Keister, "Childhood Religious Denomination and Early Adult Asset Accumulation," in Rogers, Krueger, and Hummer, *Religion, Families, and Health*, 164–185.
51. Keister, "Childhood Religious Denomination and Early Adult Asset Accumulation." See also Lisa Keister, *Faith and Money: How Religion Contributes to Wealth and Poverty* (New York: Cambridge University Press).
52. Duane Alwin and Jacob L. Felson, "Religion and Child Rearing," in Rogers, Krueger, and Hummer, *Religion, Families, and Health*, 40–60.
53. Evelyn Lehrer, "Religious Affiliation and Participation as Determinants of Women's Education Attainment and Wages," in Rogers, Krueger, and Hummer, *Religion, Families, and Health*, 186–205.
54. Lisa D. Pearce, "Religion and the Timing of First Births in the United States," in Rogers, Krueger, and Hummer, *Religion, Families, and Health*, 19–39.
55. Mark Regnerus, "Religion and Adolescent Sexual Behavior," in Rogers, Krueger, and Hummer, *Religion, Families, and Health*, 61–85.
56. Charles Blow, "Religious Outlier" [editorial], *New York Times*, September 3, 2010, http://www.gallup.com/poll/142727/religiosity-highest-world-poorest-nations.aspx.

Public Health in the Practices of the World's Faith Traditions

PART I OFFERS CLOSE-UP descriptions of religious practice from a number of the world's faith traditions. We open the book in this way because we want to draw attention to the spiritual practices that people engage in throughout their lives. Religion is much more than just what people believe and say; it is most importantly what they *do*—in many cases what they do every single day. With descriptions of some of these practices, we hope to bring a vivid material reality to what is often treated as an abstract and generic concept. In much research on religion and health, the emphasis has been on the internal, subjective aspects of religious experience, such as religious belief, intrinsic religiosity, religious coping, or simply spirituality. We attempt to refocus attention on outward manifestations of religious experience; we seek to draw attention to what religion actually looks like when people do it and experience it.

Importantly, we chose to include only the routine practices of the laity. Our concern is the health of populations, not that of religious experts, so we begin with the experiences to which most members of a faith tradition are exposed. Some of the religious groups and practices that we describe have been extensively studied for their association with health; for others, there is minimal research. But as practices they all involve the physical body to some extent, and therefore have some potential to affect public health. To encourage further study, each description concludes with a short list of resources that explore possible or identified links of the practice with public health.

Many of the religious practices described in this section are found in more than one faith tradition, and certainly every religion has many practices; we paired practices with traditions to maximize the diversity of both. We adamantly do not mean to condense any faith tradition to a single practice or even to suggest that the practice that we chose is more central to the faith than others; the practices described here are intended simply as exemplars of religious practice in that tradition.

We have grouped the practices by their cyclical timing: there are daily, weekly, and annual practices. The final practices that we describe occur only once in a life course: circumcision, puberty rites, adult baptism, and cremation. Our four examples come from Judaism, African traditional religion, Latin American Evangelical Protestantism, and Hinduism, but virtually all religions have rituals for the critical moments of birth, adolescence, and death—moments of crisis and transition in the life course, when each religious group has a heightened interest in the welfare of each of its members. At such moments, individual health and the health of the group converge.

This important feature of religious practice—its multiple manifestations in different cycles—has several implications. From a public health perspective, we might think of these regular human experiences as exposures, with predictable duration and frequency. More observant members of a faith tradition are more continually exposed to these experiences than less observant members. Some individuals may be more observant (and hence more exposed) at certain periods of their lives than at other periods or may participate more or less intensively, for example taking part in annual holiday celebrations but not weekly or daily practices.

A religious studies perspective would draw attention to the content and meaning of the practice—its narrative, teaching, and symbols. But all religious practices have a physical dimension; the body and its actions are the means of observance. Our first-person accounts emphasize the embodied experience of the practice: what it feels, sounds, looks, tastes, and even smells like. Whether it is fasting or singing, doing Taiji or being baptized in a river, the practice is experienced physically and spiritually. As we worked on this volume, the field of religious studies seems to have been moving in the same direction of emphasis—toward a focus on the materiality and practice of religion. Recent books by well-known scholars such as Robert Orsi,[1] Caroline Bynum,[2] Manuel Vásquez,[3] David Morgan,[4] and Martin Riesebrodt[5] have put forward new theories and interpretations of religion that rely primarily on practice, ritual, and worship as their entry points for understanding. Our interdisciplinary work in this volume thus seems to be converging with important trends in religious studies scholarship.

From both the public health and the religious studies perspective, the connection between these cyclical practices and the human life cycle is a profound one. From the moment of birth or even before it, to the moment of death and afterward, religions offer individuals, families, and communities a means of enacting their beliefs and telling the stories of their religious traditions. The gestures, clothing, foods, and music of religious practices are embedded in daily life and take on special importance at key turning points in the life course. For many billions of people, these are lifelong exposures whose health consequences may be direct or indirect, known or unknown. We present firsthand descriptions of religious practices here to capture the saturation of those billions of lives in religious practices that provide meaning and structure at the same time that they may affect health and well-being.

Notes

1. Robert A. Orsi, *The Cambridge Companion to Religious Studies* (Cambridge: Cambridge University Press, 2011).
2. Caroline Walker Bynum, *Christian Materiality: An Essay on Religion in Late Medieval Europe* (New York: Zone Pages, 2011).
3. Manuel Vásquez, *More Than Belief: Toward a Materialist Theory of Religion* (New York: Oxford University Press, 2010).
4. David Morgan, *The Embodied Eye: Religious Visual Culture and the Social Life of Feeling* (Berkeley: University of California Press, 2012).
5. Martin Riesebrodt, *The Promise of Salvation: A Theory of Religion* (Chicago: University of Chicago Press, 2010).

Daily Religious Practices

2 | Refuge Meditation in Contemporary Buddhism

GESHE LOBSANG TENZIN NEGI AND BRENDAN OZAWA-DE SILVA

U NDERSTOOD AS THE GATEWAY TO Buddhism, *going for refuge* is one of the most universal forms of practice for Buddhists across all traditions. Most Buddhists engage in it on a daily basis, and within the tradition, being a Buddhist means being someone who goes for refuge to the Three Precious and Sublime Jewels. These Three Jewels are the Buddhas (the enlightened beings), the Dharma (their teachings and realizations), and the Sangha (the spiritual community). Across the Buddhist world, one can encounter the familiar refuge prayer:

Buddham saranam gacchami (I go for refuge to the Buddha).
Dhammam saranam gacchami (I go for refuge to the Dharma).
Sangham saranam gacchami (I go for refuge to the Sangha).

As fundamental as it is for Buddhists, refuge is multifaceted, and the practice of it grows in richness and complexity as an individual's understanding of Buddhism deepens.

Growing up in a Buddhist family and culture in the Himalayan village of Ribba, in Kinnaur, the Indian region bordering western Tibet, I—Lobsang Tenzin Negi—don't even recall when I first learned the words of the refuge prayer. In traditional Buddhist societies, it is a natural part of the culture itself. My earliest memories of it trace back to winter, those three to four months each year when Kinnaur is snowed in and inaccessible to the outside world. Most of the work of the villages must be suspended due to the snow, so activities take place indoors. There is plenty of time for storytelling, reciting prayers, and chanting, and as is traditional in Buddhist practice, prayers always began with the verse of taking refuge.

As is probably the case for many Buddhists who have not studied the tradition in much depth, my understanding of going for refuge was rather naïve. The Buddhas or enlightened beings were to my mind beings who could be relied on in times of danger. The villages had plenty of ghost stories about spirits and unseen beings, and the Buddhas were, as I understood it, simply other beings who could protect us from these spirits. Today, I would say that this form of going for refuge is that of a person who is culturally Buddhist—that is, someone who participates in religious activities because they are part of his or her culture without necessarily understanding the underlying Buddhist principles.

For refuge practice to truly become the gateway to the Buddhist path, however, it cannot take place only on this superficial level. Genuine refuge takes shape as one becomes more deeply aware of Buddhist philosophy. Because Buddhism concentrates primarily on the transformation of the mind, refuge begins to take on psychological and spiritual dimensions. As Buddha himself said, the main content of his teaching was suffering and the way out of suffering. By this he meant not only temporary dangers and perils but more important—as identified succinctly in the Four Noble Truths—the continuing chain of suffering that unfolds on many levels in our lives, the primary causes that give rise to this physical and emotional suffering, the cessation of such suffering, and the paths that lead to the cessation of suffering.

When I became a monk at age 14, I began to pursue the study of Buddhist philosophy and its inner science of mind. It was then that the practice of refuge began to take on a whole new meaning for me. I saw that the Buddhas were not unseen beings who would protect me if I called upon them, but rather physicians whose teachings, like the medicines offered by doctors, could lead to the elimination of suffering if I put them into practice with the help of the spiritual community. As the Buddha Maitreya wrote in his *Uttaratantra*, or *Sublime Continuum*:

> Just as the disease needs to be diagnosed, its cause eliminated, a healthy state achieved, and the remedy implemented, so also should suffering, its causes, its cessation and the path be known, removed, attained and undertaken.

A patient who is manifesting symptoms of illness first needs to recognize that he or she is ill and find a doctor who can offer a diagnosis and prescription and then take the medicine prescribed. In the same way, going for refuge requires first understanding that one's suffering is primarily caused by one's own deeply embedded unhealthy karmic patterns or behavioral dispositions as well as destructive emotions and emotional dispositions and then turning to the enlightened beings and the spiritual community for help in changing those destructive patterns and dispositions. It is the enlightened beings whose teachings and instructions must be incorporated into one's heart and life if suffering and its causes are to be overcome and genuine happiness achieved, and it is the spiritual community that supports and assists along the way, as nurses support the work of physicians.

In a psychospiritual context, going for refuge requires a twofold mindset. The first is a sense of concern for one's future well-being arising from an awareness that the conditions that give rise to suffering—namely, deeply conditioned destructive behavioral and emotional dispositions—are ingrained in one's body and mind. The second is a deep confidence in the Buddha, the Dharma, and the Sangha and their abilities to bring about inner transformation.

It's important to note that the Three Jewels do not have the ability to release us from suffering and its causes without any effort on our part. Rather, just as it is by taking the medicine that the patient finds relief from illness, it is only by incorporating the Dharma into one's life that suffering and its causes can be transcended. As a famous Buddhist verse says:

Buddhas do not wash away sins with water,
Nor remove the suffering of beings with their hands.
They cannot transfer their realizations into others.
Rather, they liberate others by showing the truth of reality.

As I began to understand this, the practice of refuge took on a different dimension for me. It became clear to me that the main source on which one needs to rely to transform the inner causes of suffering and achieve greater happiness and well-being is the medicine of the Dharma, which must be integrated into one's life. Dharma, from a Buddhist point of view, is not merely the scriptural teachings; rather, the actual Dharma is the transformative qualities conveyed by these scriptures, such as mindfulness, love, compassion, forgiveness, tolerance, and insight into reality.

Approaching refuge in this way primarily yields personal well-being and flourishing, which is a perfectly legitimate pursuit, as each of us seeks to find happiness and avoid suffering. The practice of refuge can become even richer, however, when the practitioner gives greater importance to the welfare of all sentient beings than to his or her individual welfare. Reflecting on how others share the same fundamental aspiration to genuine happiness and freedom from suffering and on how one's individual well-being is deeply interconnected with that of others, the practitioner develops a strong sense of concern not only for him- or herself but for all. In this context, the practitioner turns to the Buddha, Dharma, and Sangha not merely for him- or herself but for the benefit of all sentient beings. This is like when a mother who has contracted an apparently fatal virus learns that her children have acquired it also. She turns to the doctors, the nurses, and the medicine that they prescribe not just for herself but also for her children. In a similar fashion, embracing others with compassion makes those others naturally a part of one's own going for refuge. For me, therefore, the practice of refuge takes on a much deeper significance when it is engaged in the context of the teachings on compassion for all sentient beings.

All Buddhist practices, even the most advanced, begin with going for refuge in the Three Jewels, individually or communally. To deepen the sense of reliance so that it infuses the mind, Buddhist practitioners often engage in meditations that involve repeated recitation of the refuge verse together with visualization. These meditations can take many forms, some of which are very elaborate. One simple form is described here.

First, the practitioner visualizes him- or herself surrounded by all sentient beings and begins with a brief reflection on his or her present condition in the context of the Four Noble Truths, namely, suffering and its causes, to give rise to a strong sense of concern. This consideration is then extended to include all other sentient beings, recognizing how they share the practitioner's aspiration for genuine happiness and freedom from suffering and how interconnected one is with them. Reflecting on the situation of these others, the practitioner develops a strong sense of concern for their suffering, which is compassion. Asking to whom he or she can turn for assistance, the practitioner reflects on the nature and qualities of the Buddha, Dharma, and Sangha, developing a deep sense of confidence in their ability to effect inner transformation.

To establish a firmer sense of their presence, the practitioner visualizes the Three Jewels: the Buddha seated on a beautiful throne with cushions of lotus, moon, and sun with the teachings in the form of texts on a beautiful table in front of him and the assembly of advanced practitioners surrounding him. The practitioner goes for refuge by developing a heartfelt sense of reliance on the Buddha, Dharma, and Sangha, and to deepen this sense of reliance, the refuge verse is repeated many times.

Simultaneously with the recitation, the practitioner engages in a three-stage process. In the first stage, from the heart of the Buddha, the texts, and the surrounding Sangha, white wisdom lights, which are understood to be the essence of the Three Jewels, emanate to reach the practitioner and all the sentient beings surrounding him or her. They enter in, soaking him or her in wisdom lights and infusing every cell and aspect of being and, in the course of that, dispelling suffering and its causes, that of all sentient beings and that of the practitioner. This leads to a deep sense of being cleansed from suffering and its causes. Second, golden lights emanate from the Three Jewels, entering into the practitioner and all other sentient beings, completely saturating the body and mind. These golden lights enhance the positive qualities of body, speech, and mind, bringing about greater physical, emotional, and spiritual flourishing. The visualization of these white and golden lights creates a vivid sensory and embodied experience that facilitates inner transformation. Finally, the practitioner cultivates a strong sense of being placed under the secure protection of the Three Jewels.

Within the context of tantric practice, refuge practice becomes even more profound, because the Buddhas are not seen as distant beings; rather, the enlightened state referred to as *Dharmakāya* ("Truth Body") is understood as manifesting as a living presence in the form of one's own spiritual teacher. This way of seeing enlightenment embodied in the teacher helps to give tremendous inspiration and impetus to the spiritual practitioner.

The psychological and spiritual purpose of refuge practice is to bring about a deeper resolve in the practitioner to overcome what is destructive in his or her body, speech, and mind and to enhance what is constructive, while strengthening compassion for others and bringing about a deep sense of security and confidence that is conducive to spiritual development. Other practices can follow after a meditation on refuge, but even engaging in this practice by itself can yield great benefits from a Buddhist perspective—not only spiritually but also in terms of physical and psychological health, relationships, and ethical conduct. As the seventh-century Buddhist sage Chandrakirti said in his *60 Verses on Going for Refuge*:

If the merit of going for refuge had physical form,
The entire multiverse would be too small to contain it.

For Further Reading

Beyer, Stephan. *The Cult of Tara: Magic and Ritual in Tibet*. Berkeley: University of California Press, 1978.

Gethin, Rupert. *The Foundations of Buddhism*. New York: Oxford University Press, 1998.
Gyatso, Tenzin (H. H. the Dalai Lama). *The World of Tibetan Buddhism: An Overview of Its Philosophy and Practice*. Somerville, MA: Wisdom Publications, 1995.
Harvey, Peter. *An Introduction to Buddhism: Teachings, History, and Practices*, 2d ed. Cambridge, UK: Cambridge University Press, 2013.
Lopez, Donald. *Buddhism in Practice*. Princeton, NJ: Princeton University Press, 1995.
Prebish, Charles S. *Luminous Passage: The Practice and Study of Buddhism in America*. Berkeley: University of California Press, 1999.

Editor's Note

The health research literature related to the specific practice of refuge meditation in Tibetan Buddhism is minimal. However, there is a substantial body of scientific literature on Buddhist meditation. Beginning in the late 1970s and at an increasing pace since, meditation has been studied in observational and survey research, interventions, and experimental designs. A wide range of outcomes and clinical populations has been studied; the greatest interest has come from neuroscience and clinical psychology. Research is reported from the United States, but more comes from other countries, including Thailand, Sri Lanka, India, Japan, and Hong Kong. Some of the most frequent topics for research have been neuro-imaging of the brain in meditative states, the correspondence between the practice of Buddhist meditation and psychological/psychoanalytic concepts, and the development of mindfulness-based cognitive psychotherapy. Populations in which interventions have been reported include patients with cancer, addiction, suicide risk, diabetes, and depression.

Resources for Public Health Research

Bushell, William C. "New Beginnings: Evidence That the Meditational Regimen Can Lead to Optimization of Perception, Attention, Cognition, and Other Functions." *Annals of the New York Academy of Sciences* 1172, no. 1 (2009): 348–361.
Chiesa, Alberto, and Alessandro Serretti. "A Systematic Review of Neurobiological and Clinical Features of Mindfulness Meditations." *Psychological Medicine* 40, no. 8 (2010): 1239–1252.
Dakwar, Elias, and Frances R. Levin. "The Emerging Role of Meditation in Addressing Psychiatric Illness, with a Focus on Substance Use Disorders." *Harvard Review of Psychiatry* 17, no. 4 (2009): 254–267.
Huynh, Thanh V., Carolyn Gotay, Gabriela Layi, and Susan Garrard. "Mindfulness Meditation and Its Medical and Non-Medical Applications." *Hawaii Medical Journal* 66, no. 12 (2007): 328–330.
Jevning, R., R. K. Wallace, and M. Beidebach. "The Physiology of Meditation: A Review. A Wakeful Hypometabolic Integrated Response." *Neuroscience & Biobehavioral Reviews* 16, no. 3 (1992): 415–424.

Kelly, Brendan D. "Buddhist Psychology, Psychotherapy and the Brain: A Critical Introduction." *Transcultural Psychiatry* 45, no. 1 (2008): 5–30.

Keng, Shian-Ling, Moria J. Smoski, and Clive J. Robins. "Effects of Mindfulness on
Psychological Health: A Review of Empirical Studies." *Clinical Psychology Review*
31, no. 6 (2011): 1041–1056.

Marchand, William R. "Mindfulness-Based Stress Reduction, Mindfulness-Based Cognitive Therapy, and Zen Meditation for Depression, Anxiety, Pain, and Psychological
Distress." *Journal of Psychiatric Practice* 18, no. 4 (2012): 233–252.

Rapgay, Lobsang, Ven Lati Rinpoche, and Rhonda Jessum. "Exploring the Nature and
Functions of the Mind: A Tibetan Buddhist Meditative Perspective." *Progress in
Brain Research* 122 (1999): 507–515.

Weaver, Andrew J., Adam Vane, and Kevin J. Flannelly. "A Review of Research on Buddhism and Health: 1980–2003." *Journal of Health Care Chaplaincy* 14, no. 2 (2008):
118–132.

Wiist, W. H., B. M. Sullivan, D. M. St. George, and H. A. Wayment. "Buddhists' Religious and Health Practices." *Journal of Religion and Health* 51, no. 1 (2012):
132–147.

3 | Taiji (T'ai-chi) in Taoism

ERIC REINDERS

E VERY WEEK, FORTY TO SIXTY adults of all ages, mostly Caucasian, gather in a large dance studio in Santa Barbara, California. The group forms into a grid pattern. More experienced practitioners are positioned in the four corners of the group, so that whichever way the group turns, beginners always have in sight a competent body to mimic. The first collective action is signaled by the call *jingli* (obeisance), and everyone bows to the teacher. Then the whole group begins the basic set, a slow series of pushes, weight shifts, and turns. During the set, new students step out of the grid to watch. After that, smaller groups practice at different levels. Some of the more experienced members act as instructors, helping new students with lower levels. Groups like this gather all over the United States, in church halls, YMCAs, public parks, and senior centers to practice Taiji.

My own group, in Atlanta, Georgia, meets in one of the studios of the Decatur School of Ballet. Here, six to eight of us practice for an hour and a half each Sunday. We have all been practicing for many years, so we focus on increasing our level of awareness during the forms. Our teacher also offers Taiji instruction to both beginners and continuing practitioners through Emory University's Continuing Education program. The students in these classes tend to be middle-aged or older and are often drawn from the staff of the university and the nearby hospitals. Most have seen Taiji on television; a few have had some rudimentary experience or have done another martial art.

Where yoga increases flexibility and muscle tone, Taiji improves balance and circulation. When we walk normally, we engage in a controlled falling forward, with the weight moving forward before the heel even touches the ground. In Taiji, typically, the weight always remains stable—the heel touches the ground but weight does not immediately follow; instead, weight moves forward only when the foot is on firm ground. In Taiji, almost at any point in a form, we could freeze and not fall over. Sustaining awareness of one's balance at all times gives us the sense of being centered even while in motion.

Balance is also improved through a strong sense of rootedness. Doing Taiji, we develop a feeling of the power of the earth coming up through the legs and hips, the sense of force traveling through the body. When the hand goes forward for a hand strike, for instance, it feel like a matter not of the arm but of the whole body. Ideally, it feels like the blow pushes *down into* the earth as the kinetic energy of the torso drives the hand. Anything meeting with the hand would then seem to be striking not the arm but the ground itself.

The energy spoken of in Taiji and Qigong is *qi* (ch'i). Definitions of qi range widely, including some that are relatively scientific (heat, kinesis) and others that are more psychological (qi as mental attention) or cosmic (qi as the life force of the universe). Qi is the basic concept in acupuncture and in fengshui; it implies that nothing is truly inanimate. The idea that the energetic flow of the body is somehow the same as the flow of energy in the landscape (and the weather, and even commerce) gives rise to a sense of connection in contrast to the isolation of the body imagined as a self-contained unit, animate in an inanimate world. Setting aside any empirical questions of the existence of qi, it is something that can be experienced. It may feel like (or be imagined as) a kind of magnetism or light, circulating in and extending around the body.

Most Taiji forms are executed without weapons, but there are sword (*jian*), saber (*dao*), staff, and fan forms. The most common form in America is a Yang-style series without weapons called the Twenty-Four Form. Describing any of the motions takes longer by far than the action itself. But let us examine the move called "part the horse's mane."

We begin with a position called "hold the ball." Weight is mostly on the right foot, with the ball of the left foot resting on the ground for balance—this is the "empty stance." The right arm is raised before the chest, the left arm below, with the two palms facing each other, as if holding a large beach ball. The sense of energetic connection between the two palms is very tangible. The waist turns to the right very slightly, and the right hand reaches toward the left shoulder. Here the body feels coiled. Then the left foot steps out, not directly ahead but at a wide angle. The torso completes the turn to the left, and most of the weight of the body shifts forward. This power in the torso drives the left hand forward and up, as if effortlessly. At the same time, the right hand pushes back and down. In martial terms, you have just grabbed an opponent's oncoming fist with your right hand, not meeting it but adding to its force and directing it downward; meanwhile, you have driven the edge of your left hand into your opponent's throat. In energetic terms, you have developed a ball of qi and then extended it. Without a sense of rootedness, all this feels like waving our arms around. With a sense of rootedness, our hands feel the power of the earth channeled up through the legs and hips.

These movements might take four seconds. No matter how eloquent, any description of them ends up sounding convoluted. The description gives little impression of the apparent simplicity of the movements. In fact, when teaching Taiji, you have to get students to do the right move, but the hardest part is getting them to stop doing all the *other* moves that are *not* part of the form. New students frequently make movements without thinking: shifting weight too quickly, dropping the arms for no reason, bending forward, and so on. Much of the sense of stillness that practitioners report is due to the sustained focus on certain bodily movements and the suppression of any others. Taiji is described as "moving meditation" because it constantly calls the attention back to a focus. In this sense, it is comparable to *vipassana*, which brings the mind always back to the breath, or mantra recitation, which brings the mind back to a word. But in Taiji, the focus includes the motion of the whole body.

Another aspect of early Taiji training is the experience of moving from self-conscious inability (fixated on rules, making frequent errors) to unself-conscious mastery; yet once formal mastery is attained, the mind still should not wander off. Those of us who have practiced a form for a long time would seem to "know" it, but there are always nuances that are missed, sloppy habits that creep back in, and ever more subtle refinements to be discovered. Each time I do a form, it is a unique experience.

Some students see the practice as a martial art. The martial roots of Taiji may be emphasized more or less, according to the teacher. At times an explanation in terms of the self-defensive aspect can help a student grasp the point of the movement, but clearly the training has limited efficacy in combat. The forms include blows with the hand, elbow, or foot, but the emphasis is rarely on attacking. The moves imply an imagined opponent striking from various angles. In response, we channel the opposing force down or to the sides, using opponents' own aggressive energy against them. In other words, the force that an opponent exerts to strike is not met with an opposing force but rather coaxed onward, so that the opponent is rendered off balance. This basic lesson, common to many martial arts, can be extended into daily life and applied in social situations. The practice of Taiji may encourage a habit of directing aggression away from the self, of manifesting an ideal interplay of force and yielding. Taiji teachers commonly encourage students to extrapolate the experience of this "power of yielding" as a way of being or an art of life.

In such experiences, one finds explicit connections to Daoist philosophy. There are, nonetheless, legitimate questions about the association of Taiji and Daoism. In what sense is Taiji a religious practice? Certain passages from the Daoist classic the *Daodejing* (*Tao Te Ching*) seem to be speaking directly of Taiji, especially in terms of the deflection of harm rather than direct opposition to it, the strategic use of weakness (yielding) to defeat the opponent, the emphasis on rootedness and concentration of energy in the core. In chapter 39, for example, the *Daodejing* advises, "Turning back is how the way moves; Weakness is the means the way employs." And in chapter 68:

> One who excels as a warrior does not appear formidable; one who excels in fighting is never roused in anger; one who excels in defeating his enemy does not join issue; one who excels in employing others humbles himself before them. . . . This is known as making use of others.

Quotations such as these become particularly vivid during the Taiji exercise called "push hands." In this practice, two people stand facing each other, and (in a formal, stylized manner) attempt to push each other over; each remains standing only by twisting the torso and redirecting the pushes to one side. Precisely at the moment when the other person's shove is at its furthest extent, the one receiving the push is most able to topple him or her.

Both Taiji and Daoist cultivation focus on the directed circulation of internal energies. But serious Daoist cultivation involves a vastly more complex set of visualizations and internal energy manipulations rarely taught in popular Taiji classes. In this sense, Taiji is similar to yoga, a physical practice that may or may not be associated with a religion—both yoga and Taiji are taught in YMCAs. In modern America, *Daoist* can mean all sorts of things, ranging from an institutional religion to a mellow, "go with the flow" attitude.

For Further Reading

Chiu, Milton M. *The Tao of Chinese Religion*. Lanham, MD: University Press of America, 1984.

Clarke, J. J. *The Tao of the West: Western Transformations of Taoist Thought*. London: Routledge, 2000.

Kohn, Livia, Editor. *Taoist Meditation and Longevity Techniques*. Ann Arbor: University of Michigan Press, 1989.

Kohn, Livia, Editor. *The Taoist Experience: An Anthology*. Albany: State University of New York Press, 1993.

Maspero, Henri. *Taoism and Chinese Religion*. Amherst: University of Massachusetts Press, 1981.

Editor's Note

The health research literature related to the practice of Taiji (T'ai-chi) is extensive. Beginning in the 1980s, Taiji has been studied in observational research, interventions, and randomized controlled trials. A wide range of outcomes and clinical populations has been studied. Some of the most frequent topics of research are musculoskeletal pain, balance, fall prevention, bone density, diabetes, coronary heart disease, cognitive impairment, quality of life, and aerobic capacity. The impact of Taiji on depression, insomnia, anxiety, stress, stroke, cancer, blood pressure, Parkinson's disease, obesity, asthma, immune response, and kidney disease have also been studied.

Resources for Public Health Research

Alperson, Sunny Y., and Vance W. Berger. "Opposing Systematic Reviews: The Effects of Two Quality Rating Instruments on Evidence Regarding T'ai Chi and Bone Mineral Density in Postmenopausal Women." *Journal of Alternative and Complementary Medicine* 17, no. 5 (2011): 389–395.

Birdee, Gurjeet S., Peter M. Wayne, Roger B. Davis, Russell S. Phillips, and Gloria Y. Yeh. "T'ai Chi and Qigong for Health: Patterns of Use in the United States." *Journal of Alternative and Complementary Medicine* 15, no. 9 (2009): 969–973.

Dalusung-Angosta, Alona. "The Impact of Tai Chi Exercise on Coronary Heart Disease: A Systematic Review." *Journal of the American Academy of Nurse Practitioners* 23, no. 7 (2011): 376–381.

Ho, Tsung-Jung, David C. Christiani, Tso-Chiang Ma, Tsong-Rong Jang, Chih-Hui Lieng, Yi-Chun Yeh, et al. "Effect of Qigong on Quality of Life: A Cross–Sectional Population–Based Comparison Study in Taiwan." *BMC Public Health* 11, no. 1 (2011): 546.

Jahnke, Roger, Linda Larkey, Carol Rogers, Jennifer Etnier, and Fang Lin. "A Comprehensive Review of Health Benefits of Qigong and Tai Chi." *American Journal of Health Promotion* 24, no. 6 (2010): e1–e25.

Lee, Myeong Soo, Paul Lam, and Edzard Ernst. "Effectiveness of Tai Chi for Parkinson's Disease: A Critical Review." *Parkinsonism & Related Disorders* 14, no. 8 (2008): 589–594.

Li, Fuzhong, Peter Harmer, K. John Fisher, Edward McAuley, Nigel Chaumeton, Elizabeth Eckstrom, and Nicole L. Wilson. "Tai Chi and Fall Reductions in Older Adults: A Randomized Controlled Trial." *Journals of Gerontology Series A: Biological Sciences and Medical Sciences* 60, no. 2 (2005): 187–194.

Liu, Hao, and Adam Frank. "Tai Chi as a Balance Improvement Exercise for Older Adults: A Systematic Review." *Journal of Geriatric Physical Therapy* 33, no. 3 (2010): 103–109.

Rand, Debbie, William C. Miller, Jeanne Yiu, and Janice J. Eng. "Interventions for Addressing Low Balance Confidence in Older Adults: A Systematic Review and Meta-Analysis." *Age and Ageing* 40, no. 3 (2011): 297–306.

Reid, M. Carrington, Maria Papaleontiou, Anthony Ong, Risa Breckman, Elaine Wethington, and Karl Pillemer. "Self-Management Strategies to Reduce Pain and Improve Function among Older Adults in Community Settings: A Review of the Evidence." *Pain Medicine* 9, no. 4 (2008): 409–424.

Sarris, Jerome, and Gerard J. Byrne. "A Systematic Review of Insomnia and Complementary Medicine." *Sleep Medicine Reviews* 15, no. 2 (2011): 99–106.

Wang, Chenchen. "Tai Chi and Rheumatic Diseases." *Rheumatic Diseases Clinics of North America* 37, no. 1 (2011): 19–32.

Yeh, Gloria Y., Chenchen Wang, Peter M. Wayne, and Russell S. Phillips. "The Effect of Tai Chi Exercise on Blood Pressure: A Systematic Review." *Preventive Cardiology* 11, no. 2 (2008): 82–89.

Yeh, Gloria Y., Chenchen Wang, Peter M. Wayne, and Russell Phillips. "Tai Chi Exercise for Patients with Cardiovascular Conditions and Risk Factors: A Systematic Review." *Journal of Cardiopulmonary Rehabilitation and Prevention* 29, no. 3 (2009): 152–160.

4 | Veiling in Islam: A Western Feminist Outsider's Perspective

KATHRYN M. YOUNT

W ITH AMBIVALENCE, I SHARE MY perspective, based on personal experiences, on the meaning of veiling as a daily religious practice. To start, I will situate myself as a feminist European American of Christian heritage. I also am a longtime resident of the southern United States, with no cultural, religious, or ancestral ties to the geographies where veiling has a prominent history. Many scholars and lay experts who have these ties might assert that I am not ideally positioned to offer insights about veiling as a daily religious practice. I respect these views and considered them soberly before putting pen to paper for this invited essay. At the same time, I lived in Cairo for more than two years (1995–1997) and have worked for almost twenty years in various parts of the Middle East and South Asia, where veiling is a visible part of daily public life. Finally, I am a researcher of gender in cross-cultural contexts, and I believe that cross-cultural dialogues are fundamental for transformation. From this standpoint as an "informed outsider," I share my observations and experiences of the daily practice of veiling.[1]

In the space that I have, I will share some personal recollections of veiling, as I encountered it in the settings where I have lived and worked and where I have been privileged to know both veiled and unveiled women. I was invited to write exclusively from "lived experiences," but I will bend these parameters and share some thoughts about scholarship on veiling and its representation in the West. This departure is necessary, as scholarship on veiling and Western media have shaped the lens through which I view this daily practice. Finally, I will end my essay with a veiled woman's story and a call to take such voices as the point of departure in future conversations about veiling as a daily practice.

The one observation I will relay up front is that veiling is one of the most diverse daily practices that one can imagine. Note that I use the phrase "daily practice" rather than "daily religious practice." My choice of words is intentional, as I believe that the meanings of veiling extend well beyond religious ritual. For some women, veiling is a devoted, public expression of religious faith. For others, it also is the symbolic essence of feminine modesty, simplicity, and discretion—a "portable seclusion"[2] and an expression of dedication to a "moral way of life in which families are paramount . . . and the home is associated with the sanctity of women."[3] For others, it *also* is a marker of social status—of the *balady* or déclassé woman and of the educated urbanite.[4] For others, the veil is such a usual form of dress that it provokes little reflection on its meaning for the wearer.

In Cairo in the 1990s, these multiple meanings were apparent to me on summer evenings, when I was a newcomer to the city and strolled the banks of the Nile alone for entertainment. Invariably, the promenade was crowded and bustling with passersby, many of whom were chatting and laughing while walking arm in arm to their destinations. On more than one of these walks, I encountered women adorned in vibrant and contemporary *hijab* (head scarves), thoughtfully tucked in to loose-fitting, matching dress suits. Intermingled were women dressed in earthen-tone skirts that dusted the pavement, loose-fitting shirts extending below the wrists, and *khimars* or waist-length veils. On some nights, entire groups of women would approach, whom I presumed—correctly or incorrectly—to be family members from a location in the Gulf. In many cases, these women were *Munaqabat* (face-veiled women), dressed entirely in black with only narrow openings for the eyes. Finally, there were women who wore no veil at all, and without knowing them by name or having some deeper acquaintance, I was left with no clue about their religious affiliations.

These impressions of diversity in daily veiling frame my observations of veiling and unveiling at various life stages by closer Egyptian colleagues. One colleague was distinct for *not* being veiled, as she was a resident of Upper (southern) Egypt, where veiling by Muslim women was all but universal. Sahar (I will call her) was remarkable for her physical beauty, her strong intellect, and her animated personality, which carried a note of youthful rebellion. For most of my time in Egypt, I knew Sahar as an unmarried, unveiled Muslim woman. Around the time of her engagement and marriage, virtually overnight, she took up the hijab and the loose-fitting dress suits. We never discussed the reasons for her decision, as I left this conversation to her discretion. In our ongoing projects, she retains her energetic charm and somewhat distinctive ability, for an Upper Egyptian woman, to travel unaccompanied for her waged work.

These "on-the-ground" images of diversity in daily veiling contrast sharply with the Western media's portrayal of the "downtrodden hijabi (veiled) woman"[5] as well as *Vogue* magazine's "appropriation of the burqa as haute couture."[6] Sadly, even impersonal, public impressions of diversity in daily veiling remain inaccessible to most Westerners. As a result, the richer layers of diversity in meaning are shrouded from Western view by stereotype, fear, avoidance, and ethnocentrism.

Some of these more hidden meanings of the practice are proposed in the writings of (often Western) anthropologists. Many such scholars have made veiling a focus of inquiry, often as a counterpoint to prevailing media stereotypes. My reading of these ethnographies has shaped the lens through which I interpret daily veiling, and the work of Arlene Elowe MacLeod,[7] among others, is influential. In her account of the "new veiling" among lower middle-class women in Cairo, MacLeod describes veiling not only as a daily religious ritual but also as an "ambiguous political struggle" under local and global patriarchies. Namely, some Cairean women have taken up the veil as a public symbol of conformity to respectable woman-hood as they transgress the boundaries of gendered spaces to work outside the home. On the one hand, daily veiling has enabled some lower middle-class women to enter historically proscribed spaces. On the other hand, it reveals the "ambivalent ways in which women react to their inequality and try to struggle against it."[8] MacLeod's argument, which frames my inter-pretation of Sahar's adoption of the veil, is that this act is a complex, per-sonal political project of strategic conformity. By maintaining the public appearance of the "good woman," veiling enables women to access spaces once reserved for men. Yet, it poses "the problem of understanding wom-en's . . . paradoxical participation in relations of power."[9]

Some Muslim women who have taken up the veil attach very different meanings to their daily practice. Ayesha Nusrat, a 23-year-old Muslim Indian and women's rights activist from New Delhi, clarified her own de-cision to become a "hijabi woman" in a *New York Times* op-ed piece:

It's been over two months since I decided to become a hijabi. . . . I see this as the most liberating experience ever. . . . In a society that embraces uncov-ering . . . I see hijab as the freedom to regard my body as my own concern and as a way to secure personal liberty in a world that objectifies women. . . .

I look forward to . . . when true equality will be had with women not needing to display themselves to get attention nor needing to defend their decision to keep their bodies to themselves. . . . My hijab is a visual religious
marker that makes it very easy . . . to spot me in a crowd as a separate entity
representing or adhering to a particular religion. . . . Being a hijabi in the
public arena . . . drives me to work in ways that would help break the undig-
nified stereotypes, barriers and prejudices that my Islamic faith is relent-
lessly and irrationally associated with. As an extension of my personality
and identity, it instigates me to challenge the misconception that Muslim
women lack the bravery, intellect and resilience to challenge authority and
fight for their own rights.[10]

Thus, the daily practice of veiling for women becomes political in the
context of local *and* global patriarchies as well as the commodification of
the practice in the Western media. The "practice" might better be understood as a mosaic of practices and motivations, of the mundane, of morality, of strategic conformity, and of Muslim feminist emancipation. In full
acknowledgement of my own narrow perspective, I would call on scholars
and laypeople alike to centralize women's voices in evolving definitions of
this daily practice. I also would call on scholars and laypeople to care
about its social, emotional, and psychic significance for women alongside
any implications for their physical health.

Editor's Note

Research on the health consequences of the wearing of hijab or veils by
Muslim women is not extensive, but work has been reported by researchers in the United States, United Kingdom, Denmark, Sweden, Nigeria,
Iran, Lebanon, Italy, Jordan, and Turkey. Topics of investigation have
included vitamin D deficiency and associated osteoporosis, rickets, and
fractures, and the accidental ingestion or inhalation of "turban pins" by
adolescent girls. There are also studies of positive psychological effects in
terms of increased well-being and self-esteem associated with veiling as
well as incidence of psychological disorders, including eating disorders,
body dissatisfaction, and depression, among veiled women.

Resources for Public Health Research

el-Sonbaty, M. R., and N. U. Abdul-Ghaffar. "Vitamin Deficiency in Veiled Kuwaiti
    Women." *European Journal of Clinical Nutrition* 50 (1996): 315–318.

Gannagé-Yared, Marie-Hélène, Rana Chemali, Najwa Yaacoub, and Georges Halaby. "Hypovitaminosis D in a Sunny Country: Relation to Lifestyle and Bone Markers." *Journal of Bone and Mineral Research* 15, no. 9 (2000): 1856–1862.

Glew, Robert H., Michael J. Crossey, Jup Polanams, Henry I. Okolie, and Dorothy J. VanderJagt. "Vitamin D Status of Seminomadic Fulani Men and Women." *Journal of the National Medical Association* 102, no. 6 (2010): 485–490.

Guzel, R., E. Kozanuglu, F. Guler-Uysal, S. Soyupak, and T. Sarpel. "Vitamin D Status and Bone Mineral Density of Veiled and Unveiled Turkish Women." *Journal of Women's Health & Gender-Based Medicine* 10, no. 8 (2001): 765–770.

Hasdiraz, L., C. Bicer, M. Bilgin, and F. Oguzkaya. "Turban Pin Aspiration: Non-Asphyxiating Tracheobronchial Foreign Body in Young Islamic Women." *Thoracic & Cardiovascular Surgeon* 54, no. 4 (2006): 273–275.

Mishal, A. A. "Effects of Different Dress Styles on Vitamin D Levels in Healthy Young Jordanian Women." *Osteoporosis International* 12 (2001): 931–935.

Rastamesh, Reza, Marci E. Gluck, and Zhaleh Shadman. "Comparison of Body Dissatisfaction and Cosmetic Rhinoplasty with Levels of Veil Practicing in Islamic Women." *International Journal of Eating Disorders* 42, no. 4 (2009): 339–345.

Tolyamat, Lana D., and Bonnie Moradi. "US Muslim Women and Body Image: Links among Objectification Theory Constructs and the Hijab." *Journal of Counseling Psychology* 58, no. 3 (2011): 383–392.

Notes

1. I am most grateful to Dr. Rania Salem for her thoughtful comments on a prior version of this essay.
2. Hanna Papanek, "Purdah in Pakistan: Seclusion and Modern Occupations for Women," in *Separate Worlds: Studies of Purdah in South Asia*, ed. Hanna Papanek and Gail Minault (Columbus, MO: South Asia Books/Chanakya Publications, 1982), 190–216.
3. Lila Abu Lughod, "Do Muslim Women Really Need Saving? Anthropological Reflections on Cultural Relativism and Its Others," *American Anthropologist* 104, no. 3 (2002): 785.
4. Lughod, "Do Muslim Women Really Need Saving?"
5. Ayesha Nusrat, "The Freedom of the Hijab," *New York Times*, July 13, 2012.
6. Ellen McLarney, "The Burqa in Vogue: Fashioning Afghanistan," *Journal of Middle East Women's Studies* 5, no. 1 (2009): 1.
7. Arlene Elowe MacLeod, *Accommodating Protest: Working Women, the New Veiling, and Change in Cairo* (New York: Columbia University Press, 1993).
8. MacLeod, *Accommodating Protest*, xiv.
9. MacLeod, *Accommodating Protest*, 3.
10. Nusrat, "Freedom of the Hijab."

5 | Vegetarianism in Seventh-day Adventism

GEORGE H. GRANT AND JOSE MONTENEGRO

THE SEVENTH-DAY ADVENTIST CHURCH (SDA), a Christian faith tradition, is known for its emphasis on physical health and its community-based, spiritually holistic lifestyle. Diet is a particularly important component that often involves traditions of ethnicity, family, and the religious doctrines of the SDA faith. Above all, the commitment to a healthy vegetarian or semivegetarian diet must be seen as a religious practice. Our family table and the food we eat are at the core of a belief system that as Adventists we are physically and spiritually prepared for service to God, to ourselves, to each other, and to the earth.

For devout SDA members, food is a key part of Sabbath celebrations. In the SDA tradition, the Sabbath begins at sunset on Friday and ends at sunset on Saturday. During the Sabbath hours, we rest from all work and make it a special day distinctive from the rest of the week. We assemble as a family an hour before sunset on Friday for worship, songs, games, and a short devotional thought. After we begin the Sabbath, we gather around the table and eat challah bread, some cut fruits, and almond milk. On the next day, we gather with other family members for the main Sabbath meal. The Sabbath lunch varies based on family background and culture. One of us comes from a Hispanic SDA family and our meals on the Sabbath—as every day—typically consist of beans, rice (whole grain or white), meat substitutes, and a good amount of salad. The salads are the favorites at my house; they are made with cucumber, spinach, red radish, romaine lettuce, tomatoes, avocados, and a dressing of extra-virgin olive oil, lemon, and salt.

During the week, family meals tend to be less formal, although food choices are still driven by our beliefs. Breakfast usually consists of cereal and granola with almond milk. For dinner, the foods we most enjoy are whole-wheat spaghetti, steamed broccoli, and salad (the salad can be just lettuce and tomato with extra-virgin olive oil, lemon, and salt as dressing); traditional Venezuelan *arepas* (made from corn flour; my wife adds oatmeal for fiber and protein) are also a favorite. The arepa is a small, circular bread, almost like pita bread, and it is cut open and filled with cheese, lettuce, tomato, and avocado. During the week, we do not have lunch at home because the children are in school and my wife and I are at work. For snacks we have fruits, such as apples, grapes, bananas, oranges, tangerines, and mangos. One of our personal favorite snacks is homemade popcorn with olive oil and salt.

Members of the SDA church are not required to be vegetarian, but it is strongly encouraged. Those who advocate a religious commitment to vegetarianism or semivegetarianism base their argument in the Genesis 9:3–6 account of the period after the great flood, which says that consumption of plants and some animals was permitted during that difficult time, although God's original plan for the types of food humankind should eat, given in Genesis 1:29, included only nuts, grains, and fruits.[1]

Individuals are free to decide which path is most appropriate, but most who religiously commit follow a vegetarian diet of some kind. There are several paths to a vegetarian or semivegetarian lifestyle: lacto vegetarianism, lacto-ovo vegetarianism, full veganism, and clean-meat semivegetarianism. The lacto vegetarian consumes plant life and dairy products; lacto-ovo vegetarians consume dairy products and eggs, while vegans will not consume any product derived from animals. Semivegetarians eat dairy products, eggs, and meat that follows kosher restrictions that are very similar to the Jewish tradition. The church follows the guidelines given in the Hebrew scripture book of Leviticus (Lev. 7:19, 23–24; 8:31) for clean and unclean meat. There can be no consumption of unclean meat such as pork, lobster, or shellfish.

The most prominent voice in the origination of the SDA's health commitment was Ellen G. White (*ca.* 1860s). White drew upon her knowledge of Hebrew and Christian scripture to offer visions that greatly influenced the religious practice of the SDA: "Let none who profess godliness regard with indifference the health of the body, and flatter themselves that intemperance is no sin, and will not affect their spirituality. A close sympathy exists between the physical and the moral nature."[2] White became known as an advocate for bodily health at a time when hygienic and nutritional principles were just beginning to be understood. She wrote and preached a message that evokes the modern phrase "you are what you eat." If you eat animals, she argued, then your animalistic nature will have to face the consequences of the diseases and other harmful outcomes associated with eating flesh. White's premise, based on scripture, was that there was only one time on the earth when it was absolutely necessary for humans to consume flesh, and that was after the great flood when plants were struggling to replenish. Her dietary health message was respectful of food availability and region but could generally be understood as vegetarian:

> God has furnished man with abundant means for the gratification of an un-perverted appetite. He has spread before him the products of the earth, a bountiful variety of food that is palatable to the taste and nutritious to the system. Of these our benevolent heavenly Father says we may freely eat. Fruits, grains, and vegetables, prepared in a simple way, free from spice and grease of all kinds, make, with milk or cream, the most healthful diet. They impart nourishment to the body, and give a power of endurance and a vigor of intellect that are not produced by a stimulating diet.[3]

These pre-scientific visions were certainly prescient, reflecting many ideas that have come to be accepted as central to the health regimens of today. What has evolved from these original messages has been adapted to the present-day context. For instance, the moderate use of herbs and spices is an accepted food choice for today's Adventist. However, the influence of White's teaching is still felt across the tradition.

In fact, various cultural tensions in the international spread of the nutrition message have spurred reassessments of the early diet "counsels." There are today seventeen million Seventh-day Adventists in virtually every corner of the globe; less than 10 percent live in the United States, where the movement began. The nutritional needs of and the food products available to SDA communities vary from place to place and culture to culture. The SDA church recognizes that in some parts of the world the primary foods available are meats, and rice, beans, or vegetables are difficult to obtain or prohibitively expensive. For some in the SDA (including co-author J. M.), it would be "un-Christian" to require a vegetarian lifestyle for these communities. Nevertheless, even allowing for cultural and regional diversity with regard to vegetarianism, an SDA person abstains from eating unclean meats as well as using tobacco, alcohol, or drugs.

The universally accepted recommendation of White is that one should strive for a balanced lifestyle. A person must take into consideration his or her own health and environment. Within the SDA community, there is the belief that the best form of nutrition will be found in what the earth provides for consumption. Overall, one should strive for healthy, moderate eating, or, better yet, seek to eliminate anything that could be harmful to one's future safety and health, by adopting a vegetarian lifestyle:

> Along with adequate exercise and rest, we are to adopt the most healthful diet possible and abstain from the unclean foods identified in the Scriptures. Since alcoholic beverages, tobacco, and the irresponsible use of drugs and narcotics are harmful to our bodies, we are to abstain from them as well. Instead, we are to engage in whatever brings our thoughts and bodies into the discipline of Christ, who desires our wholesomeness, joy, and goodness.[4]

The health message of the SDA church is much broader than the recommendation of vegetarianism. Health is a product of all aspects of life, including exercise, rest, and participation in a community of worshipers. James Bates, a sea captain and one of the founding fathers of the SDA church, observed on one of his trips that many of the things he put energy and money into, such as alcohol, were things that would not help him secure salvation. He subsequently became engaged in the temperance and abolition movements and began to incorporate the seventh-day Sabbath as his faith practice. His influence, along with that of the younger Ellen White, led to the strong religious commitment to treat the body as a holy sanctuary that is today characteristic of SDA members. The overall concentration on and consciousness of what we put into our bodies is the observance by which SDA members grow closer in their relationship with God in the present and in turn are more prepared for the second coming of God in the future.

The SDA people are diverse in terms of culture, ethnicity, and region, but they share religiously driven commitments to a common health message. The health message is key to the core beliefs of the SDA church, but it is important to remember that Seventh-day Adventism is much more than a simple commitment to a healthy lifestyle; it is a religious faith. The religious underpinnings that encourage and support the people of this faith tradition have often been overlooked in the public attention that has come to the SDA church and its practices. Although the church's regimens are becoming accepted in the mainstream secular world as fundamental components of a healthy lifestyle, for the SDA people, they originated as—and remain—*religious* practices and expressions of faith.

Editor's Note

There is substantial research literature on the health of Seventh-day Adventists in the United States and around the world. The Adventist Health Studies, begun at Loma Linda University in the late 1950s, have enrolled more than one hundred thousand Adventists in research on lifestyle and health outcomes. Specific areas of investigation undertaken by these and researchers at other centers include the impact of SDA vegetarianism on mortality from all causes, particularly ischemic heart disease, stroke, and cancers of the prostate, breast, colon, lung, and ovaries; cardiovascular disease risk factors including hypertension and lipids; obesity; respiratory symptoms due to environmental exposure in this nonsmoking population; and the role of SDA hospitals and health professionals in missions around the world. The Adventist Health Studies website (http://www.llu.edu/public-health/health/index.page?) lists more than four hundred publications in scientific journals. The following are some recent examples of such research.

Resources for Public Health Research

Beezhold, Bonnie L., Carol S. Johnston, and Deanna R. Daigle. "Vegetarian Diets Are Associated with Healthy Mood States: A Cross–Sectional Study in Seventh-day Adventist Adults." *Nutrition Journal* 9 (2010): 26.

Feldbush, Martin W., and Jeffrey T. Mitchell. "A Time for Renewal: A Lessons-Learned Review on the Role of the CISM in Caring for Missionaries after the Rwandan Genocide." *International Journal of Emergency Mental Health* 12, no. 1 (2010): 51–56.

Fonnebo, Vinjar. "The Healthy Seventh-day Adventist Lifestyle: What Is the Norwegian Experience?" *American Journal of Clinical Nutrition* 59, no. 5 Suppl. (1994): 1124S–1129S.

Heuch, Ivar, Bjarne Jacobsen, and Gary E. Fraser. "A Cohort Study Found That Earlier and Longer Seventh-day Adventist Church Membership Was Associated with Reduced Male Mortality." *Journal of Clinical Epidemiology* 58, no. 1 (2005): 83–91.

Pawlak, Roman, and Marta Sovyanhadi. "Prevalence of Overweight and Obesity among Seventh-day Adventist African American and Caucasian College Students." *Ethnicity & Disease* 19, no. 2 (2009): 111–114.

Rouse, I. L., B. K. Armstrong, and L. J. Beilin. "Vegetarian Diet, Lifestyle and Blood Pressure in Two Religious Populations." *Clinical and Experimental Pharmacology and Physiology* 9, no. 3 (2007): 327–330.

Willett, Walter. "Lessons from Dietary Studies in Adventists and Questions for the Future." *American Journal of Clinical Nutrition* 78, no. 3 Suppl. (2003): 539S–543S.

Notes

1. David C. Nieman, *The Adventist Healthstyle: Why It Works* (Hagerstown, MD: Review and Herald, 1992), 59–60.
2. Ellen G. White, *Counsels on Diet and Foods* (Washington, DC: Review and Herald, 1938), 43.1, chapter 2.
3. White, *Counsels on Diet and Foods*, 92.1, chapter 4.
4. Seventh-day Adventist Church, "Fundamental Beliefs," http://www.adventist.org/beliefs/fundamental/index.html.

Weekly Religious Practices

6 | The Eucharist in Roman Catholicism

PHILLIP M. THOMPSON

N *THE MOVIEGOER*, THE CATHOLIC novelist Walker Percy has his protagonist, Binx Bolling, observe a businessman leaving a celebration of the Mass in New Orleans on Ash Wednesday. The businessman has gone to church not for spiritual transformation but to maintain his social status. But Binx speculates that he receives transformation anyway through "God's own importunate bonus." It is a good thing that the grace operating through the Eucharist, or holy communion, is importunate—that is, annoyingly persistent—because we Catholics are too often captives to the world, its demands, its assumptions, and its idols. It is not easy to extract ourselves from these snares through the rituals of our faith. For me, the Mass always provides timely help, although admittedly not in the same way or to the same degree each time.

So how does this happen? Let me share one particular experience of attending a celebration of the Mass. My own thoughts when entering the church for this Mass are scattered and disjointed. I have spent a week being battered by the demands of relentless multitasking. How then to renew myself? The process begins with not eating or drinking for an hour before the Mass as I try to calm my body and mind. Then, my wife and son and I rush to the car as I wonder, "Did I get the money to put in the offertory envelope?" We enter the church in haste, along with a number of other procrastinators. Walking into the nave, I put my fingers in a bowl of holy water and quickly make the sign of the cross, moving my right hand from my forehead to my chest to my left shoulder then crossing back to my right shoulder, touching at each point with my fingertips, to trace the form of a cross on my body. To find seats, we have to squeeze past fellow parishioners. More than a little agitated, I kneel and try to pray, but what I am thinking is, "Did I turn off my cell phone?" I hear an announcement to greet my fellow parishioners. I reluctantly oblige.

A hymn begins and the priest, wearing the green vestments of Ordinary Time, enters slowly, followed by a deacon holding up the Book of the Gospels and young altar servers carrying a processional cross and candles. The priest turns and faces us; he smiles slightly while making the sign of the cross and then proclaims, "The Lord be with you." We respond, "And with your spirit.[1]" After the greeting, the congregation asks forgiveness for their sins, praises God, and then listens to three scripture readings, separated by brief responses from the Psalms. There is a short homily based on the readings that offers insights on our daily challenges as people of faith.

We sense through the readings, the homily, and even the vestments where we are in the ebb and flow of the annual liturgical cycle. The Mass has its regularities across all cycles, which provide a sense of continuity, but there is also change as we move through the year. The season of Lent starts with Ash Wednesday, which is usually in February. The black smudge of a cross on our foreheads is a visible symbol of our mortality and our fallen natures. Lent reminds us that we need a spiritual assessment and cleansing. We reflect on what have we done wrong to our friends, neighbors, and even to God. On Maundy Thursday, on the cusp of Easter but still in Lent, the priest washes parishioners' feet in the front of the church to reenact Jesus's symbolic command to his apostles to follow a life of service. On Good Friday, just before Easter, we remember that Jesus suffered for us and with us on the cross. In one church that I attended, Father Ed would dim the lights on Good Friday so that a beam of light fell on the steps to the altar. On the steps, he placed a large wooden cross with nails on the arms. The parishioners would then silently process to the front of the church. The only sound to be heard was when each person picked up a hammer and hit the metal spikes. Through this ritual, we were vividly reminded of the consequences of our choices.

Having reached the bottom, we then arise and are reborn. With Easter Sunday, the bonds of death are broken. Life spills forth in a torrent of renewal. Where I live, plants and trees bloom with the unstoppable and sublime power of creation. The priests' white vestments embroidered with gold herald spiritual renewal. For the forty days of the Easter season, we are vividly reminded of the living Christ, a presence that walks intimately with us on our pilgrimage.

Following Easter, we enter Ordinary Time, a liturgical period not marked by a special period of repentance, reflection, and renewal. In this time, we must rediscover the holy, the extraordinary, in the ordinary.

Let us return to the Mass of the Ordinary Time. After the homily, we recite in unison the Nicene Creed—the basic truths that we accept as Christians and that connect us in the mystical body of Christ. The parishioners then pray for the Church, its leadership, and those suffering and in need. We place our offerings in wicker baskets that are briskly passed down the aisles.

So we have praised God, sung hymns, listened to inspired words of scripture, received a life lesson, proclaimed our common beliefs, and provided for the needs of the church. This is all preparation for the Eucharist; we are ready to change bread and wine into the real presence of Jesus. The altar is prepared with the placing of linen, on which a flat circular metal plate or paten holding the Eucharistic wafer and a golden chalice or goblet for the wine are placed. The priest reminds us of the source of this sustenance as he raises a large wafer above the alter: "Blessed are you, Lord, God of all creation. Through your goodness we have this bread to offer, which earth has given and human hands have made. It will become for us the bread of life." Similarly, he raises the chalice of wine above his head: "Blessed are you, Lord, God of all creation. Through your goodness we have this wine to offer, fruit of the vine and work of human hands. It will become our spiritual drink." We are thus reminded that the work of human hands operates in concert with the bounty of nature to bring us the bread and wine. We are active participants in the process of divine creation.

We continue with another round of prayer, hymns, invocation, and praise of God. The priest then washes his hands as a ritual cleansing of his sins, and we are now ready for the consecration of the bread and wine. There is a pause; the church is silent. We must now employ a variety of elements in a Eucharistic prayer to enact the transformation. We begin with prayers that lift our hearts to God and ask that the bread and wine be blessed. The priest prays for the spiritual and physical healing of the faithful, "for the redemption of their souls and in hope of health and well-being." He then holds his hands over the wine and bread and invites the material to become spiritual: "Be pleased, O God, we pray, to bless, acknowledge, and approve this offering in every respect; make it spiritual and acceptable, so that it may become for us the Body and Blood of your most beloved Son, our Lord Jesus Christ."

The priest then recounts the story of the Last Supper and praises the salvific power and glory of God. The Eucharistic prayer ends with the priest lifting the bread and wine and proclaiming, "Through him, and with him, and in him, O God, almighty Father, in the unity of the Holy Spirit, all glory and honor is yours, for ever and ever." We respond, "Amen."

Having invited Christ among us, we then recognize his holy gifts and our need for his constant help in the prayer given us by Jesus, the our Father. We are now connected to one another in the mystical body of Christ, and we recognize our solidarity by offering each other a sign of peace. My wife, son, and I hug each other, and then we gladly shake the hands of our fellow communicants saying, "Peace be with you."

We ask for the healing of our sins and for peace as we pray in unison twice, "Lamb of God, you take away the sins of the world, have mercy on us." This is concluded with "Lamb of God you take away the sins of the world, grant us peace." The priest then joins his hands and quietly requests God's mercy, which will bring "protection in mind and body and a healing remedy." The congregation kneels.

The priest holds up the communion host and proclaims, "This is the Lamb of God who takes away the sins of the world. Happy are those who are called to his supper."

We respond, "Lord, I am not worthy that you should enter under my roof, but only say the word and my soul shall be healed."

With that plea, we rise and process to the altar, seeking God's mercy and our healing. Taking in the real presence of Jesus in the Eucharistic wafer and wine, we join ourselves to one another and to God. I bow and then receive from the Eucharistic ministers first the thin, round consecrated wafer of unleavened bread and then a sip of wine from the chalice. I would like to describe this moment, but there is no analogy that captures it. I feel clarity, love, connection. I am with everyone and everything. But it is more, so much more.

My hands clasped together in front of my chest, I slowly return to my seat, letting a mystical presence soak into me. Things are slower now, calmer. At our seats, we kneel and pray until all have been served, and the remaining hosts are placed in a tabernacle or liturgical case behind the altar. The last words spoken from the altar remind us that our transformation must extend beyond the church: "The Peace of the Lord be with you always. Let us offer the sign of peace." We end as we began, with music and a procession of the priest, deacon, and altar servers as they depart the nave of the church.

So ends our story. But not quite. In the narthex, or entrance area, I shake hands with the priest. As I leave the church, I joke with my son and kiss my wife. There is a sense of something new. Peace? Joy? Healing? I am more relaxed, more alive both spiritually and physically. Amidst the music and prayers, the candles, the kneeling and shaking hands, there has been a transformation in me. I remember why our participation in the celebration of the Mass is so crucial to our faith. As the late Cardinal Joseph Bernardin reminds us:

> Liturgy is not an option nor merely an obligation, not a bonus, but a need— like food and drink, like sleep and work, like friends. We need to gather, listen, give praise and thanks, and share communion. Otherwise we forget who we are and whose we are; and we can have neither the strength nor the joy to be Christ's body—present in the world today.[2]

For Further Reading

Johannes H. Emminghaus. *The Eucharist: Essence, Form, Celebration.* Translated by Linda M. Maloney. Collegeville, MN: Liturgical Press, 1978.
Romano Guardini. *Preparing Yourself for Mass.* Manchester, NH: Sophia Press, 1997.
Edward J. Kilmartin. *The Eucharist in the West: History and Theology.* Collegeville, MN: Liturgical Press, 1999.
Margaret Scott. *The Eucharist and Social Justice.* Mahwah, NJ: Paulist Press, 2009.
Robert Skolowski. *Eucharistic Presence: A Study in the Theology of Disclosure.* Washington, DC: Catholic University Press, 1994.

Editor's Note

Health research on the Roman Catholic Eucharist is extremely limited and has not focused on the social support functions of the ritual. What research there is has focused on the potential for transmission of infections through use of the common cup; this topic has been mentioned, if not carefully studied, in religious and medical journals since the early twentieth century. More recent topics have included celiac disease and the health implications of intinction—dipping the consecrated wafer into the wine—versus drinking from the common cup.

Resources for Public Health Research

Furlow, T. G., and Mark J. Dougherty. "Bacteria on the Common Communion Cup." *Annals of Internal Medicine* 118, no. 7 (1993): 572–573.
Gill, O Noël. "The Hazard of Infection from the Shared Communion Cup." *Journal of Infection* 16, no. 1 (1988): 3–23.
Loving, A. L. "A Controlled Study on Intinction: A Safer Alternative Method for Receiving Holy Communion." *Journal of Environment and Health* 56, no. 1 (1995): 24–28.

Loving, LaGrange. "The Effects of Receiving Holy Communion on Health." *Journal of Environmental Health* 60, no. 1 (1997): 6–10.

Moriarty, Kieran J., Duncan Loft, Michael N. Marsh, Steven T. Brooks, Derek Gordon, and G. Victor Garner. "Holy Communion Wafers and Celiac Disease." *New England Journal of Medicine* 321, no. 5 (1989): 332.

Notes

1. All cited liturgy come from Catholic Church, International Committee on English in the Liturgy, *Chants of the Roman Missal* (Collegeville, MN: Liturgical Press, 2011).
2. Cardinal Joseph Bernardin, *Guide for the Assembly* (Chicago: Archdiocese of Chicago Liturgy Training Publications, 1997), 16.

7 | Congregational Hymn Singing in Mainline Protestantism

DON E. SALIERS

THE EMOTIONAL POWER OF MUSIC is well attested from ancient times. The Greek physician Galen wrote in his medical treatises about the role of music and drama on those whom he observed at the *Asklepieion* (his treatment center in Pergamum). He observed the psychosomatic effects of music, voice, and instruments. Plato, too, understood the emotional power of music, banning flute players from his ideal republic because of the psychic and erotic distraction that they offered. At the same time, religious rituals have from ancient times employed music to express praise and lament as well as to induce alternate states of consciousness, from the purgative to the ecstatic. The Hebrew psalms, for example, are filled with musical references and were performed musically. Various forms of sacred music can offer far more than entertainment or even a particular kind of pleasure. Even particular kinds of pleasure (the "aesthetics" of song)—especially with respect to ritual and social singing in religious traditions—are relevant to questions of sickness and health, including the healing power of song in religious conversion.

Recently, the literature studying relationships between singing and the brain has expanded greatly. Oliver Sacks's *Musicophilia* presents a number of examples that confirm my own experience. Music is more than auditory vibrations that reach the ear. *Hearing* and *listening* (attentively) involve different aspects of the brain and of human intention. Listening requires a wide range of associative and imaginative skills that mere hearing does not. The act of singing involves an even wider mental and physiological range of human capacities; it involves breath, formed musculature, pulse and pitch discrimination, memory skills, and the ability to listen to others as well as a sense of disciplined coordination with a social body. The phenomenon of group singing presents a distinctive opportunity for understanding the relationship between music and human health.

One of the most powerful examples of group singing that I have experienced is with shape-note singing, known also as sacred harp singing, in Georgia. On one occasion, nearly eighty people gathered in an old Baptist church for a whole day of singing. We sang for nearly three hours in the morning, stopped for "dinner on the grounds," and sang again for three hours into the afternoon. The sound, often raw and boisterous, composed of four parts without any accompanying instruments, made the space and our bodies vibrate. Divided into four sections in a box arrangement, we faced one another so that the sound and the sight of one another's faces and bodies fused together.

While singing with force—especially with the vigorous "fuguing" tunes, in which voices followed one another in fugue style—I found myself becoming "lost" in the collective sound. The harmonies were not refined, nor were the voices, but a remarkable sense of physical solidarity emerged. Sustaining such singing over many hours was at once exhilarating and demanding. The words, from eighteenth- and nineteenth-century hymn texts, ranged from deep lament to ecstatic praise. The whole experience created a kind of collective shout or a deep common lament. These group sings are social and ritual occasions, featuring a common meal of foods brought by the participants. This is a full-bodied context for singing in every sense of the word.

A famous case of a monastic community in southern France, documented by Alfred Tomatis in *The Conscious Ear*, provides a fascinating counterpoint to my experience. After Vatican II, the abbot of the community streamlined the monks' daily pattern of sung prayer to render their day more efficient, eliminating some of the eight sung prayer offices in which they had customarily engaged. Over time, the monks became depressed and ill and began sleeping more. The efforts of several physicians and medicines proved fruitless. As a last resort, Dr. Tomatis proposed that the monks had lost a source of order and well-being in the chanting of the eight daily prayer offices. He reasoned that their bodies and minds were affected by the loss of the older chant forms and the distinctive rhythms of sung prayer, and he ordered that these be restored. Within a few weeks, the monks had regained energy and health. Tomatis claimed that the regular rhythm of communal sung prayer throughout the day was a principal factor in their rejuvenation.

Recovering their familiar patterns may have been important in the monks' return to health, but consider the distinctive features of the chant form: the long breathing, the somatic features of sound production and reception in tune with the heartbeat, the long vowel sounds, the extended meditation of sacred texts, all resulting from practices of communal monophonic listening over days, weeks, months, and years. These features of chanting require direct psycho-physical engagement over time. Yet for Tomatis, this particular singing practice has both evident physiological and spiritual benefits.

In my extensive observations of congregational singing in many churches and in talking with fellow singers, I find evidence of strongly emotive, cognitive, and physical effects in the acts of common song, in the contexts both of worship and of social singing. I have been involved as a participant or leader in several congregations. Singing with these different groups gave me a bodily experience of the emotional value of song, which the members of these groups knew intimately from long-shared experience. After leading informal hymn sings with them, I listened for stories from the choirs, the pastors, the musicians, Sunday school classes, youth groups, children, and other members.

One particularly interesting interview began with older members of a women's class in a Charleston, South Carolina, church. We spoke first of hymns learned in childhood from repetitive singing, such as "Amazing Grace," "Blessed Assurance," and "How Great Thou Art." When I asked what those hymns meant to these women, an unexpected set of stories followed. They remembered sounds of their grandmothers' or grandfathers' voices or the comforting feeling of having sung beside their mothers. They remembered prayer meetings and church socials, summer camps and family singing at holiday time. One recounted how a particular hymn brought to her the smell of the church basement and the meals shared there. They were offering descriptions of embodied memory of text and tune. More significantly, they were evoking my own experience of the performative dimensions of singing. This was much more than a casual or one-time association, I realized as the conversation developed. Their understanding of their own mental and physical processes had been altered by the experience and continued practice of singing together, linking other senses to the sense of hearing.

The women also spoke of times of crisis in which singing together (whether in the congregation's worship space or in their homes) was more than comforting, "it was healing," several women said. One group had gathered around hospital bed of a fellow church member who was in acute pain. The friend, according to the women's description, was disturbed by the fact that four of them were crowded into the room. Together the visitors and the patient began to sing familiar hymns. To the surprise of the patient as well as the attending nurse, after a period of ten minutes, the pain gradually diminished. The hospitalized patient and her friends were members of the same singing congregation, and those hymns were part of the repertoire that they had shared on many occasions. Both the actual sonic experience and the deeply associative memory worked together to work a bodily change in the woman. Pastoral experience in several churches has yielded similar stories of the power of shared singing to release stress, if not to heal acute medical conditions.

More stories confirmed my own experiences of the dynamics of shared sound. Following an informal hymn sing in a church in Georgia, several congregational members shared accounts of their long-term practices of singing together. An 80-year-old man spoke of how, when he sang with the choir in Wednesday-night practices and Sunday-morning worship, his Parkinson's disease symptoms were often simply "overruled": "My disease hasn't gone away, but when we sing . . . I don't understand it . . . my hands stop shaking and I don't feel strange." A middle-aged woman spoke of how singing "Amazing Grace" alleviated her chronic arthritic pain over time. Another person told me that singing with the community was a significant part of her recovery from an abusive relationship. These reports were often added to general descriptions of how certain hymns—both known "by heart" and recently learned—allowed the singers to enter into the joy and the pathos of the poetry of the words. As one person put it, "When we sing the spirituals—especially songs like 'Sometimes I Feel Like a Motherless Child'—I am expressing in a healing way my own traumatic history."

In one of the churches, I was told about a family whose father had slipped into dementia after one of their daughters had gone to college. Her second Christmas holiday home from school, she requested that they all go to church during her December break. The mother strongly cautioned against taking the father, warning that he could be confused or even disruptive. The daughter insisted. Once in the church sanctuary, he did become quite confused and restless, to the point that the family was about to take him out. Just then, the congregation stood to sing the Doxology ("Praise God from Whom All Blessings Flow"). Suddenly, the father stood and sang every word in a strong, melodious voice the family had not heard for several years. The power of a song that he had learned from childhood brought him back to his surroundings, if only for a brief period. He was able to stay through the remainder of the worship service, even singing part of the concluding hymn at the end.

These bodily effects must play into our understanding of the embodied power of congregational singing. Even outside of singing in the context of services designed for healing through prayer, anointing, and laying on of hands, sung hymns have the effect of focusing attention on religious symbolism and teachings, which may, over the long run, affect both mind and body. Because gathered congregations sing regularly, music comes to inscribe tunes and words on the body. Regular congregational singing may thus allow a significant number of hymns to be "learned by heart." Singing a hymn once may be striking, but singing the same hymn over years installs it in a person's inner repertoire. Such bodily memory provides a storehouse of emotional and cognitive resources that can be called upon in various life circumstances. Longitudinal studies of singing groups will thus reveal how singing practices create and sustain communities of well-being.

The ancient physician Galen knew something that we cannot neglect in the contemporary studies of human health. From my own experience as a singer and director of singing, I have seen convincing evidence of the health-giving benefits of shared practice. Active singing communities, from synagogues and churches to whole cultures, may carry the promise of such benefits and are thus to be fostered and studied more attentively.

For Further Reading

Campbell, Don. *The Mozart Effect*. New York: Harper Collins, 2001.
Sacks, Oliver. *Musicophillia: Tales of Music and the Brain*. New York: Knopf, 2007.
Tomatis, Alfred A. *The Conscious Ear*. Barrytown, NY: Station Hill Press, 1991.

Editor's Note

There is considerable research in the scientific literature on singing and health and a substantial amount on choral or group singing, but little of it is in the context of religious practice. The health effects of singing that have been studied include the impact of caregiver singing on dementia patients, the therapeutic effects of singing in older persons with Parkinson's disease and other chronic conditions, and the impact of singing on mental health and well-being in healthy adults.

Resources for Public Health Research

Bygren, Lars Olov, Gösta Weissglas, Britt-Maj Wikström, Boinkum Benson Konlaan, Andrej Grjibovski, Ann-Brith Karlsson, Sven-Olof Andersson, and Michael Sjöström. "Cultural Participation and Health: A Randomized Controlled Trial among Medical Care Staff." *Psychosomatic Medicine* 71, no. 4 (2009): 469–473.

Chatterton, Wendy, Felicity Baker, and Kylie Morgan. "The Singer or the Singing: Who Sings Individually to Persons with Dementia and What Are the Effects?" *American Journal of Alzheimer's Disease and Other Dementias* 25, no. 8 (2010): 641–649.

Clift, Stephen. "Creative Arts as a Public Health Resource: Moving from Practice-Based Research to Evidence-Based Practice." *Perspectives in Public Health* 132, no. 3 (2012): 120–127.

Grocke, Denise, Sidney Bloch, and David Castle. "The Effect of Group Music Therapy on Quality of Life for Participants Living with a Severe and Enduring Mental Illness." *Journal of Music Therapy* 46, no. 2 (Summer 2009): 90–104.

Müller, Viktor, and Ulman Lindenberger. "Cardiac and Respiratory Patterns Synchronize between Persons during Choir Singing." *PloS ONE* 6, no. 9 (2011): e24893. doi:10.1371/journal.pone.0024893.

Skingley, Ann, and Trish Vella-Burrows. "Therapeutic Effects of Music and Singing for Older People." *Nursing Standard* 24, no. 19 (2010): 35–41.

Annual Religious Practices

8 | *Hatsumōde*, the Visitation of Shinto Shrines: Religion and Culture in the Japanese Context

CHIKAKO OZAWA-DE SILVA

A S I APPROACHED THE SHRINE, the appetizing smell of fresh stall food enveloped me. I made my way along the street vendors' stalls, pushing through the huge crowd. Only the weather made it feel different from the summer shrine festivals that I had often attended—it was bitterly cold. But this was my first time doing *hatsumōde*, the practice of making a first visit of the year to a shrine.

I passed under the tall red-colored *torii*, the traditional arched gateway; walking through it cleanses the pollution one has accumulated since the last visit. Despite the crowd, something felt different once I crossed under the *torii*: there was something peaceful and calming about the atmosphere within the shrine's precincts. Perhaps it was due to the carefully cultivated landscaping and the many trees around the grounds, which gave it a sheltered and protected feel.

Ahead of me stood a long line of at least a hundred people. I joined the line, waiting in the cold. Fortunately, it moved swiftly, and I soon approached the *temizuya*, where people were rinsing their mouths and hands with water in ritual purification. Like the others before me, I scooped the cold water with a dipper and poured it into my hand and then rinsed my mouth with it. Then I took more water and rinsed both hands, starting with the right. I continued in the line of people along the *sandō*, the main path to the *haiden* or hall of worship, where people make their prayers. Despite the cold, people were patiently waiting in the line for their turn. Many women were dressed in traditional Japanese kimono, which added to the sense of this being a special event, since kimonos are worn only on special occasions in Japan.

After an hour in line, I finally came to the hall of worship, a large wooden building. The hall of worship is the most typical building of a shrine, the one shown on television programs and in other such representations of shrines. In this shrine in Kagoshima, the hall of worship was the most prominent building. I could barely see the center of it due to the crowds of people around me, but I could tell that everyone was headed there. The crowd split into four lines, and I entered one of them, eventually being pushed forward to the front center of the building. Before me stood a large rectangular wooden offertory box, an *osaisenbako*, and above it was a large round bell with a long, thick string. I tossed some small change into the box—another act that removes bodily pollution— stood upright, and performed two bows. I clapped my hands twice, keeping my hands in front of my chest. I then bowed one more time and made a silent wish for good health for my family and friends. With so many people around, everything was rushed; my performance was over in a matter of seconds, and as I stepped aside, the next person quickly took my place.

In the shrine courtyard, some people were tying this year's *omikuji*, fortunes written on strips of white paper, onto the branches of a tree. At the nearby shrine shop, others were buying protective *omamori* amulets. Since I didn't feel like joining another long line to buy an amulet or tie an *omikuji* to the tree, I decided my *hatsumōde* visit was finished. After looking around a bit more at the activities around me, I made my way out of the shrine and left the festive atmosphere behind.

New Year's or *oshōgatsu*, which comprises the first three days of January, is the most celebrated national holiday in Japan. People often return to their hometowns to spend the holiday with their families, just as I was doing with mine. Roughly half of the Japanese population participates in *hatsumōde* during this time, making a visit that would in most cases be identical to the one that I described above. I had not participated before because my parents were Christian (something quite unusual in Japan), and they considered *hatsumōde* a practice from another religious tradition and therefore not appropriate for us to participate in.

When I interviewed twenty people in Japan about their *hatsumōde* practices, all but one said they did *hatsumōde* regularly each year; that one exception was again due to Christianity—in this case a young woman married to a Christian husband. While Christians often do not participate in *hatsumōde* because they see it as conflicting with their religious beliefs, there has traditionally been no such tension for Buddhists, who may choose to practice *hatsumōde* by visiting either a Buddhist temple or a Shinto shrine.

Technically, although *hatsumōde* is considered a religious event in both the Shinto and Buddhist traditions, it comes from the practice of *toshikomori*, which is a part of the Shinto practice of welcoming the new year's *kami* to each household. The word "*kami*" is often translated as "gods," "deities," or "spirits," but ancestors also become *kami* upon their deaths, spirits who protect their descendants, and even inanimate objects and places have *kami*, so the term "god" is probably more misleading than helpful. Terms like "god" or "deity" also imply a religious dimension that may not be present in the understanding of Japanese people. It seems that most laypeople, including those whom I interviewed, do not associate *hatsumōde* with religion at all. As far as they are concerned, going to *hatsumōde* does not involve participation in a religion or religious ritual. Rather, it is simply a good thing to do to welcome in the new year and to make prayers for the well-being of oneself and one's family.

So *hatsumōde*, originally a Shinto practice, is no longer associated with religion or even with Shinto for many Japanese (few of whom would ever self-identify as Shinto believers or adherents). Why then do so many people participate? Those with whom I spoke often employed the expression *nantonaku*, "for no particular reason." When questioned further, one person said that she would feel anxious if she didn't go, as if she were being left alone while others were doing something. When she goes, she feels good that she has done "one of the things I'm supposed to do for this year." Others said similar things: that it is one of the events that one should participate in and that it is one of the several "new year's-related activities" one should do. They didn't delve into exactly why one should; it seemed to be just a general feeling of traditional and social norms. Many people said they go to *hatsumōde* because others do. Remarkably, not a single person I spoke with said they went to *hatsumōde* for any religious reason.

Wishing to know more about how the Shinto tradition itself views *hatsumōde*, I arranged for an interview with a Shinto priest at a popular shrine in Yokohama. Dressed in the white ceremonial robes of a priest, he emphasized that people at *hatsumōde* almost always pray for *buji*, which means "safety" but also "good health," "peace," and "quiet." This term captures the importance of health in Shinto belief as the foundation for a safe, peaceful, and calm life. The priest clarified that "being healthy itself may not be the primary purpose of people's new year's wish itself, but health is the foundation for being able to spend the new coming year safely and to do anything at all, such as helping others." He confirmed that although *hatsumōde* is indeed a Shinto practice, most people do not think that what they are doing has anything to do with religion. He also confirmed that Shinto was in fact a religion in his opinion, although he acknowledged that most people might not see it that way. For him, Shinto serves as a foundation for many aspects of the Japanese way of life and its values. He also felt that *hatsumōde* practice should continue into the future; for it to fade would be like losing an important part of Japanese culture, since it is a national custom and tradition.

It has been argued that because the Japanese have traditionally lived in an agricultural society based on rice cultivation such an environment required people to be unified and harmonized, since it took a unified collective to reap the harvest properly. Individual health was only possible when there was communal health and a successful harvest. A strong sense of cooperation among people and with the natural world evolved into the numerous Shinto rites that include prayers to bring a rich harvest and to dispel or prevent unexpected misfortune. There was little point in praying for an individual's health, since such a thing did not exist independently of the community and nature. The fact that most participants' primary wish is for the good health of their family and themselves reflects this traditional emphasis on communal well-being, even though nowadays it may be as small a unit as a family, rather than a village or clan.

Investigating the practice of *hatsumōde*, which is ostensibly a religious practice but in practice is perhaps not at all so, and the broader question of whether Shinto is a religion or rather a part of Japanese culture, highlights the way in which concepts like "religion" and "culture" have been framed in Western discourse, where the terms have arisen principally in relation to the large monotheistic traditions and secondarily around the other "world religions," of which Shinto is not one. When seen in this light, it should not surprise us that many Shinto scholars find it hard to define Shinto as a religion, and even Shinto priests are happy to equate Shinto with Japanese culture, rather than as a separate religion apart from Buddhism, Christianity, and other traditions practiced in Japan.

Hatsumōde ultimately provides a special opportunity for the Japanese to be aware of the importance of being healthy and being part of a larger community—whether it is religious is immaterial to most of those who go to the temple. In places such as Japan, religion and culture are much more mutually implicated, and the consequences for health are correspondingly complicated by a strongly communal conception of health and well-being, all of which is evident in *hatsumōde*, a practice that has become deeply embedded in the life of many Japanese.

For Further Reading

Kawano, Satsuki. *Ritual Practice in Modern Japan: Ordering Place, People, and Action.* Honolulu: University of Hawaii Press, 2005.

Nelson, John K. *A Year in the Life of a Shinto Shrine.* Seattle: University of Washington Press, 1996.

Picken, Stuart D. B. *Essentials of Shinto: An Analytical Guide to Principal Teachings.* Westport, CT: Greenwood Press, 1994.

Plutschow, Herbert. *Matsuri: The Festivals of Japan.* Richmond, UK: Curzon Press, 1996.

Editor's Note

While there is substantial research on pilgrimages, especially to Mecca and Lourdes, there is little health-related research on this popular annual practice in Japan. There are small numbers of papers on the influence of Shinto on bioethics and on beliefs and practices related to hygiene, on problems in survey methods and measurement with the concept of religion in Japan, on the performance of ritual as a means of facilitating social control and social support, and on the links between religious practice in Japan and mental health and well-being, rather than on physical health.

Resources for Public Health Research

Hansen, Wilburn. "Eye on Religion: Shinto and the Japanese Attitude toward Healing." *Southern Medical Journal* 100, no. 1 (2007): 118–119.

Kaneko, Satoru. "Dimensions of Religiosity among Believers in Japanese Folk Religion." *Journal for the Scientific Study of Religion* 32, no. 1 (1990): 1–18.

Krause, Neal, Berit Ingersoll-Dayton, Jersey Liang, and Hidehiro Sugisawa. "Religion, Social Support, and Health among the Japanese Elderly." *Journal of Health and Social Behavior* 40, no. 4 (1999): 405–421.

Mitsuhashi, Takeshi. "A Study of the Health of the Elderly from the Standpoint of Shinto." *Journal of Religion & Aging* 4, nos. 3–4 (1989): 127–131.

Mizuno, Toshinari, and Brian Taylor Slingsby. "Eye on Religion: Considering the Influence of Buddhist and Shinto Thought on Contemporary Japanese Bioethics." *Southern Medical Journal* 100, no. 1 (2007): 115–117.

Roemer, Michael K. "Ritual Participation and Social Support in a Major Japanese Festival." *Journal for the Scientific Study of Religion* 46, no. 2 (2007): 185–200.

Roemer, Michael K. "Religion and Psychological Distress in Japan." *Social Forces* 89, no. 2 (2010): 559–583.

Roemer, Michael K. "Shinto Festival Involvement and Sense of Self in Contemporary Japan." *Japan Forum* 22, no. 3–4 (2010): 491–512.

Schnell, Scott. "Sanctity and Sanction in Communal Ritual: A Reconsideration of Shinto Festival Processions." *Ethnology* 36, no. 1 (1997): 1–12.

9 | Fasting in Islam

ABDULLAHI AN-NA'IM

I N A BASIC, FORMAL SENSE, fasting for a Muslim means total abstention from eating, drinking, and having sex from dawn to sunset, in addition to some personal and social etiquette for perfecting the fast. Those who are too weak due to sickness or old age are excused from fasting, but those who are able to fast at a subsequent stage are expected to make up for the Ramadan days that they were unable to fast. A person may seek religious and medical advice as to whether he or she qualifies for this license to break the fast of Ramadan, but the decision and ultimate responsibility remain personal.

The meaning, resonance, and significance of fasting is a profound and evolving spiritual, emotional, and social experience that frames the cycle of a lifetime, from early childhood to old age. Reflecting back on my own Ramadan experience, I see the constant play of cycles of life in the coming and going of Ramadan: birth and death, earning the privilege of fasting as we approach puberty and losing that privilege when we are too sick or old to fast.

Apprehensive anticipation is my first recollection of Ramadan as a child growing up in a village on the Nile two hundred kilometers north of Khartoum, as grown-ups around me counted the months and then days until Ramadan, anticipating it like a long-awaited traveler returning home. For us children, Ramadan held the excitement of special activities, different foods, and unusual drinks in the evenings, with slight apprehension for our own disrupted meals during the day, as grown-ups were too dehydrated and hungry to cook for us while they fasted. Children are not allowed to fast until they reach puberty; we couldn't wait to be old enough to fast and make our rite of passage into adulthood. Children would dare each other to fast a few days, but they often broke the fast by mid-morning or early afternoon, when the hunger and thirst become too much to bear. Our parents were torn between encouraging us to finish the day of fasting that we had started and tolerating our breaking the fast, fearing that we would make a habit of it.

Grown-ups also struggled to hide their worry about the approaching hardship of fasting for the whole day for a month, and their apprehensions mounted as each day brought Ramadan closer. It is unthinkable for adults to speak of their ambivalence about fasting for Ramadan, as the faithful are expected to be eager for the blessings that it brings, of forgiveness for all sins and multiplied rewards for every act of charity or kindness. These mixed feelings were so deeply engrained into our consciousness as children that we grew up with a complex combination of love and apprehension of Ramadan; we were socialized into the values of self-discipline and management of ambiguity required by the fast as well as the ambivalent relationship between religious piety and social conformity. When our time to fast regularly finally came, failing to observe the fast was alien and abhorrent to us. This aversion to failure to observe Ramadan is reflected in our struggle with whether to take the license to break the fast because of sickness or old age. The dilemma is whether one is committing a sin in harming one's health by fasting to keep social appearances or is taking the license to break the fast without really qualifying for it. We know that God knows what is best for us to do, but how do we know?

As Ramadan approaches each year, the women of the village start preparing the special drinks of Ramadan (*sorej*, *aabri abyad*, and *hul-mur*), made from fermented and intensely spiced sorghum (a drought-resistant cereal). I recall my excitement and eagerness when I was sent on errands to prepare for the day when the women of several households would gather to prepare the drinks together, the tasting of the first cooked drinks, and the scents of the spices that lingered in the house for days. Then there was the excitement of the sighting of the new moon, marking the beginning of the lunar month of fasting.

Preparations for Eid al-Fitr, the festival of the breaking of the fast, started a week before the end of Ramadan, when our fathers took us shopping for new clothing and our mothers gathered to bake special cookies and sweets for the intense social activities during the three days of Eid al-Fitr. After four weeks of fasting, the men and women of the village began to look for the new moon, which marks the beginning of the next month

(Shawal) in the Islamic calendar. There were also annual ritual comments about whether we started or ended Ramadan correctly, as the size of the new moon a few days later confirmed our initial announcements of the sighting of a new moon. As we started to go to school in the town and return to the village, we began to "instruct" our elders on the values of the scientific calculation of the lunar calendar. Yet as grownups ourselves, we are now reluctant to substitute more modern methods for the physical sighting of the new moon, which is stated in the Qu'ran and Hadith of the Prophet to be the astronomical determination of the coming and going of Ramadan.

Muslims may fast almost any day of the year, and some follow various protocols set by the practice of the Prophet (Sunna) or some Sufi masters for "volunteer" (tataw^c) fasting. The strict religious obligation, as one of the essential requirements of being a Muslim, is limited to fasting every day of the month of Ramadan. The other four essential requirements of the Muslim faith are confessing the faith, praying five times each day, giving alms according to specific requirements, and making the pilgrimage to Mecca once in a lifetime, if possible. These religious practices are supposed to be interactive and mutually reinforcing. For instance, in its initial meaning, affirmation that there is no god but God and Muhammad is God's messenger is the entry point, the threshold to membership in the community of believers. But the object of saying is doing and ultimately being— moving from verbal affirmation to daily practice to actual realization in lived experience. This progression from verbal to behavioral affirmation of the unity and wholeness of God (twhid) is to be realized through perfecting required and volunteer practices, striving for deeper and more sincere prayer and fasting, charity, and self-discipline. So, verbal affirmation of the faith is the prerequisite for all religious practice, and perfecting religious practice is the means to realizing the true significance and value of that affirmation.

Religiously valid fasting requires a completely voluntary and deliberate decision and intent (niya) to fast that is formed prior to the dawn of the fast day. This intent to fast is entirely a matter of internal consciousness and free choice and need not be spoken aloud or made in any particular manner or location. Abstention from food, drink, and sex without that voluntary and deliberate intent to fast does not count as Islamic fasting. In the case of continuous fasting, like in Ramadan, the deliberate intent can be formed for the duration of the month or any number of days that a believer wishes.

Such abstention, with the required intent, must also be accompanied by the maintenance of appropriate decorum by avoiding harming other people, hurting their feelings, or using abusive language. Finally, the more affirmative good that a person does while fasting, as opposed to simply refraining from causing, the more religious benefit that he or she realizes. Reported traditions (*Hadith*) of the Prophet repeatedly caution against futile fasting, in which the person achieves nothing but deprivation because of failure to observe the etiquettes (*adab*) of fasting. But the biggest danger to the religious value of fasting arises when a person feels pride and moral superiority for having fulfilled all the requirements of fasting. To the contrary, the best fast is one accompanied by a constant feeling of inadequacy and shortcoming, a sense that "Yes, I am keeping all the rituals but not quite up to the degree of essence and spirituality that I should."

My understanding of Ramadan has evolved since childhood. I remember religious instruction classes telling us about the moral and social benefits of fasting. Teachers at each stage told us to appreciate what we had, to be compassionate with the disadvantaged, and to share our privilege. They told us about the values of endurance, self-discipline, and solidarity with community. In my personal experience, however, Ramadan fasting touches my soul from where the Qu'ran comes, beyond human comprehension. Now that I believe that I am excused from the Ramadan fast for health reasons, I miss the experience of fasting with my family. Still, I feel the blessings of Ramadan in its smells, sights, and sounds at home and seek its touch in the company of those who are fasting and in reciting the Qu'ran in my prayers.

For Further Reading

Brown, Kerry, and Martin Palmer. *Essential Teachings of Islam*. London: Century Hutchinson, 1989.

Levy, Reuben. *The Social Structure of Islam*. Cambridge: Cambridge University Press, 1957.

Smith, Huston. *The World's Religions: Our Great Wisdom Traditions*. New York: HarperOne, 1991.

Editor's Note

There is a substantial research literature on the health effects of fasting during Ramadan. Specific areas of investigation include the effects of Ramadan fasting on Type 2 diabetes; cholesterol and serum lipids; pregnancy-related issues including fertility, birth frequency, and nursing; chronic kidney disease, particularly the effects on kidney transplant patients;

stroke; physical endurance and athletic training; intraocular pressure, tear secretion, and the frequency of migraines; sleep patterns; and the use of health services.

Resources for Public Health Research

Azizi, Fereidoun. "Islamic Fasting and Health." *Annals of Nutrition and Metabolism* 56, no. 4 (2010): 273–282.

Dikensoy, Ebru, Ozcan Balat, Bahar Cebesoy, Ayhan Ozkur, Hulya Cicek, and Gunay Can. "Effect of Fasting During Ramadan on Fetal Development and Maternal Health." *Journal of Obstetrics and Gynaecology Research* 34, no. 4 (2008): 494–498.

Friger, Michael, Ilana Shoham-Vardi, and Kathleen Abu-Saad. "Trends and Seasonality in Birth Frequency: A Comparison of Muslim and Jewish Populations in Southern Israel: Daily Time Series Analysis of 200,009 Births, 1988–2005." *Human Reproduction* 24, no. 6 (2009): 1492–1500.

Lamri-Senhadji, M. Y., B. El Kebir, J. Belleville, and M. Bouchenak. "Assessment of Dietary Consumption and Time-Course of Changes in Serum Lipids and Lipoproteins before, during and after Ramadan in Young Algerian Adults." *Singapore Medical Journal* 50, no. 3 (2009): 288–294.

Najafizadeh, K., F. Ghorbani, S. Hamidinia, M. A. Emamhadi, M. A. Moinfar, O. Ghobadi, et al. "Holy Month of Ramadan and Increase in Organ Donation Willingness." *Saudi Journal of Kidney Diseases and Transplantation* 21, no. 3 (2010): 443–446.

One-Time Religious Practices

10 | Circumcision in Judaism: The Sign of the Covenant

DON SEEMAN

> As for me, behold my covenant is with you . . . Neither shall your name any more be Abram, but Abraham you shall be called, for I have set you as the father for a multitude of nations.
>
> *Genesis 17: 4–5*

MY SON WAS NAMED AT his circumcision ceremony (*brit*) when he was eight days old. We gave him a name that means "pleasantness" because that is what we wished him and also because that is how we perceived him. We also named him for his grandmother, who was taken from us far too young. Names carry both descriptive and prescriptive weight in Jewish tradition. History and destiny, the promise of new life, and the intractable bonds of collective and personal fate are all so thickly intertwined. Circumcision itself harks seamlessly both forward and back. It is the sign of the covenant between God and Abraham with which the Jewish story traditionally begins, and it is sealed in the organ of generation that carries human life forward. Tied by a biblical text (Genesis 17) to the inheritance of the land, circumcision also helped to convey rootedness to a people in exile.

The festivities that traditionally surround circumcision celebrate new birth and new horizons, but they also promote public reflection upon chains of meaningful continuity that transcend mere choice or volition. Circumcision and the covenantal relation to which it points both rely upon the complex relationship between foundational acts of choice and the no longer wholly free consequences and responsibilities invoked by such acts: Judaism is a covenantal relation. It is therefore no accident that contemporary debates over infant circumcision and worrying attempts to ban the practice in some jurisdictions have focused inevitably on our culture's anxiety over the tensions between religious freedom for families (who wish to honor the covenant) and claims about the importance of personal autonomy for children.

Circumcision as Religious Practice

Despite some controversy in non-Orthodox circles, circumcision is still one of the most widely observed Jewish customs today. One fascinating recent trend has been the voluntary circumcision in adulthood by Jewish émigrés from the former Soviet Union, where religious practice was heavily suppressed. As a matter of Jewish law, circumcision is incumbent upon the father of an eight-day-old boy, or upon an adult convert or other Jewish man whose father did not fulfill this obligation. The operation, which can take place in a synagogue or home or at a doctor's office, involves the removal of the foreskin followed by the peeling back or removal of the epithelium, which is called *priah*, or uncovering. Ancient practice also requires that a small amount of blood be drawn through the wound, which may help to prevent infection as long as it is performed in a sterile manner. Nowadays, almost all fathers appoint a specialized agent or mohel to perform the ritual on their behalf: a religiously valid circumcision must be performed by an adult Jewish person who can stand in legally for the father, and it must be performed with the specific intent of entering the covenant of Abraham.[1]

There are many different practices associated with circumcision in different Jewish communities. Many families invite friends and relatives to a public celebration on the Friday night preceding a circumcision and some, like my wife's family, insist—for reasons that are unclear even to them—that beer and chickpeas should be served. Chickpeas are known as *arbis* in Yiddish, which may sound like a Hebrew word for fruitfulness, but the reasons matter less to most participants than the chance to gather in celebration with friends and relatives the way that their ancestors once did. At the brit itself, the baby is carried in on a pillow by a relative or friend and passed to the *sandek* (a Greek word for godfather), who holds the child during the ritual. Sandek and baby are seated on a high, ornate seat known as Elijah's Chair, in recognition of a tradition that holds that this biblical prophet, who never died but went up to heaven in a fiery chariot, attends every brit to testify that the ancient covenant is still observed. Typically, circumcision is a public liturgical event that includes responsive readings and prayers for the well-being of mother and child as well as a public naming of the baby.[2]

Anxieties about the physical act of circumcision—including the pain caused to children—vary. At one recent brit that I attended, an older sibling of the infant broke the tension by calling to his friend at the back of the synagogue, "Mendl, do you want to come see the cutting part?" People laughed in part because he had named the one thing that nobody wanted to talk about.

Circumcision, Body, and Text

Jewish cultures have historically been textual cultures, and it is impossible to consider a ritual like circumcision without at least some attention to its complex elaboration in Jewish literary tradition. The ritual itself is accompanied by references to a variety of biblical and rabbinic texts, like the one from Ezekiel 16: "And I said to you, 'In your blood, live!'" There is also a very long history of Jewish ethical and exegetical reflection upon circumcision, which helps to shape the meaning of the ritual for some participants. The twelfth-century physician and philosopher Moses Maimonides, for example, classed circumcision along with devotional practices like prayer that encourage constant reflection upon the love and unity of God. In his philosophical work *Guide for the Perplexed*, he adds that circumcision helps to signal the importance of sexual restraint and also instills values of friendship and solidarity among members of the covenant. Yet despite his interest in the putative reasons for divine commandments, Maimonides never entertained the possibility raised by some modern Jews that the commandment itself was optional upon assent to the reasons that he had suggested. Like other traditionalists, Maimonides affirmed the force of religious law as a binding covenantal obligation that transcends (though it is not opposed to) individual assent and understanding.

Maimonides's philosophical approach was contested by his more mystical near-contemporary Nahmanides, who pointed out that biblical texts are more likely to associate male circumcision with themes of fertility and fruitfulness; he notes that fruit trees as well as men can be described as "uncircumcised" in biblical Hebrew and argues that this has something to do with "opening up" an organ for its proper use. It is no accident, therefore, that Abraham's covenant of circumcision is accompanied by a divine promise that he will become the "father of many nations." Following this logic, many later mystical writers treated circumcision as a vital prerequisite for certain kinds of divine blessing.

Circumcision also came to be an important point of contention between early Christian and Jewish communities. The Christian church's ultimate rejection of obligatory circumcision for Gentile converts was understood by both sides as a rejection of Jewish law and peoplehood or what some Christian writers referred to as "Israel according to the flesh."

Covenant, Moral History, and the Burdens of Kinship

Ancient controversies resonate with contemporary moral burdens. The 1990 German film *Europa, Europa* tells the true story of a German Jewish boy named Solomon Perel (Solek) who comes of age in Lodz Poland just as the Nazis come to power. When Solek's sister is killed in anti-Jewish riots, the family sends Solek and his older brother eastward into Poland, but they are separated in the chaos of the Soviet invasion. Solek finds himself in a Soviet orphanage, where he is indoctrinated into rejecting his Jewishness. Later, when Germany invades the Soviet Union, Solek survives by convincing an SS officer that he is an ethnic German who can serve as a translator for German troops. The officer mentors and then adopts Solek, sending him back to school in Berlin. Yet Solek lives in terror that his circumcision and hence his Jewishness will be discovered. He must never shower with the other boys or become intimate with girls. When he is sent back to the front as a German soldier, he is saved from being shot as a spy only by a chance encounter with his long-lost brother, only recently liberated by the Soviets from a Nazi death camp. Sole survivors of their extended family, we know that they are saved when they are able to pee together behind the bushes in amicable silence, free from terror that they will be discovered.

Europa, Europa says something important about the place of circumcision in the contemporary Jewish imagination. During the ancient Seleucid persecutions commemorated by the Hanukkah festival, some Jews became martyrs by defying the edict against circumcision. Yet despite the apparent continuities, Solek's experience is quite different from those of the ancient martyrs. The victims of twentieth-century genocide were targeted not for acts of religious fidelity but for a putative racial identity that was neither chosen nor subject to exchange. In a context characterized precisely by this horrible erasure of all real agency, circumcision has come to stand for some as an expression of the mysterious and indelible *difference* in which modern Jewishness sometimes seems to reside. Such conditions might evoke either shame or pride, but they cannot be ignored, and they are intimately related to histories of resistance and persecution.

At the end of *Europa, Europa,* the real Solomon Perel appears on screen against the landscape of the kibbutz that he and other survivors helped to build after the war. The scene signifies both homecoming and new beginnings, as Perel tells us laconically that he did not hesitate when the time came to circumcise his own son. But what are we to make of this avowal? Certainly not all Holocaust survivors made the choice that Perel made. Nor can this ritual be reduced to a single register of significance for the people who practice it. Yet Perel's account resonates with me as a profound enactment of modern Jewishness on a variety of levels. It is not just an act of loyalty to the God and people of Abraham; it is also an act of resistance to those forces of death, entropy, and genocide that have characterized our modernity. On some fundamental phenomenological level, it is also an enactment of our appreciation for the sheer moral weight of those features of the human condition—like Jewishness—that are not chosen but with which we must nevertheless reckon as moral agents.

For Further Reading

Cohen, Shaye J. D. *Why Aren't Jewish Women Circumcised? Gender and Covenant in Judaism.* Berkeley: University of California Press, 2005.

Hoffman, L. A. "Rituals of Birth in Judaism." In *Life Cycles in Jewish and Christian Worship,* edited by P. F. Bradshaw and L. A. Hoffman, 32–54. Notre Dame, IN: University of Notre Dame Press, 1996.

Krohn, P. J., ed. *Bris milah: Circumcision, the Covenant of Abraham: A Compendium of Laws, Rituals, and Customs from Birth to Bris, Anthologized from the Talmudic and Traditional Sources.* New York: Mesorah, 1985.

Maimonides, Moses. "Fourteenth Class, Marriage Laws." In *Guide for the Perplexed.* Part 3, Translated by Shlomo Pines. Chicago: University of Chicago Press, 1973

Seeman, Don. "'Where Is Sarah Your Wife?' Cultural Poetics of Gender and Nationhood in the Hebrew Bible." *Harvard Theological Review* 91, no. 2 (1998): 103–125.

Seeman, Don. "Pentecostal Judaism and Ethiopian-Israelis." In *Religious Conversions in the Mediterranean World,* edited by Nadia Marzouki and Olivier Roy (New York: Palgrave-Macmillan, 2013), 66–83.

Editor's Note

There is a great deal of literature on the health consequences of circumcision, including its role in the prevention of HIV, herpes simplex, human papilloma virus, and penile and cervical cancer. Much of this research pertains to developing countries, Muslim and Christian populations, and adult circumcision. Research literature pertaining particularly to infant circumcision addresses surgical techniques, complications, the traditional practice of the mohel, and health insurance coverage.

Resources for Public Health Research

Addanki, Krishna C., D. Gene Pace, and Omar Bagasra. "A Practice for All Seasons: Male Circumcision and the Prevention of HIV Transmission." *Journal of Infection in Developing Countries* 2, no. 5 (2008): 328–334.

Brusa, Margherita, and Y. Michael Barilan. "Cultural Circumcision in EU Public Hospitals: An Ethical Discussion." *Bioethics* 23, no. 8 (2009): 470–482.

Chaim, J. Ben, Pinhas M. Livne, J. Binyamini, Benyamin Hardak, David Ben-Meir, and Yoram Mor. "Complications of Circumcision in Israel: A One-Year Multicenter Survey." *Israel Medical Association Journal* 7 (2005): 368–370.

Drain, Paul K., Daniel T. Halperin, James P. Hughes, Jeffrey D. Klausner, and Robert C. Bailey. "Male Circumcision, Religion, and Infectious Diseases: An Ecologic Analysis of 118 Developing Countries." *BMC Infectious Diseases* 6, no. 1 (2006). doi: 10.1 186/1471-2334-6-172

Menczer, Joseph. "The Low Incidence of Cervical Cancer in Jewish Women: Has the Puzzle Finally Been Solved?" *Israeli Medical Association Journal* 5, no. 2 (2003): 120–123.

Prais, Dario, Rachel Shoov-Furman, and Jacob Amir. "Is Ritual Circumcision a Risk Factor for Neonatal Urinary Tract Infections?" *Archives of Disease in Childhood* 94, no. 3 (2009): 191–194.

Schenker, Inon, and Eitan Gross. "Male Circumcision and HIV/AIDS: Convincing Evidence and Their Implication for the State of Israel." *Harefuah* 146, no. 12 (2007): 957–963.

Notes

1. Though the matter is disputed in the Talmud, liberal Jewish movements have recently begun allowing both men and women to conduct circumcisions.
2. It should be said that while traditional Judaism mandates no equivalent of circumcision for girls, different communities have adopted a variety of ceremonies to mark the naming and welcome of a girl child at around this age.

11 | Puberty Rites in African Religious Traditions: *Kloyo Peemi*

EMMANUEL YARTEKWEI AMUGI LARTEY

THE KROBO PEOPLE, GHANA'S FOURTH largest ethnic group, live in the fertile plains between the coastal town of Somanya and the mountains just inland near the central town of Odumasi, in the eastern region of the country. The Krobo and their ethnic relations, the Shai, mark the passage of girls into womanhood by performing a series of rituals popularly known as *Dipo* or, less commonly but perhaps more descriptively, *kloyo peemi* (literally meaning "making a Krobo woman"). Through these rites, girls at or near the age of puberty are inculcated with the traditional ideals and practices of Krobo womanhood.

Despite modern intrusions into traditional Ghanaian culture, especially Western Christian incursions that have generally been disparaging of traditional African religiocultural practices, the popularity of Dipo rites, which have been practiced since the eleventh century, has not waned. Changes have been introduced to the ritual to reflect national educational developments, and social and cultural transformations such as the introduction of formal education and employment for women have had an effect on the practices—for instance, where in the past the training could last several months, girls are now confined for only a few days—but the essence and significance of the various rites and rituals have been largely preserved.

Sociologist of religion Kofi Asare Opoku points out that the Dipo initiation season usually begins in the fourth month of the traditional Krobo calendar, that is, in February.[1] Originally, the period of enculturation into womanhood lasted for an entire year, but today the rituals are conducted over periods of ten to twelve days. The ceremony has distinct stages. In the first, the young woman engages in a series of cleansing rituals to prepare for her education as a woman and prove her virginity. Then, she enters into a period of education. Finally, she is returned to society and presented to her family and potential suitors as a woman.

Leaving Childhood Behind

The Dipo enculturation session begins with a declaration announcing that Nene Kloweki, the Krobo Earth Goddess, queen of the gods, and wife of Mawu (The Creator), will preside over the training and the ceremonies. It concludes with a summons to "every Krobo to come and make [his or her] daughter a Krobo woman."[2]

Each initiate is set apart as a *Dipoyo* (Dipo-girl). She enters the designated ritual house, where she sheds her clothing, symbolizing her childhood, and is given new clothes by her ritual mother. Ritual mothers are experienced Krobo women who act as godmothers and instructors for the Dipo-girls. Each ritual mother has custody of two to five girls, depending on the total number in a cohort. A string of carnelian beads is tied around the girl's waist, to which is attached a red loincloth that reaches nearly to the ground in front and behind her. According to Carol Beckwith and Angela Fisher, "The color of the beads and the cloth symbolize the blood of menstruation and offer protection from evil spirits."[3] Raffia fibers are also tied around their necks. Opoku includes at this point in his account "the killing of the goat," a ceremony in which a sacrificial goat is killed and its blood allowed to flow upon the feet of each initiate "to cleanse her of any harm that may stand in her way and impede her growth towards full womanhood and motherhood."[4]

The following morning the cleansing rituals continue. Shaving their heads, the initiates carry calabashes—gourds used as cups—to the river to bathe. The washing ceremony is a purification rite to cleanse the body and spirit. After their ritual bathing, the girls partake of a common meal called *ho fufui* (Saturday's fufu), consisting of cooked yam pounded into dumplings and palm-oil soup prepared by their ritual mothers, the priestesses of Nene Kloweki, and the Dipo guardians.

Climbing the Sacred Stone of Virginity

The climax of the Dipo initiation ceremony is called "the blessing of Tek-pete," referring to a legendary sacred stone that the Krobo carried down from Krobo Mountain when the British evicted them from their place of origin in the nineteenth century. In preparation for the ritual, each initiate changes into a white loincloth and carries a small pot of millet beer. The girls are led to the sanctuary of Nene Kloweki. There, they have spots marked on their foreheads, temples, shoulders, legs, and arms with white clay. Then, they are presented to the presiding priestess, who pours a millet wine libation on the earth and says prayers of dedication and protection for the girls. The young women are then washed with water infused with medicinal herbs. Marks are made with red clay on their foreheads, temples, arms, shoulders, legs, and breasts in preparation for the final climactic ritual, the climbing of the sacred stone. In this ceremony, the initiates—smeared with various ointments and carrying long white sticks in their arms—assemble at the chief's compound. The white and red marks symbolize the girls' physical and spiritual status. Wearing white loincloths between their legs, beads around their waists, and white strips of calico around their heads and chests, they maintain contemplative silence, each pressing a single sacred medicinal leaf between her lips. Beckwith and Fisher describe what happens next:

> One by one, the girls are greeted by the priestesses who will lower each in turn three times onto the sacred Tekpete stone. The priestesses study each girl as she touches the stone. Only when they are satisfied that the girl is a virgin will they pronounce her to be worthy of Dipo. The sanctity of the ritual depends on the initiate being pure of mind and body.[5]

As each girl is placed on the sacred stone, the priestesses command her, "Sit down! Stand up! We are making you a Krobo woman!" Opoku outlines the significance of this ritual:

> So important was the ideal of the *Dipo* in former times that its violation constituted a crime which was surpassed only by willful murder. Thus, a girl who became pregnant before the performance of the custom was banished together with the man who was responsible for it. This calamity even affected the families of both. . . . The breaking of the *Dipo* was such a taboo that the whole compound occupied by the girl would have to be cleansed by the performance of purification rites. The penalty for violating the *Dipo* may not be as severe today as it used to be, but the gravity of it still remains and serves as a deterrent. Today, the man who is found to be responsible for a girl breaking the *Dipo* custom is made to bear the expenses of the purification rites that have to be performed in both households.[6]

Opoku further explains that it is even believed that a girl who has not been chaste can cause the death of the woman who places her on the sacred stone or of some members of her family.

After sitting on the sacred stone of virginity, the Dipo initiate is carried out of the temple by her father or another family member, usually male, amid exultation and celebration. Each young woman is given a cylindrical *Dipo-pe* straw hat similar to those worn by priests. These hats are a sign of honor and purity.

Confinement and Training

Following this ceremony, the *Dipo-yei* enter a period of confinement. In ancient times, this time was devoted to a traditional education that could last several months. These days, initiates are confined for about a week. During the period of confinement, the young women are under the tutelage and supervision of older women well versed in Krobo culture and tradition, whose duty it is to transmit their knowledge and wisdom to the young women and thus transform them into full-fledged Krobo women. Initiates are taught about grooming, appropriate conduct, cooking, domestic and housekeeping skills, arts, crafts, singing and dancing, and sex—including the enhancement of pleasurable sexual relations. They learn the *klama* dance, which they will perform at their Outdooring Ceremony. They are also introduced to the religious culture and spiritual traditions of their people. The entire exercise is geared toward the acquisition of the physical, spiritual, and social graces deemed necessary for a full life as an adult Krobo woman.

The confinement period closes with a rite that includes the making of nine small cuts between the thumb and the wrist of each initiate as permanent signs that she has undergone Dipo and is now a full-fledged Krobo woman and the putting of a broom into the right hand of each young woman, signifying her "graduation" from the domestic science school of Dipo.

The Outdooring Ceremony

The Dipo-yei are now ready for their Outdooring Ceremony, during which they will be presented to the community of family, friends, and potential suitors. The girls put on their Dipo-pe hats and perform the klama dance, which emphasizes the graceful movement of hands and feet. Tied around their necks and hips are beads that have often been passed down through a family for many generations and are of great worth to the Krobo, who are among the oldest and most famous makers of ground-glass beads in Africa. Many of the beads, known as *akori* or *aggrey*, are made locally; others have been traded from Venice since the seventeenth century as well as from Holland. Denoting family wealth and social status, each type of bead has significance. Blue beads, called *koli*, mean "something you love very much" and are associated with affection and tenderness. Yellow beads symbolize maturity and prosperity. Large yellow beads known as *bodum* are said to possess magical protective powers. White beads, worn by priestesses, signify respect for the gods and ancestors.

The movements of the dance are designed to reveal the beauty, dexterity, and gracefulness of the dancers. With small rhythmic steps and heads turned demurely downward, the dancers embody quiet elegance. The young women demonstrate their dancing skills for the chief, relatives, and the entire community that celebrates their coming of age. Prospective suitors gather to admire the women's display of feminine grace and beauty and often approach a young woman's family after the ceremony to make an offer of marriage.

The Dipo ceremonies constitute a coming-of-age ritual marking the entry of girls into adulthood, signifying physical, social, and spiritual maturity. The young women who complete the process can assume the responsibilities of adults in society.

Editor's Note

The health consequences of traditional African puberty rituals for girls have been little studied, and the specific practices of the Krobo people of Ghana have received even less attention. The public health research literature notes the continuing existence of African puberty rituals, particularly in less urbanized areas of the continent. The pressing need for sexuality education is taken as a given in the context of the HIV epidemic, and the period of puberty is seen as a largely unexploited opportunity for education and intervention. Some general readings relevant to African puberty rituals and the health of preadolescent girls follow.

Resources for Public Health Research

Chrisler, J. C., and C. B. Zittel. "Menarche Stories: Reminiscences of College Students from Lithuania, Malaysia, Sudan, and the United States." *Health Care for Women International* 19, no. 4 (1998): 303–312.

Cox, James, ed. *Rites of Passage in Contemporary Africa: Interactions between Christian and African Traditional Religions*. Cardiff, UK: Cardiff Academic Press, 1998.

Lincoln, Bruce. *Emerging from the Chrysalis: Rituals of Women's Initiation*. New York: Oxford University Press, 1991.

Pillai, V. K., T. Barton, and K. Benefo. "Sexual Activity among Junior Secondary School Girls in Zambia." *Journal of Biosocial Science* 29, no. 3 (1997): 297–301.

Sommer, Marni. "An Overlooked Priority: Puberty in Sub-Saharan Africa." *American Journal of Public Health* 104, no. 6 (2011): 979–981.

Zimba, Robert. "Indigenous Conceptions of Childhood Development and Social Realities in Southern Africa." In *Between Culture and Biology: Perspectives on Ontogenetic Development*, edited by Heidi Keller, Ypes H. Poortinga, and Axel Scholmerich, 89–115. Cambridge: Cambridge University Press, 2002.

Notes

1. Kofi Asare Opoku, *West African Traditional Religion* (Accra, Ghana: FEP International Private, 1978), 118.
2. Opoku, *West African Traditional Religion*, 119.
3. Carol Beckwith and Angela Fisher, *African Ceremonies* (New York: Harry N. Abrams, 2002), 30.
4. Opoku, *West African Traditional Religion*, 119.
5. Beckwith and Fisher, *African Ceremonies*, 32.
6. Opoku, *West African Traditional Religion*, 118.

12 | Baptism by Immersion in Latin American Pentecostalism

THE *SANTA CRUZ* CASE

L. WESLEY DE SOUZA

*T*HOUGH IMPLICITLY ACCESSING AND SUBSTANTIATING *the experience of other Latin American evangelical Christians, this chapter focuses on the ritual of baptism as shown in the last part of* Santa Cruz, *a documentary that follows the opening of a Pentecostal church in a clandestine ground share in the suburbs of Rio de Janeiro, Brazil.[1] I have chosen* Santa Cruz *as a case because the film reveals how those who face socioeconomic struggles and exclusion from the benefits of society, including access to health care, are gradually redeemed from and protected against everyday life disorder by a tiny church classified as part of a growing, strict-discipline religious movement—classical Pentecostalism.*

A bus speeds along a remote, dusty road through the evergreen mountains of Rio de Janeiro. For its passengers, this day will resound with powerful meaning for a long time to come. Setting out in full conviction that something powerful and transformative will take place, they've embarked on a rite of passage experienced by Christians throughout the ages—the sacrament of baptism. For this group of believers, this ritual is also deeply inflected with hopes for the restoration of their human dignity and implications for their holistic health.

The rite of baptism casts among those who undergo it the net of a saving, healing faith. By association and appropriation, this faith runs deep through their souls, bridging a chasm between the sources of pain and struggle in their daily lives and their new lives in Christ. In their minds, disease and suffering, fear and vulnerability, loneliness and lament, and poverty and exclusion will become things of the past. They are now on the road to a new life in which believing goes beyond mere religious aesthetics and elaborations of theology. Their expression of faith through baptism is the cure for their very humanity and the fulfillment of their part in God's story for the reconciliation of all creation.

A Communal Journey and the Running Waters

In excruciating pain from a diseased heel, 50-year-old Carmen (who stopped stealing electricity from her neighbor once she became a Christian) is assisted out of the bus by her daughter. Once out of the bus, Carmen proclaims, "Jesus Christ has said it was to be today, so we are going into the waters. I am sick, but when I leave, I shall be cured for the honor and glory of the Lord." Her faith and hope in linking the act of baptism with physical healing are not unusual in the Pentecostal expression of faith.

Others in the group also seek healing for a kaleidoscope of physical, emotional, mental, relational, and spiritual illnesses. They are part of a small, mostly Afro-Brazilian congregation located in one of the most miserable areas of Rio de Janeiro. The neighborhood where most of them live and worship has no hospitals, no clinics, no schools, no running water, no sewer system, and no jobs. They suffer from malnutrition, poverty, economic exploitation, and alcohol and drug abuse; their engagement with the church is a means not only to minister to the spirit and the mind but also to heal and renew the body. This small church is unmistakably part of classical Pentecostalism in Brazil. Pentecostalism helps people to regain their dignity by providing a new identity to individuals who face material privation, marginalization, and insecurity, along with structures that support the family and help to break patterns of destructive behavior, and by emphasizing spiritual gifts that stand in opposition to material riches.[2]

The interaction that precedes the baptism ritual is full of spirituality and permeated by a sense of the divine. "Is that the Jordan River?" asks Bianco, a 12-year-old boy who joined the baptism procession early on. "No, it's not *that* Jordan River, but it is *our* Jordan River," remarks a member. This specific river was carefully chosen both to reflect participants' spiritual expectation and to create the proper symbolic resonance. Surrounded by Serra do Mar's forest, these waters run smoothly under a blue sky; the river forms a bay of calming, transparent waters, crystalline in its perfection. A mother holding her 3-year-old daughter as she wets her feet says that the water is cold, "but it is as clean as the blood of Jesus was clean and pure." As Zahniser points out, "Water symbolism is prominent in [Christian] baptism."[3] For this group, it is also essential that this is flowing water. Many denominations baptize in still waters, but the assumption here is that still water does not take away the rotting of a fallen humanity, the sinfulness of the heart, or the illness of the body and the soul.

An Encounter with Creation and with the Healer of It

As they prepare for baptism, with a deep sense of celebration, trust, and humbleness, the faithful are singing one of their favorite songs: "Guide me always, my Lord. Guide my paces, dear Savior. You bought me upon the cross. So guide in everything, my Jesus!" As the line of singing people descends toward the riverbank, an unusual sense of attachment to and fellowship with one another begins to grow, along with a spirit of celebration and an atmosphere of transformation.[4] As their senses interact with the environment, connecting their inner world to the outer one, God's creation helps them to bond to the Gospel message that they have embraced. In this moment, creation becomes a vital part of the set of symbols that point to something and someone beyond themselves. The journey from the city to the mountains signifies a magic encounter with God's natural creation, which—like the faithful themselves—is both beautiful and damaged. This transition separates them from their old status, imposed by and experienced in an unjust society. Here, salvation is not only about saving souls; it denotes the healing of creation.[5]

As the flock gathers on the shores, the singing sharpens the moment, generating a deep sense of environmental symbolism and its encounter with the divine. The interpretation of what is sensed may vary depending on the individual's personality, education, and life story, but it is manifested by a vernacular faith that sees the need for human cure and reconciliation, so that creation may find its original health as people restore their lives. After all, these people know as few others do that "the whole creation has been groaning as in the pains of childbirth right up to the present time" (Romans 8:22).[6] Sin is a disease that must be taken away by a divine grace, a greater river that flows from God's throne, now represented by the river they now face. Running waters symbolize God's healing grace, as expressed by the modern Christian song lyrics, "Oh happy day, when Jesus washed my sins away."

The Ceremony of Being Buried and Coming Alive Again

Bianco is the first to enter the waters. "I'm Bianco Fernandes de Noronha," he declares. Pastor Jamil responds, "Bianco Fernandes de Noronha, for thou hast believed in our Lord Jesus Christ as your personal savior, I baptize thee in the name of the Father, the Son, and the Holy Spirit." Now, Bianco is completely submerged backwards by Jamil and the assistant, until the waters swallow his entire body. The former Bianco has disappeared; half a second later, a new creature in Christ comes alive as they lift him from the waters.

Tatiane, a 17-year-old Afro-Brazilian; 45-year-old Aparecida; and Maria José follow Bianco into the water. All are entirely submerged in water, wholly immersed as a symbolic burial for the remission of their sins, and immediately drawn out again. In baptism, they experience liminality, a "chaotic limbo condition of transition."[7] Their baptism takes them through the "betwixt and between"[8] stages of separation, liminality, and reintegration.

At last, it is Carmen's turn. Helped by two assistants and the pastor, she walks very slowly. The pain is excruciating, but she is determined. She follows the instructions and is immersed. As she emerges, an unexpected thing happens. She begins to jump repeatedly, going deep in the waters and rising high, her face expressing mixed emotions. Still in pain, almost falling, she is escorted to shore. Then she stops for a few seconds. Bowing her head, she looks around with a growing smile. Before the eyes of all those present, she walks through the group with no help, climbing the hill all by herself, showing no pain at all.

In the minds of Carmen and her brothers and sisters, the baptism functions as a bridge that not only seals the promise of forgiveness for their sins but also carries them through the dangers and fears of life. It works as a divine bridge, one that rises over all the chasms of a troubled, oppressed life.

A Creed of Faith, Life, and Health

Long before they passed through the healing waters, the members of Pastor Jamil's congregation memorized Psalm 91, adopting it as a creed of life and faith. "It is the most powerful text in the bible," says Veronilson, a 30-year old assistant mason, who was baptized before and now serves as one of Pastor Jamil's assistants. Though he and the vast majority of the adherents are illiterate, the psalm comes easily to their mouths. To complete the ceremony, Pastor Jamil invites them to recite it from memory, a request to which they respond enthusiastically.

This adoption of a particular part in the bible is contextually driven. Psalm 91 speaks of a countercultural perspective now consolidated by the participants' baptism—God's protection manifested in the community of faith. The communal initiation of baptism by immersion casts people toward a broader, more concrete understanding of what it means and what it takes to be healed and encourages them to look for real, holistic health. "What Christianity [gives] to its converts [is] nothing less than their humanity,"[9] and that gift is conveyed through the communal nature of baptism rituals. Faith, fully expressed through the communal journey, links adherents to a healing church that then becomes a way of re-envisioning and revolutionizing their material world.

The Latin American Pentecostal rituals of baptism have strengthened adherents to fight the sources of their socioeconomic struggles and to promote social transformation. The church has given people a structure for restoring personal dignity, strengthening microcommunity networking, and reducing illiteracy; it has also provided instruction on how to live a healthier life. After all, as a structured rite of passage, baptism offers the journey of "separation, transition, and reintegration" without which, according to Zahniser, "no social transformation can take place."[10]

Editor's Note

There is little research literature on the health consequences of baptism, particularly baptism by immersion. There are some related papers about water quality and sacred bodies of water in countries where water-related religious practices other than baptism take place frequently, and some on waterborne diseases in Latin America. There is some evidence that places with sacred bodies of water push for clean-water policies. There may be implications for public health related to river-immersion baptism based on these public health issues, but the research has not been done. We note two films, both available on the Internet, that document baptism by immersion: the first shows the events described in this chapter, while the second shows baptisms in the River Jordan in Israel.

Resources for Public Health Research

De Sam Lazaro, Fred. "Jordan River Baptisms." *Religion & Ethics Newsweekly*, October 8, 2010. http://www.pbs.org/wnet/religionandethics/2010/10/08/october-8-2010-jordan-river-baptisms/7179/.

Fisher-Ogden, Daryl, and Shelley Ross Saxer. "World Religions and Clean Water Laws." *Duke Environmental Law & Policy Forum* 17, no.1 (Fall 2006): 63–118.

Hotez P. J., M. E. Bottazzi, C. Franco-Pardes, S. K. Ault, and M. Roses Periago. "The Neglected Tropical Diseases of Latin America and the Caribbean: A Review of Disease Burden and Distribution and a Roadmap for Control and Elimination." *PLoS Neglected Tropical Diseases* 2, no. 9 (2008): e300. doi:10.1371/journal.pntd.0000300.

Semwal, N., and P. Akolkar. "Water Quality Assessment of Sacred Himalayan Rivers of Uttaranchal." *Current Science* 91, no. 4 (2006): 486–497.

Thompson, Felicity. "Water Woes in Senegal's Holy City." *Bulletin of the World Health Organization* 88, no. 1 (2010): 7–8.

Notes

1. João Moreira Salles, dir., *Santa Cruz* (Rio de Janeiro: VideoFilmes, 2000).

2. L. Wesley de Souza, *The Assemblies of God in Brazil: Lessons in Indigenization* (Ph.D. dissertation, Asbury Theological Seminary's E. Stanley Jones School of World Mission and Evangelism, 2003), 263.

3. A. H. Mathias Zahniser, *Symbol and Ceremony: Making Disciples Across Cultures* (Monrovia, CA: MARC World Vision International), 99.

4. See Zahniser, *Symbol and Ceremony*, 91.

5. Howard A. Snyder, *Salvation Means Creation Healed: The Ecology of Sin and Grace: Overcoming the Divorce between Earth and Heaven* (Eugene, OR: Wipf & Stock Publishers, 2011).

6. All biblical references are to the New International Version.

7. Zahniser, *Symbol and Ceremony*, 93.

8. Victor Turner, *The Ritual Process: Structure and Anti-Structure* (New York: Aldine de Gruyter, 1969), 95.

9. Rodney Stark, *The Rise of Christianity: How the Obscure, Marginal Jesus Movement Became the Dominant Religious Force in the Western World in a Few Centuries* (Princeton, NJ: Princeton University Press, 1996), 215.

10. Zahniser, *Symbol and Ceremony*, 93.

13 | Cremation Rites in Hinduism

DEATH, AFTER DEATH, AND THEREAFTER

BHAGIRATH MAJMUDAR

THE HINDU RELIGION ENCOMPASSES MANY diverse and ramifying traditions. Each is distinct from the others and yet, like the 108 beads of a Sanskrit *Mala*, they all are strung together by a common thread. My discussion will be based on a common and established Hindu belief system largely practiced in India. The fundamental principle of this belief system is acceptance of the cycle of life, death, and life again. The cycle is eternal and implies life after death. Death is called *dehanta* in Sanskrit, meaning the end of the body only—the soul is immortal. To grieve a death in this context is therefore an illusion of the mind. The body is subject to old age, disease, and death; the soul on the contrary is immune to physical and mental degradation and remains ever living.

Theology lays a foundation for the practice of religion and the subsequent development of its rituals. The Hindu religion bears a constant and repeated message that life invariably follows death, as morning comes after every night, while the soul remains beyond suffering and destruction. That idea is deeply engraved in every life, in everyday life, and subsequently in the society at large.

Death is incorporated as the last of the sixteen *sanskaras* or sacraments of life. The ritual that follows death serves to extinguish the fire of grief or *shokagni*, the overwhelming feeling of insurmountable loss. Through the ceremony, necrophobia, or fear of death, is curtailed and the grief is somewhat muffled. At the same time, the bereaved family receives comforting support and much needed practical help.

Rituals for an Imminent Death

The understanding and acceptance of death can begin even when the death is imminent. There is an old Sanskrit saying that when the body is besieged by multiple diseases and there is an irreparable failure of all the organ systems, the holy water of the river Ganges should be offered as the only medicine and God as the ultimate physician. The aphorism, however, must be judiciously applied in the presence of advancing technology to differentiate between salvageable life and the fruitless prolongation of an inevitable death. Such a situation can pose a difficult dilemma for an afflicted family. A joint consultation with the physician, the family, and a spiritual leader can help the family to reach a timely decision to terminate an unproductive agony. When such a decision must be made, which is becoming increasingly common in India as elsewhere in the world, the family reads from the scriptures before a lighted lamp and the physician withdraws life support systems. The family experiences a spiritual confidence in allowing their loved a death with dignity, eliminating feelings of guilt in ensuing years. The death is conquered by its inevitable acceptance.

Rituals after Death

The rituals after death are as varied as the Hindu culture itself and are greatly influenced by regional geography, societal customs, family traditions, and religious subcultures. There is, therefore, no "standard" protocol. Nearly all Hindus adopt cremation for the disposal of the dead body.[1] Babies, however, are sometimes buried. According to Hindu belief, the body is composed of five basic elements—wind, water, sky, fire, and earth, called *Panchamahabhuta*—and the lifeless body is returned to those elements. Sacred fire is a common theme running through all religious ceremonies, including the wooden pyre at the final farewell.

The most commonly observed cremation ritual is described by Pittu Laungani.[2] Except in the large cities, the cremation usually takes place at the bank of a river, far from residential areas. The holiest location for funeral ceremonies is at the bank of the river Ganges, in the holy city of Benares (Varanasi). One can see a countless number of cremations conducted continuously, day and night, at that place. After the cremation, sacred ashes are collected by the family, who usually scatter them in a river, preferably the Ganges.

Contemporary Hindu funerals, particularly in urban areas, are quite different from those in the past.[3] While older practices may have taken up to twelve hours, modern ceremonies take less than half the time. Speed and efficiency are the guiding factors. The death is announced in the obituary section of the newspaper, along with all the requisite details for those who will participate. Women usually stay at the home of the deceased. All other family members visit the bereaved family either at home or at a specially booked hall. Spiritual songs are played at the place. The visits are quick but cordial. No food or beverages are served.

The body is carried to the crematorium by a van, accompanied by intimate members of the family. The oldest son of the deceased has the privilege of conducting the final rituals and, when it is possible, setting fire on the pyre. In other cases, he pushes the body into the crematory, which is gas or electrically operated. The son or daughter of the deceased is sometimes asked to put out the fire at the end by pouring milk on the pyre. The oldest son often gets his head shaved as a part of the ceremony. The ashes are collected later.

Feasting after death has greatly diminished. In the past, people spent a luxuriant amount of money on food for a death ceremony, but this tradition has been curbed. Some families offer a feast on the thirteenth day after the death. Many families offer assistance to feed and help the poor; some donate to charity in the name of the deceased, believing that doing so will bring peace to the departed soul. The tradition of reciting from the holy scripture (especially *Bhagavatam*) for seven evenings after the death is also decreasing, as is the practice of seeking assistance from a priest for the funeral or thereafter. The traditional custom of *Sati*, in which the wife joins her husband's dead body on the pyre, is now outlawed.

Rituals That Continue after Death

It is part of the Hindu tradition to remember the departed members of the family respectfully. The anniversary of the death, called *Punya-tithi* or a sacred day, is celebrated year after year and often announced in the newspapers. The day carries the same significance as a birthday during life and is celebrated for years. It is quite common to see pictures of departed parents and grandparents hanging on the walls of homes. Children and grandchildren are trained to take a respectful bow before these pictures on all joyous, sad, and challenging occasions. One month per year is dedicated to the parental generations from both sides of the family. At weddings, the previous generations of both bride and groom are all recited by name, and a sacred fire serves as a witness, connecting the living with the dead and linking the couple to their roots. In short, the loss of a family member is given meaning by comforting and philosophical words, and the memory is retained and nurtured for years to come.

Changing Trends among Hindus in the United States

The ceremony of death among Indians settled in Western countries takes a different shape because of circumstantial needs. As a culture, Indians are known to retain their old traditions, while dynamically adopting new ones. The emerging traditions accordingly reflect a synthesis of both the new culture and the old. Some of these new practices are a result of convenience offered by modern technology. E-mail and telephones are now the most customary methods of informing friends and family about a death and the funeral service. The availability of facilities to store the body allows the family to wait for the important members of the family to arrive.

Funeral and memorial services are usually held in the hall provided by the funeral home, where the crematory is located. Unlike in India, where the body is simply wrapped in a white cloth, the anointing and dressing of the body is more common in the United States. Flowers, incense, and lighted lamps are common accompaniments. The family and the attending community can thus offer a respectful bow and a flower. An official priest will conduct the final rituals, if the family wishes. The scriptures are recited in most services, and spiritual hymns are offered from the *Bhagavadgita*. Friends and family may offer a eulogy.

The open display of grief and crying is not sanctioned, but a moment of silence always concludes the meeting. The family accompanies the staff of the funeral home to the crematory. Once the body is placed in the crematory, the switch is turned on by the oldest son or siblings. Mantras from the scriptures are recited continuously. The family comes out to show their silent gratitude to all the members waiting there. Later, ashes are collected to be dispersed in a river. A reception with food for those who attend the service may or may not be provided. All rituals end with "Om, Shanti" or "peace, peace, peace."

A broad-based definition of public health should include religious, cultural, psychological, and spiritual aspects of human wellness. It therefore must address the care of the dead. In the disposal of the dead, religion may conform to public health practices but unknowingly may violate them as well. In developing countries where infections constitute a common cause of death, no precautions are usually taken to prevent infections spreading from the dead. Protective masks and gloves are seldom worn, if at all. There is often a misconception that the disease dies with the patient. The traditional funeral ceremony, especially in India, allows intimate contact with the dead body. This can represent a threat to public health, where the dead body is often kept at home and children may be unprotected from contagious diseases. A rising incidence of AIDS in India and other developing countries may cause a particular threat to those caring for sick or dead patients with contagious diseases. The river is a symbol of sacredness in Hindu religion, and, therefore, the bank of a river is the preferred site of cremation. However, the ancient custom of leaving bodies in the Ganges, although greatly curtailed, needs to be discontinued.

For Further Reading

Flood, Gavin. *An Introduction to Hinduism*. Cambridge: Cambridge University Press, 1996.
Flood, Gavin. "Rites of Passage." In *Themes and Issues in Hinduism*, edited by Paul Bowen, 254–276. London: Continuum Publishers, 1998.
Fowler, Jeaneane. *Hinduism: Beliefs and Practices*. Eastbourne, UK: Sussex Academic Press, 1996.
Zaehner, Robert Charles. *Hinduism*. New York: Oxford University Press, 1966.

Editor's Note

Since the launching of the Ganga Action Plan in 1985 by Prime Minister Rajiv Gandhi, there has been considerable scientific attention to pollution levels in the rivers of India. There are many industrial, agricultural, and sewerage sources, but the practice of riverbank cremations is mentioned frequently in reports as a significant source of pollution. The following websites illustrate the impact of riverbank cremation and disposal; the videos may be graphic:

Bahadur, Ajeet. "Cremation Customs Pollute Ganges River." *India Unheard*, February 25, 2011. http://indiaunheard.videovolunteers.org/cremation-customs-pollute-ganges-river/.

Bhagat, Brooke, and Gaurav Bhagat. "Clean the Ganges." *Ecoworld*, December 19, 2004. http://www.ecoworld.com/animals/clean-the-ganges-2.html

Resources for Public Health Research

Alley, Kelly. *On the Banks of the Ganga: When Wastewater Meets a Sacred River*. Ann Arbor: University of Michigan Press, 2002.

Barrett, Ron. *Aghor Medicine: Pollution, Death and Healing in Northern India.* Berkeley: University of California Press, 2008.

Canning, L., and I. Szmigin. "Death and Disposal: The Universal, Environmental Dilemma." *Journal of Marketing Management* 26, no. 11–12 (2010): 1129–1142.

Ha, S. R., and D. Pokhrel. "Water Quality Management Planning Zone Development by Introducing a GIS Tool in Kathmandu Valley, Nepal." *Water Science & Technology* 44, no. 7 (2001): 209–221.

Markandya, Anil, and Maddipati Narasimha Murty. *Cleaning Up the Ganges: A Cost–Benefit Analysis of the Ganga Action Plan.* New York: Oxford University Press, 2000.

Sharma, Sudhindra. 2003. "Water in Hinduism: Continuities and Disjunctures between Scriptural Canons and Local Traditions in Nepal." *Water Nepal* 9–10, nos. 1–2 (2003): 215–247.

Notes

1. Lisa Miller, "We Are All Hindus Now," *Newsweek*, August 14, 2009, 70.
2. Pittu Laungani, "Death in a Hindu Family," in *Death and Bereavement across Cultures*, ed. Colin Murray Parkes, Pittu Laungani, and Bill Young (New York: Routledge, 1997), 52–72.
3. Siddhartha Mukherjee, "The Letting Go," *New York Times Magazine*, August 28, 2011, 58.

Religion in the History of Public Health

Part II takes an historical perspective on the mostly unknown relationship between religion and public health in England and the United States. Before the publication of Steven Johnson's *The Ghost Map*, few—including historically minded epidemiologists who are among the authors of this volume—had ever heard of the Reverend Henry Whitehead and his pivotal role in determining the cause of London's 1854 cholera epidemic.[1] Even today, John Snow, the physician who removed the handle from the Broad Street pump, continues to be known as the discoverer of the cause of cholera—although it was Whitehead who went door to door collecting data on the outbreak and wrote the initial report. In this section of the book, we build on a newly emerging historical narrative by examining three other largely untold stories of the intertwining of religion with nascent institutions of public health in England and the United States.

In the eighteenth and nineteenth centuries, religious institutions were powerful and well established, and what we think of as public health institutions were just being formed. In England and the United States, the dominant religious institutions were Christian churches. Religious leaders were in the forefront of some public health reform movements, and often they had a strong social justice orientation that linked economic and living conditions to health. Religion and public health have not always been cooperative partners, however; we take a particular look at a period in US history when religious motivations dictated reproductive health policy and law in a way that undermined women's reproductive health for decades.

We begin with the contributions of John Wesley, the Anglican clergyman who founded the Methodist Church, in a chapter by Karen Scheib. Wesley's ministry included strong elements of concern for laypersons' physical as well as spiritual well-being. He saw knowledge about health and disease and access to affordable medicines as the means of promoting health; he created dispensaries for simple medicines and wrote and distributed a manual for laypersons entitled *Primitive Physick* (1774).[2] The

second chapter in this section moves ahead a century to examine developments in the United States: the roles played by tract societies, temperance
movements, the social gospel movement, and activist laypersons such as
Robert Hartley and John Griscom in influencing the shape of public health
institutions. John Blevins details the theological undercurrents that swirled
around these reform movements, elements of which influence political
dialogues in the United States to the present day. In the final chapter, Lynn
Hogue and Carol Hogue detail the sweeping effects of the nineteenth-
century US anti-obscenity laws known as the Comstock laws, which severely limited sex education, contraceptive practice, abortion, and, by extension, women's ability to protect their reproductive health. In Part II, as
elsewhere in this volume, we see the interests of religion and those of
public health aligned in some times and places and at odds in others.

Several important themes emerge from these discussions. One thread
that runs through all three chapters is the concern for children and their
welfare. Wesley's *Primitive Physick* contains extensive recommendations
for the care of sick children in the home; Robert Hartley's concern about
the effect of the liquor trade on the milk supply—the primary source of
nourishment for small children—emerged from his investigations of high
infant mortality levels in New York City; and Anthony Comstock justified
his crusade against obscenity on the basis that the minds of young children
could be corrupted by exposure to such materials. The social determinants
of health perspective starts from the influence of social forces on health
and well-being in early life. For the historic figures that we profile here, a
major point of impact for their efforts was in infancy and childhood.

A second thread running through these chapters is the importance of
literacy and the dissemination of information related to health. Given
our focus on Protestantism, with its emphasis on scripture and the priesthood of all believers, this is not surprising. The millions of pamphlets on
health topics distributed by the American Tract Society and the seventeen editions of *Primitive Physick* printed in England between 1747 and
1774 reflect a rising level of literacy in England and the United States
and receptive audiences for health messages. But, ironically, it was precisely the distribution of sex (health) education materials through the
US mail that the Comstock laws prosecuted. Education and health literacy were key social determinants of health then as they are now, and
while religion has supported their spread in some contexts, there are
clearly counterexamples.

A final thread is the awareness these reformers had of the influence of
poverty on health. Henry Whitehead was "on the ground" during the

cholera epidemic of 1854, as were all of the reformers that we profile—in the streets and houses of the poorest districts of the growing urban centers of London, New York, and Chicago. They knew firsthand the living conditions of the most impoverished and spoke directly to the effects of material deprivation on the health of those who were most deprived. John Griscom and Robert Hartley had complex thoughts on the underlying causes of "pauperism," but they clearly saw it as a force with the power to shorten lives and create misery. John Wesley promoted the use of simple remedies and made knowledge freely available so that people could help themselves and their neighbors without resorting to physicians; his dispensaries were set up to distribute basic medicines to those who could not afford expensive physician-produced "compound medicines." They saw that health had social determinants before there was a language for it.

Our authors represent the professions of the law and the clergy and the disciplines of epidemiology, global health, and theology. Sometimes they find that religious institutions are powerful vehicles through which improvements in public health are advanced, and in other cases they find that religion was up to no good. We highlight this small sampling of stories in hope that future scholarship will further reveal the complex history of the relationship between these two important social institutions.

14 | Christian Commitment to Public Well-Being: John Wesley's "Sensible Regimen" and *Primitive Physick*

KAREN D. SCHEIB

ESPITE CLEAR BLUE SKIES, THE air in Carlisle, Pennsylvania, was making people sick, and in 2004 Reverend Jennifer McKenna decided to do something about it. The result, as Ellen Idler describes in chapter 1 of this volume, was Pennsylvania's 2008 Diesel-Powered Motor Vehicle Idling Act, which was signed into law largely due to the efforts of an ecumenical group established by Reverend McKenna. When asked what motivated her to take action to ensure cleaner air for the inhabitants of Carlisle, McKenna replied, "I believe that we are supposed to be good stewards of the earth and take care of it. And certainly it would be immoral to know that this air is hurting our children and not do anything."[3] Reverend McKenna is but one example of a Christian minister whose religiously based moral commitment to the most vulnerable among us resulted in policies to improve public health and well-being. She may or may not have been aware that a little more than two hundred and sixty years earlier another cleric across the Atlantic had been motivated by a similar commitment.

Inhabitants of eighteenth-century London also suffered from bad air, though the primary causes were wood and coal fires and the stink from open cesspools rather than idling trucks. The poor of London, who often lived in overcrowded neighborhoods, were the most likely to be affected by the lack of clean air or water.[4] Reverend John Wesley, an Anglican cleric who was deeply committed to serving the poor, took note of the health conditions of those he served. In 1746, in addition to his work forming small groups (known as societies) dedicated to fostering spiritual growth, he opened a medical clinic for poor residents of London. A year later, as his clinic became overwhelmed by the needs of the community, Wesley published *Primitive Physick*, a small, inexpensive tract that made the best current medical knowledge available to people who did not otherwise have access to care.[5] This little volume became one of the most popular medical tracts in eighteenth- and nineteenth-century England: twenty-three editions were published during Wesley's lifetime, and the thirty-seventh and last edition was published in 1859, a little over a century after its first publication.[6]

Wesley's concern for the physical well-being of his followers was not unusual; indeed, most eighteenth-century Anglican priests were trained in medicine and provided basic medical care to parishioners, particularly in villages lacking a physician.[7] However, Wesley's efforts to care for the body as well as the soul went well beyond common expectations of clergy. His medical practice cannot be separated from his ministry; both were founded on deeply held theological convictions. Until recently however, the importance of Wesley's efforts to care for the health of his followers, particularly through *Primitive Physick*, have been largely undervalued.[8] The impact of Wesley's work on public health has received even less attention.

Even though public health did not emerge as a separate discipline until more than a century after Wesley, his practices foreshadow contemporary commitments to health promotion, attention to the effect of social determinants such as poverty on health, and concern for equal access to health care. Wesley promoted a set of practices and beliefs that, although he pursued them for theological and religious reasons, had a significant impact on public health, including an active concern for the poor, which led to awareness of the relationship between living conditions and health; a focus on a "sensible regimen," designed to encourage personal practices that promote and maintain health; and an intent to provide accessible medical care that rose to accepted standards of care. Wesley's work illustrates that religiously motivated concern for public health like that demonstrated by Reverend McKenna is not only a contemporary phenomenon; rather, it is part of a long-standing, though perhaps little known, strand of the Christian tradition.

John Wesley and the Methodist Movement

John Wesley (1703–1791) was the founder of what became known as the Methodist movement, which began as an effort to reform the Anglican

Church. The Methodist movement arose during a time of religious and social ferment in England, in the midst of the Enlightenment and during a larger Evangelical revival. Though Wesley remained a priest in the Anglican Church throughout his life, he spent little time in pulpits; most of his ministry occurred as a field preacher among the poor, who were often not welcomed by more respectable, affluent congregations. At the time, poverty was construed as a moral as well as a financial condition, and the church often did not welcome those judged to be lacking in moral, spiritual, or financial resources. By contrast, Wesley declared "the world is my parish" and actively engaged in ministry with the poor of England.[9]

Wesley called his followers to individual salvation and personal piety as well as "practical holiness," which required putting faith into action in daily relationships and in one's life in the world as a way of expressing the transformation brought about through God's grace.[10] The continual growth in grace expected of Methodists was fostered through societies for spiritual formation whose mission was to spread "holiness of heart and life."[11] The societies, for which Wesley drew up rules in 1738, were each concentrated in a particular city or neighborhood. Members met several times each week for Bible study, hymn singing, preaching, and mutual encouragement. Society members retained their membership in the Anglican Church and typically attended church services regularly to receive the sacraments. The societies were divided into smaller groups of bands and classes, membership in which was voluntary. These small groups were the heart of the early Methodist movement and the crucible for spiritual growth through preaching, religious education, and accountability of members to each other for progress in their spiritual lives. Classes, which formed somewhat later than the bands, were made up of twelve people and a class leader; over time, classes became the primary communities in which members grew spiritually and cared for one another. In fact, societies, bands, and classes often provided material as well as spiritual support to their members.

Class leaders enforced or at least encouraged accountability among class members by issuing tickets for entrance to society meetings to those who followed the rules of the society and withholding them from those they judged unworthy of being called Methodists.[12] The class leaders were, in turn, accountable to Wesley, who provided oversight and established the rules for the societies. Wesley had high expectations of society members. While the primary requirement for joining the society was "the desire to flee the wrath to come," Wesley expected members to manifest this desire in outward holiness marked by a disciplined life. Members of the societies were to eschew "softness and needless indulgence" and exhibit decency and cleanliness.[13]

Historian Phillip Ott asserts that Wesley understood the disciplined life as "the norm or standard of the Christian life" and proposed as part of this discipline a regimen for both spiritual and physical health that included moderation in food and drink as well as spiritual practice.[14] Wesley believed that "the issues of health and medicine were profoundly interwoven into the texture of religious faith."[15] As a consequence, these practices were deeply embedded in the life of the Methodist movement and evident in the practices of the classes and societies. Although Wesley is most often remembered as a priest and church reformer, concern for the physical health of his followers, which he saw as inseparable from spiritual health, was central to his theology and ministry.

Wesley and the Tradition of Clerical Medicine

Like most Anglican clergy candidates in the eighteenth century, Wesley studied basic medicine as part of his education at Oxford. The parish priest was often the most educated person in the villages that dotted the English countryside, and priests were expected by bishops and parishioners alike to "offer informed advice about treatment of ailments and promotion of health as part of their overall ministry."[16] This practice was officially supported, as evidenced by the "church's willingness to dispense medical licenses."[17] Additional evidence is found in Robert Boyle's remark, included in the preface to his *Medicinal Experiments* (1692), that Anglican bishops had approved his publication for use by clergy and that the remedies in it were intended for the poor, who often could not afford a physician, if one could be found at all.[18]

Priests functioned as what Henry D. Rack called "benevolent amateurs," providing parental care and oversight to their communities, practices that continued well into the Enlightenment period.[19] A number of texts, such as *The Family Guide to Health* (1767), advised clergy to provide such care as part of the obligation of their profession: "The world has been long since admonished of the expediency of having recourse in sickness to a physician in Holy Orders. To call a clergyman, who has study physic, is just equivalent."[20] Given this heritage of clerical medical knowledge and care, it was not unusual that Wesley studied "anatomy and physic" when he began his studies at Christ Church College, Oxford, in 1720.[21] He soon discovered that he had a deep interest in science and particularly medicine, an interest that continued throughout his life.[22] He revived this interest in preparation for a missionary trip to Georgia in 1735, as he not only desired to bring Christianity to the native population and colonists there but also hoped to "be of some service to those who had no regular physician among them."[23] While his missionary activities were less than successful, his view of healing was affected by his sojourn in Georgia, where he was deeply impressed by the healing practices of the native population. In the preface to *Primitive Physick*, he observes of the country's population:

> Their diseases are exceedingly few; nor do they occur by reason of their continual exercise and (till of late) universal temperance. But if any are sick, or bit by a serpent, or torn by a wild beast, the fathers immediately tell their children what remedy to apply. And it is rare that the patient suffers long; those medicines being quick, as well as generally infallible.[24]

Wesley's spiritual development was also influenced by his encounter with German Moravians during his work in Georgia. While he was disappointed with his ministry among the colonists and natives, the Moravians' spiritual practices left a lasting impression on him and reinforced his desire to return to the practices of the early church or what he called "primitive Christianity."

Wesley's View of Healing

Wesley's theology was significantly influenced by his intent to revive primitive Christianity, which he revered as the pure essence of Christianity represented in the early church, the apostolic age, and the writings of the early church fathers.[25] His conviction of the superiority of primitivism also shaped his view of medicine, leading him to prefer simple remedies to compound medicines and empirically proven healing practices to those based on speculative philosophy, which had gained popularity in the medical practice of Wesley's time.[26] Historian Deborah Madden asserts that primitivism "provided a holist framework for Wesley's thinking and praxis" in both religion and medicine:

> This was his *modus operandi* and the ideals of Primitivism, whether it applied to the apostolic age or an ancient standard in physic, are intricately woven into The Preface of Wesley's medical volume. The theme of whole-

ness was central to his theology and structured all his work, in its written, oral, and practical forms.[27]

Within this structure, Wesley understood health not only as the restoration of individual physical soundness but also as part of God's plan for the redemption of the whole of creation. Illness was a manifestation of human brokenness and occasionally an opportunity for spiritual growth, while physical health was a good, though not the ultimate good, and a part of God's plan for salvation.

Wesley's broad understanding of healing is revealed in his letters, such as one in which he admonished Alexander Knox, "It will be a double blessing if you give yourself up to the Great Physician, that he may heal soul and body together."[28] Wesley was convinced that God intended both "inward and outward health," and, distinctively, that "*both* dimensions of divine healing can be experienced in the present," rather than only after the resurrection.[29] He was convinced that "the way of love brought healing to the soul" and that it also brought health to the mind and body.[30]

Health and healing, in other words, were divine gifts, although the means by which these gifts were administered were not only supernatural. Wesley expended considerable effort to help his followers experience God's "present saving work" as "nurturing both their souls and bodies," offering the means for this through his preaching, the spiritual guidance of the societies, and the provision of accessible health advice and care.[31] He expected his followers to preserve their health by following a "sensible regimen," and he expected his lay preachers to care for their people by offering sound medical advice. He also noted the effect of economic and social conditions on the health of the poor and advocated for social and political reforms.[32] These practical actions reflect his belief that healing is possible in this world and that Christians are called to participate in the transformation of individual lives and the larger culture.

Wesley's Concern for the Poor and Sick

Wesley's theological convictions shaped his deep commitment to providing medical care for the poor. Thus, as historian Randy Maddox states, Wesley attributed "the mediocrity of moral life and the ineffectiveness in social impact of Christianity in eighteenth-century England" to "an inadequate understanding of salvation."[33] Understanding salvation as "not barely . . . deliverance from hell, or going to heaven, but a present deliverance from sin, a restoration of the soul to its primitive health,"[34] he rejected a view of salvation as primarily concerned with guilt and the forgiveness of sin and instead advocated what Maddox calls a "*truly holistic salvation*, where God's forgiveness of sin is interwoven with God's gracious healing of the damages that sin has wrought."[35]

On a practical level, Wesley engaged with the needs of the poor and sick throughout his ministry and encouraged the members of Methodist societies to do the same, addressing this issue in his 1786 sermon "On Visiting the Sick." All Methodists were expected to "do good to all persons" through "works of mercy" and visiting the sick was one way to do so.[36] In both London and Oxford, members of the societies engaged in programs of regular visitation of the sick and by 1744 the office of "visitor of the sick" was established in all the Methodist societies.[37] The official visitor was expected to visit ill members in their area three times a week, "inquire into the state of their souls and their bodies, and to offer or procure advice for them in both regards."[38]

The lay preachers who assisted Wesley and rode all around England to visit the various Methodist societies were also expected to visit the sick and, from 1745 on, offer medical and health advice as well as spiritual advice.[39] To facilitate their fulfillment of this duty, the required training for lay preachers included basic medical texts. Aware that even the most committed lay preachers and visitors would have little or no medical knowledge, Wesley published pamphlets offering basic medical advice to provide more systematic medical knowledge to those with little or no training. The earliest pamphlet, produced in 1745, was a *Collection of Receipts* (prescriptions) that sold for two pence.[40] Through the training of these itinerant lay preachers, according to Maddox, "Wesley was clearly trying to expand the holistic care of the pastoral office within the Methodist movement."[41]

In 1746, moved by widespread illness and a desire to expand the availability of medical advice and care for the poor, Wesley opened a free dispensary in London. He described the motivation for his decision:

I was still in pain for many of the poor that were sick; there was so great expense and so little profit. . . . I saw poor people pining away, and several families ruined, and that without remedy. At length, I thought of a kind of desperate expedient. "I will prepare, and give them physic myself." . . . I took into my assistance an apothecary, and an experienced surgeon; resolving at the same time not to go out of my depth, but to leave all complicated cases to such physicians as the patients should choose. I gave notice of this to the society; telling them that all who were ill of chronical distempers (for I did not care to venture upon *acute*) might, if they pleased, come to me at such a time; and I would give them the best advice I could and the best medicines I had.[42]

The expense of running a clinic soon became unsustainable, however, and Wesley was forced to close it. That decision did not represent a change in heart, but a redirection of his commitment. His subsequent publication, *Primitive Physick*, was an expanded pamphlet of understandable and accessible medical advice that sold for a shilling, making it affordable for every family.[43]

Wesley's commitment to the poor went beyond his personal efforts; it was a deeply held value of the Methodist movement. Although Wesley's ministry was largely among the poor, a number of influential citizens joined the Methodist movement and extended its work with the poor within England and beyond. One of the people influenced by Wesley was Arthur Guinness, who encountered Wesley through his relative William Smith.[44] Although historical records do not make clear the extent of the connection between Wesley and Guinness, we do know that Guinness was deeply influenced by Wesley's social values and sought to put these into practice. Guinness, of course, is most well known as beer brewer, an occupation he took up in part to offer a healthier drink than was then available to Ireland's citizens. Because water was generally unclean and drinking it frequently led to illness, whiskey was often preferred, resulting in widespread drunkenness on the streets of Ireland. Guinness, a deeply religious man, committed himself to do something about this situation. There is no doubt his brewery also made him a successful and wealthy man, but his initial motivation was rooted in public health concerns traceable to Wesley and the values of the Methodist movement.

Deeply influenced by Wesley's admonition to his followers to "do all the good you can," Guinness further committed his wealth and talents to a wide effort to improve the lot of his countrymen.[45] He supported efforts to ban dueling, served as the chair of the board for a hospital for the poor, and promoted basic education for poor children through the Sunday schools being established under the guidance of educational reformer Robert Raikes. The Guinness brewery was known for treating its workers well, often paying higher than average wages. Arthur's heirs continued Guinness's commitment to the welfare of his workers and, as a result, Guinness workers in the 1920s—not an enlightened time for most laborers—enjoyed full medical and dental care, funded pensions, and educational benefits.[46] Wesley's influence on Guinness produced results that extended benefits for the health and well-being of the poor well beyond the lifetime of either Wesley or Arthur Guinness.

Preventive Health Care: Wesley's "Sensible Regimen"

Wesley was concerned not only with restoring health but also with preserving it. He was convinced that, while illness clearly affected physical well-being, it could also impair the ability to attend to the disciplines of faith that fostered spiritual growth. Through his sermons and other writing, he advocated what we would now consider preventive health practices. As with other health-related matters, Wesley's concern for physical health and preventive health care was a dimension of his holistic understanding of salvation. For Wesley, the "well-working of the whole was the hallmark of the original created order."[47] Good health, in this theology, was one of God's gifts, for it is God "who has all the power in heaven and earth . . . , gives life and breath and all good things, and . . . cannot withhold from them that seek him any manner of thing that is good."[48]

Health and wholeness, for Wesley, were both a gift and a discipline. In his sermon "The Good Steward" (1768), Wesley proclaimed that a healthy body is one of the gifts that we have received from God and that we are responsible for its care. He admonished his followers, "We are not at liberty to use what he has lodged in our hands as we please, but as he pleases."[49] The maintenance of that gift requires a "responsible lifestyle" that provides proper care for that "exquisitely wrought machine," the physical body.[50]

Wesley articulated his concern for the prevention of illness in his sermons, but the specifics of the discipline required for maintaining health were presented most clearly in *Primitive Physick*, where he laid out the details of his "sensible regimen":

> Observe at all times the greatest exactness in your regimen or manner of living. Abstain from all mixed, all high-seasoned food. Use plain diet, easy of digestion; and this sparingly as you can, consistent with ease and strength. Drink only water, if it agrees with your stomach, if not, good clean small beer. Use as much exercise daily in the open air, as you can without weariness. Sup at six or seven, on the lightest food; go to bed early and rise betimes. To persevere with steadiness in this course is more than half the cure. Above all, add to the rest, (for it is not labor lost) that old fashionable medicine, prayer.[51]

Wesley believed that following such a regimen would resolve the tension between contradictory forces and restore harmony between the mind, the body, and the spirit, an ideal he held as "the golden mean."[52] Achieving such harmony extended beyond the medical realm into morality, healing, and wholeness.

Primitive Physick, while written for common folk, was not folk medicine. It drew on the work of a number of well-known and respected eighteenth-century physicians who shared a similar commitment to the preservation of health, including George Cheyne. Like Wesley, Cheyne believed that health was a God-given gift that required careful tending and emphasized hygiene as a means to care for this gift.[53] In *An Essay on Regimen, Together with Five Discourses, Medical, Moral, and Philosophical*, Cheyne declared that preserving one's health was a moral duty and insisted that a person who neglects his or her health commits a crime "against the author of his being . . . despising the noblest gift he could bestow upon him."[54] Cheyne's admonition reminds us that physicians at the time were as likely to give moral and philosophical advice as clergy were to give medical advice.

Cheyne, like other physicians at the time, was influenced by the eighteenth-century revival of the Galenic and Hippocratic traditions, which divided the practice of medicine into physiology, hygiene, and pathology.[55] The seven naturals, which were the province of physiology, were defined by the constitution of the body; they included:

1. the elements (earth, water, fire, and air);
2. the qualities (hot, cold, dry, moist);
3. the humors (blood, phlegm, yellow bile, black bile);
4. the members (brain, internal bodily organs, bones, muscles, circulatory system, further classified as fundamental, subservient, specific, or dependent);
5. the faculties (natural, spiritual, animal);
6. the spirits (natural, vital, animal); and
7. the operations (hunger, digestion, retention, expulsion).[56]

Hygiene was concerned with the non-naturals, which included air, food and drink, motion and rest, sleep and waking, retentions and evacuations, and the passions of the soul.[57] These dimensions of health did not depend on nature but could have a profound impact on the health of the body. It is with these elements that Wesley is concerned in his sensible regimen. Finally, pathology dealt with the contra-naturals—diseases and their causes and consequences.[58]

The Non-Naturals and Wesley's "Sensible Regimen"

While physicians such as Cheyne may have felt that individuals had a moral obligation to preserve health, Wesley brought a more thoroughly articulated theological argument to his approach to preserving health. The elements of Wesley's "sensible regime" focused on the non-natural dimensions of health—those within an individual's control—and included an emphasis on lots of fresh air; moderation in diet and consumption of plenty of fresh, clean water; vigorous exercise; a proper amount of sleep and an early-to-bed, early-to-rise routine; and personal cleanliness.[59] Wesley believed his regimen provided both a "divinely ordained pattern for the preservation of wholeness" and a safe, cost-effective way to improve health by emphasizing strategies to prevent illness.[60] Wesley dealt with each of these elements of his regimen extensively in his sermons, letters, and other publications, including *Primitive Physick*.

Air. Wesley accepted Robert Boyle's argument that plagues and other epidemic diseases were most likely the result of noxious subterranean fumes being released into the air. These convictions were backed up by firsthand empirical observations such as those of John Locke, who reported his investigations into the occupational hazards facing lead miners in a 1666 letter to Richard Boyle. Locke reported that miners caught in the "fire damp" could "fall into a swoon and die" unless brought into open air.[61] Boyle's and Locke's influence on Wesley is evident in the advice he gives in *Primitive Physick* to those exposed to noxious fumes; to be "preserved from the poisonous fumes around them," he says, they should protect themselves by covering their nose or mouth.[62] Mechanical explanations of how atmospheric conditions contributed to disease and illness, like Boyle's and Locke's, were widely held in the eighteenth century, and they are reflected in *Primitive Physick*, which details how different types of atmospheric conditions produced different diseases. For example, cold, moist air could result in asthma, while dry, hot air was responsible for fevers or cholera.[63]

Wesley was also influenced by the work of Stephen Hales, an English clergyman whose life spanned the seventeenth and eighteenth centuries and who made significant contributions to a number of scientific fields, including physiology.[64] Wesley respected Hales for his ability to meld his "espoused mechanical explanations" and the results of his many experiments in physiology with his "deeply held pious beliefs."[65] Hales also subscribed to the belief that noxious air was responsible for disease; he even invented an "artificial ventilator" to bring fresh air into the confined spaces of ships, hospitals, and prisons to prevent diseases such as diphtheria, influenza, measles, and tuberculosis, which were believed to be airborne.

Deborah Madden argues that Wesley combined his theological beliefs that God was the divine author of nature with Boyle's and Locke's corpuscular theories. This led to Wesley's development of "a holistic model of corpuscular activity, which could explain function and malfunction in both divine and physical terms."[66] He explained this model in his sermons, which were his primary means of communicating his ideas about health. In the 1787 sermon "What Is Man?" we find this lengthy reflection on air:

> Circulation of a considerable quantity of air is necessary. And this is continually taken into habit by an engine [the lungs] fitted for that very purpose. But as a particle of ethereal *fire* is connected with every particle of air (and a particle of water too), so both air, water, and fire, are received into the lungs together, where the fire is separated from the air and water, both of which are continually thrown out, while the fire is extracted from them and mingled with the bold . . . is not the primary use of the lungs to administer fire to the body, which is continuously extracted from the air that curious fire pump? By inspiration, it takes in the air, water, and fire together. . . . Without this spring of life, this vital fire, there could be no circulation of the blood; consequently no motion of any of the fluids . . . therefore no muscular motion.[67]

While a sermon may seem an unlikely context for a scientific explanation of the functioning of the body, we must not forget that Wesley understood healing to encompass body and soul. The spiritual healing of the body occurred not in some metaphorical sense but in its physicality.

Wesley believed that that God intended both inward (spiritual) and outward (physical) health, which could be experienced in the present and not just in some future resurrected state, a belief he held alongside his conviction that Christians were required to tend to the physical body to maintain God's gift of health. He provided his followers with extensive instruction on bodily processes and practices of healthy living. For example, the advice Wesley gives in *Primitive Physick* for treating a patient with fever includes not breathing near the face of the sick person "nor swallowing your spittle whilst in the room."[68] This advice reflects a combination of miasmatic and contagion theories of illness, which overlapped in Wesley's lifetime. Bad air was thought to emanate from fetid conditions in particular areas, and environmental remedies were often recommended, such as getting plenty of fresh air.

Getting fresh air did not simply mean going outside, especially since the air in London at this time was not particularly fresh. Rather, this admonition referred to the quality of air inside one's home, which required attention to hygiene, to keep the home and body clean and free of stench. Although the adage "cleanliness is next to Godliness," often ascribed to Wesley, was a familiar saying long before his time,[69] we do see his concern with hygiene in a 1769 letter to a preacher named Richard Steele, reprinted in the Armininan Magazine in 1784. In the letter, Wesley urged Steele to keep himself and his family free of lice and itch and advised:

> Be cleanly. . . . Avoid all nastiness, dirt, and slovenliness, both in your person, clothes, house and all about you. Do not stink above ground. This is a bad fruit of laziness; use all diligence to be clean. . . . Clean yourselves of lice. These are a proof of your uncleanness and laziness; take pains in this. Do not cut off your hair, but clean it and keep it clean.[70]

Attention to hygiene was another way to maintain the gift of health and care for one's body, as was concern for one's diet.

Diet. Wesley's extensive advice on diet in *Primitive Physick*, adapted largely from Cheyne's recommendations, includes admonishments to adhere to moderation in diet, eat plain food, consume more vegetables than meat, and avoid strong liquor.[71] Above all, Wesley advocated moderation, and he warned his followers not to "use any kind of food, or such a quantity of any, either meat or drink, as in any degrees impairs his health . . . " and not to "eat more than nature requires."[72] He addressed the issue of temperance in eating in his sermon "The More Excellent Way" (1787), urging his listeners to eat with gratitude and avoid making "themselves sick with meat, or . . . intoxicat[ing] themselves with drink."[73] He believed that "in all areas of living, one must be diligent, but sensible and not endanger one's health."[74]

Sleep and Exercise. Wesley addressed the need for an adequate amount of sleep with some zeal,[75] advocating for six to eight hours of sleep as adequate for most people.[76] He was convinced that determining and assuring the proper amount of sleep was one of the disciplines of preventive health and played a role in maintaining the link between body, mind, and soul.[77] It was a topic that Wesley felt had not received the proper attention, which he addressed in his sermon "The Redeeming of Time" (1782):

> Many that have been eminently conscientious in other respects have not been so in this. They seemed to think it an indifferent thing whether they

sleep more or less, and never saw it in the true point of view, as an important branch of Christian temperance.[78]

Wesley believed that sleep was the means through which "the springs of nature are unbent." Too much sleep was as much a danger as too little: if the "springs" are relaxed too much, he warned, we "grow weaker and weaker."[79]

Vigorous and frequent exercise was also a part of Wesley's regimen for maintaining the gift of health. He advocated walking every day, "not less than an hour before dinner or after supper," and promoted horseback riding as a means of exercise. When Wesley himself could do neither, he would make use of a "wooden horse," a board between barrels, jumping up and down on it as a form of exercise.[80]

When preventive measures were not enough to maintain health, Wesley encouraged his followers to seek medical care. He did not rule out the possibility of divine healing, but neither did he advocate relying on divine healing alone. At the same time, he preferred simple remedies, advising the use of "common roots and plants over chemical, exotic, and artificial compound medicines."[81] He counseled Philothea Briggs, a member of one of the Methodist societies with whom he corresponded, "to use all possible means of recovering and confirming your health" but to avoid "taking many medicines."[82]

Wesley's publication of *Primitive Physick* was a means to make available to the general population a "plain and easy way of curing most diseases"; it "set down, cheap, safe, and easy medicines, easy to be known, and easy to be procured, and easy to be applied by plain, unlettered men."[83] His preference for the "natural cures" that "God had placed in creation" was balanced by a reliance on current medical advice, reflecting his recognition that maintaining the divine gift of health sometimes requires the intervention of science, itself also a gift of God, who had given human beings the capacities to develop it.[84]

Ease and Access to Care: Wesley's *Primitive Physick*

Much to Wesley's surprise, *Primitive Physick* soon became one of the most enduringly popular medical books in England; it even survived Wesley himself, with the last edition published 102 years after the first.[85] For many years, historians of medicine dismissed the book as a populist document with few roots in serious medicine. Likewise, religious historians, including those particularly concerned with Wesleyan history, were embarrassed by the odd-sounding remedies, like that of rubbing onion and raw egg on one's head to cure baldness, remedies that now sound like quackery. Consequently, scholars paid little attention to the work and largely overlooked the theological convictions motivating it, convictions consistent with those Wesley presented in his theological work.

Though many of Wesley's remedies appear quaint if not useless today, he drew on the standard medical texts of his time, including, in addition to Cheyne's work, those by "authors [such] as Hermann Boerhaave, Kenelm Digby, Thomas Dover, John Huxham, Richard Mead, Lazarus Riverius, Thomas Short, Thomas Sydenham, and Thomas Willis."[86] He made sure that the book was widely distributed, sending out copies to the societies scattered about England via his itinerant lay preachers. At the same time, he continued to publish other works that provided health advice, including *A Letter to a Friend Concerning Tea* (1748), *The Desideratum on Electricity Made Plain and Useful* (1760), *Advices with Respect to Health, Extracted from [Tissot]*(1769), *Extract from William Cadogan on the Gout* (1774), and *An Estimate of the Manners of Present Times* (1782). It was *Primitive Physick,* however, that people used most widely.[87]

Though Wesley's efforts to provide accessible health advice were motivated by his theological convictions, these efforts also occurred within a particular social context, one devoid of systematic health care. Medical guilds were beginning to emerge, and they would establish a professional monopoly on medicine that was well in place by the end of the century. In Wesley's time, however, an active "interplay between 'professional' physicians and lay medical practitioners" still existed.[88] Wesley was concerned about the quality and cost of care available from the professional physicians of his time; he was particularly critical of physicians who "unnecessarily protracted the cure of patient's bodies in order to derive the maximum fee," and he stressed the importance of "finding 'honest' or 'God-fearing' physicians."[89]

As the medical profession established itself, Wesley resisted efforts to restrict the authority to provide medical advice to those approved by the Royal College of Physicians. The basis of his concern was access to care. In 1746, when Wesley opened his own clinic, "there were only 80 fellows and licentiates on the College's catalogue, a ratio of about 1 to 10,000 for London alone."[90] These realities, in addition to Wesley's theological convictions about the interconnected nature of physical and spiritual health, fueled his efforts to make sound medical advice available to all, especially the poor and those in remote areas.

Wesley's Influence on Public Health

Much of the research on the impact of *Primitive Physick* has explored the intersections of religion, medicine, and individual health care. However, Wesley was concerned not only with the spiritual and physical welfare of individuals but also with that of communities. His reform movement was founded on the establishment of "societies," groups that tended to the spiritual and material well-being of their members as well as the larger communities of which they were a part. Wesley was deeply committed to holding personal piety or individual renewal in creative tension with "social holiness," which would include what we now call social transformation, and he expected his followers to share this commitment. Through his societies, Wesley "provided an effective blend of social and public health practice with a sense of individual responsibility for oneself and others."[91]

Through his attention to the impact of poverty on health, his concern for the prevention of health, and his efforts to make health care advice, if not direct care, accessible, Wesley prefigured practices we now consider part of public health. His influence on health practices in England has been noted by Robert S. Morrison, a physician and Cornell University emeritus scholar, who declared that John Wesley was "one of the formative influences on middle-class England" with regard to health. In addition to his concern for health maintenance, Wesley also "awakened an interest in sanitation (long absent from the Christian world) with the revival of the ancient Hebrew dictum that cleanliness is next to Godliness."[92]

Though it is difficult to know exactly how Wesley's concern for and influence on practices affecting the health of the public extended beyond his death, we do know that *Primitive Physick* was still in print a hundred years after its first publication. Two years before the last edition was printed, another Anglican cleric, Reverend Henry Whitehead, would have a profound impact on public health in London and help lay the foundation for the development of the discipline of public health. The tale of Reverend Henry Whitehead's role in helping John Snow prove the waterborne contagion theory of cholera is told elsewhere.[93] While we cannot draw direct links between Wesley and Whitehead, we do know that both shared a commitment to the poor and a concern for their physical and spiritual well-being. Wesley and Whitehead are but two of the more visible forebears of people such as Reverend McKenna whose religiously based moral commitment to the most vulnerable among us results in efforts to improve public health and well-being. These tales of the relationship between religious practice and public health and, more specifically, the role of clergy in forging this relationship are well worth remembering.

Notes

1. Steven Johnson, *The Ghost Map: The Story of London's Most Terrifying Epidemic—and How It Changed Science, Cities, and the Modern World* (New York: Riverhead Books, 2006).
2. John Wesley, *Primitive Physick: Or, An Easy and Natural Method of Curing Most Diseases*, 17th ed. (London: R. Hawes, 1776).
3. Ellen Simon, "Interview with Reverend Jennifer McKenna," October 26, 2007, http://carlislehistory.dickinson.edu/?page_id=154. For the enactment of the Diesel-Powered Motor Vehicle Idling Act, see Pennsylvania Business Association, "Act 124 (Idling Restrictions) and Motorcoaches," *PBA Reporter*, November 2008, http://www.pabus.org/documents/Bulletins/2008%20November%20%20Reporter%20Idling%20ACT%20124.pdf.
4. Kirstin Olsen, *Daily Life in 18th-Century England* (Westport, CT: Greenwood Press, 1999), 18, 58, 268.
5. E. Brooks Holifield, *Health and Medicine in the Methodist Tradition* (New York: Crossroad, 1986), 30.
6. Deborah Madden, *"A Cheap, Safe, and Natural Medicine": Religion, Medicine, and Culture in John Wesley's Primitive Physic* (Amsterdam: Rodopi B. V., 2007), 11.
7. Madden, *"A Cheap, Safe, and Natural Medicine,"* 48.
8. Indeed, Wesley's work in what can be seen as the foundations of public health has been neglected on both the medical and theological fronts. Deborah Madden discusses some of the reasons historians of medicine have overlooked Wesley in *"A Cheap Safe, and Natural Medicine"*; Randy Maddox, "A Heritage Reclaimed: John Wesley on Holistic Health and Healing," *Methodist History* 46, no. 1 (2007): 4–33, discusses the reasons theologians have overlooked his contributions to medicine and health.
9. Kenneth Wilson, *Methodist Theology (Doing Theology)* (New York: T & T Clark, 2011), 31.
10. Richard P. Heitzenrater, *Wesley and the People Called Methodist* (Nashville: Abingdon Press, 1995), 30.
11. Heitzenrater, *Wesley and the People Called Methodist*, 30.
12. Heitzenrater, *Wesley and the People Called Methodist*, 103–106.
13. Phillip Ott, "John Wesley on Health: A Word For Sensible Regimen," *Methodist History* 18, no. 3. (April 1980): 193–204.
14. Ott, "John Wesley on Health."
15. Holifield, *Health and Medicine in the Methodist Tradition*, xiii.
16. Randy Maddox, "Reclaiming the Eccentric Parent," in *Inward and Outward Health: John Wesley's Holistic Concept of Medical Sciences, The Environment, and Holy Living*, ed. Deborah Madden (London: Epworth Press, 2008), 16. Such training was introduced in the seventeenth century.
17. Cited in Madden, *"A Cheap, Safe and Natural Medicine,"* 47.
18. Cited in Madden, *"A Cheap, Safe and Natural Medicine,"* 47.

19. Henry Rack, "Doctors, Demons and Early Methodist Healing," in *The Church and Healing*, ed. W. J. Sheils (Studies in Church History 19; Oxford: Oxford University Press, 1982), 139, cited in Madden, *"A Cheap Safe and Natural Medicine,"* 47.

20. Anonymous, "Dedication to the Parochial Clergy of this Kingdom," in *The Family Guide to Health, Or a Practice of Physic: In a Familiar Way*, 1st ed. (London: J. Fletcher, 1767), iii–iv, cited in Madden, *"A Cheap, Safe and Natural Medicine,"* 48.

21. Madden, *"A Cheap, Safe and Natural Medicine,"* 47.

22. Holifield, *Health and Medicine in the Methodist Tradition*, 29.

23. Wesley to Vincent Perronet, December 1748, in John Wesley, *The Letters of Reverend Wesley*, ed. John Telford (London: Epworth Press, 1931), cited in Holifield, *Health and Medicine in the Methodist Tradition*, 29.

24. John Wesley, *Primitive Physick*, cited in Madden, *"A Cheap, Safe and Natural Medicine,"* 100.

25. Madden, *"A Cheap, Safe and Natural Medicine,"* 31.

26. Madden, *"A Cheap, Safe and Natural Medicine,"* 66–70.

27. Madden, *"A Cheap, Safe and Natural Medicine,"* 31.

28. Wesley, cited in Maddox, "Reclaiming the Eccentric Parent," 17.

29. Maddox, "Reclaiming the Eccentric Parent," 17; emphasis in original.

30. Holifield, *Health and Medicine in the Methodist Tradition*, 20.

31. Maddox, "Reclaiming the Eccentric Parent," 21.

32. Holifield, *Health and Medicine in the Methodist Tradition*, 20.

33. Maddox, "Reclaiming the Eccentric Parent," 16.

34. John Wesley, "Farther Appeal to Men of Reason and Religion," in *The Works of John Wesley*, ed. A. C. Outler (26 vols. Nashville: Abington Press, 1984–), Vol. 11, 106, cited in Maddox, "Reclaiming the Eccentric Parent," 16.

35. Maddox, "Reclaiming the Eccentric Parent," 17; emphasis in original.

36. Maddox, "Reclaiming the Eccentric Parent," 18.

37. Ott, "John Wesley on Health," 194.

38. Maddox, "Reclaiming the Eccentric Parent," 18.

39. Maddox, "Reclaiming the Eccentric Parent."

40. Maddox, "Reclaiming the Eccentric Parent," 48.

41. Maddox, "Reclaiming the Eccentric Parent," 18.

42. John Wesley, "A Plain Account of the People Called Methodist," in Outer, *The Works of John Wesley*, vol. 9, 275–276. See also Wesley's Journal (4 December 1746), Outer, *The Works of John Wesley*, vol. 20, 150–151.

43. Maddox, "Reclaiming the Eccentric Parent," 19.

44. Stephen Mansfield, *The Search for God and Guinness* (Nashville: Thomas Nelson, 2009), 62. Further details about Guinness in this section are taken from this work.

45. Mansfield, *The Search for God and Guinness*, xv. "Do all the good you can" was one of the general rules of the Methodist societies. This rule, along with the two other general rules, "Do no harm" and "Attend the ordinances of God," are still included in the United Methodist Book of Discipline.

46. Mansfield, *The Search for God and Guinness*, xxviii.

47. Ott, "John Wesley on Health," 204.

48. John Wesley, Preface to *Advice With Respect to Health*, Outer, *The Works of John Wesley*, vol. 14, 258–259, cited in Ott, "John Wesley on Health," 198.

49. John Wesley, "The Good Steward," in Outer, *The Works of John Wesley*, vol. 6, 138, cited in Ott, "John Wesley on Health," 198.

50. Ott, "John Wesley on Health," 198.

51. John Wesley, Preface to *The Primitive Physic*, cited in Madden, *"A Cheap, Safe and Natural Medicine,"* 155.

52. Madden, *"A Cheap, Safe and Natural Medicine,"* 155.

53. Madden, *"A Cheap, Safe and Natural Medicine."*

54. G. Cheyne, *An Essay on Regimen, Together with Fine Discourses, Medical, Moral, and Philosophical: Serving to Illustrate the Principles and Theory of Philosophical Medicine, and Point Out Some of Its Moral Consequences*, 1st ed. (London: C. Rivington, 1740), vi, cited in Madden, *"A Cheap, Safe and Natural Medicine,"* 156.

55. Roy Porter, ed., *The Popularization of Medicine 1650–1850* (New York: Routledge, 1992), cited in Madden, *"A Cheap, Safe and Natural Medicine,"* 159.

56. Madden, *"A Cheap, Safe and Natural Medicine,"* 159.

57. Madden, *"A Cheap, Safe and Natural Medicine,"* 156.

58. John Wesley, *Primitive Physick*, 24th ed. (London: G. Paramore, 1792), i, cited in Madden, *"A Cheap, Safe and Natural Medicine,"* 161.

59. Madden, *"A Cheap, Safe and Natural Medicine,"* 156; Ott, "John Wesley on Health," 200.

60. Ott, "John Wesley on Health," 204.

61. Madden, "A Cheap, Safe and Natural Medicine," 161.

62. Wesley, *Primitive Physick*, i, cited in Madden, "A Cheap, Safe and Natural Medicine," 161.

63. Madden, "A Cheap, Safe and Natural Medicine," 162.

64. Robert E. Schofield, *Stephen Hales, Scientist and Philanthropist* (London: Scholar's Press, 1980).

65. Madden, *"A Cheap, Safe and Natural Medicine,"* 163.

66. Madden, *"A Cheap, Safe and Natural Medicine,"* 162.

67. John Wesley, "What Is Man?," in *The Works of John Wesley*, ed. A. C. Outler (26 vols.; Nashville: Abington Press, 1984–), vol. 4, 20–27; see 20, cited in Madden, *"A Cheap, Safe and Natural Medicine,"* 164.

68. Wesley, *Primitive Physick*, i, cited in Madden, *"A Cheap, Safe and Natural Medicine,"* 164.

69. John Wesley, "On Dress" (1786), in Outler, *The Works of John Wesley*, vol. 3, 248–259; see 249; A. W. Hill, *John Wesley among the Physicians: A Study of Eighteenth-Century Medicine* (London: Epworth Press, 1958), 118, cited in Madden, *"A Cheap, Safe and Natural Medicine,"* 167.

70. Wesley, *On Dress* (1786), cited in Madden, *"A Cheap, Safe and Natural Medicine,"* 168.

71. Madden, *"A Cheap, Safe and Natural Medicine,"* 170.

72. Ott, "John Wesley on Health," 202.

73. John Wesley, "The More Excellent Way," Outler, *The Works of John Wesely*, vol. 7, 37, cited in Ott, "John Wesley on Health," 202.

74. Ott, "John Wesley on Health," 201.

75. Ott, "John Wesley on Health," cited in Madden, *"A Cheap, Safe and Natural Medicine,"* 171.

76. Ott, "John Wesley on Health," 201.
77. Madden, *A Cheap, Safe and Natural Medicine,* 180.
78. John Wesley, "On Redeeming the Time (1782)," cited in Madden, *A Cheap, Safe and Natural Medicine,* 180.
79. Ott, "John Wesley on Health," 200, quoting Wesley.
80. Ott, "John Wesley on Health," 202.
81. Maddox, "Reclaiming the Eccentric Parent," 20.
82. Ott, "John Wesley on Health," 204.
83. John Wesley, "Primitive Remedies," 5, cited in Ott, "John Wesley on Health," 203.
84. Maddox, "Reclaiming the Eccentric Parent," 20.
85. Madden, *A Cheap, Safe, and Natural Medicine.*
86. Maddox, "Reclaiming the Eccentric Parent," 18.
87. Maddox, "Reclaiming the Eccentric Parent," 19.
88. Maddox, "Reclaiming the Eccentric Parent," 21.
89. Maddox, "Reclaiming the Eccentric Parent," 21.
90. Maddox, "Reclaiming the Eccentric Parent," 21.
91. John Shorb, "The Holistic Vision of John Wesley: Q&A with Randy Maddox, Part I," *Church Health Reader*, October 25, 2010, http://www.chreader.org/contentPage.aspx?resource_id=580.
92. Robert S. Morrison, "Rights and Responsibilities: Redressing the Uneasy Balance," *Hastings Center Report* 4 (April 1974): 3.
93. Steven Johnson, *The Ghost Map.*

15 | US Public Health Reform Movements and the Social Gospel

JOHN BLEVINS

I N THE FALL OF 2010, Jim Curran, the Dean of the Rollins School of Public Health at Emory University, attended the blessing of the new offices of the Interfaith Health Program (IHP) at Rollins. The IHP was founded in 1992 by William Foege and former president Jimmy Carter, and the Carter Center was its first home. The IHP moved to Rollins in 1999 and into its new offices in 2010. The day after the blessing, Dean Curran dropped by the IHP's offices to offer his perspective on the previous night's events: "You know, I don't always know what to do with religion and I admit that some religious rituals make me nervous. But last night's blessing was grounded in social justice, in the social gospel. I can affirm that message" (personal communication, October 2010).

The founding of the IHP and the reaction of Jim Curran to the blessing of IHP's offices raise a number of interesting questions that help to illumine the historical connections between religion and public health: Why would Foege—a former director of the Centers for Disease Control and Prevention, a public health researcher who played a central role in the global elimination of smallpox, and the son of a Lutheran minister[1]— found an organization like the IHP? Why would Jim Curran, a former epidemiologist at the Centers for Disease Control and Prevention, have expressed an affinity for this particular kind of religious event, grounded in a commitment to social justice and to the legacy of the social gospel movement? Any attempt to answer these questions requires us to look backward to the early decades of the nineteenth century and examine the role of Christianity in the social movements of the United States.

That backward glance settles on two forces in American history: first, the role of American Protestantism in the founding of modern public health movements in the 1800s and, second, the multiple and contentious debates within Protestantism on the proper relation between Christianity and American society in the wake of the seismic social changes of the late nineteenth and early twentieth centuries. In the nineteenth century, many American Protestants shared a conviction that America could offer an example of a society guided by the highest Christian moral teachings and that these teachings carried with them a responsibility on the part of religious leaders to address the societal ills facing the country. While efforts to address those ills were marked by a certain kind of religious piety that has since been criticized, they were also marked by a commitment to address the social forces that contributed to poor health.

This unified vision of a Christianized America did not survive the societal changes of the late nineteenth and early twentieth century. No longer was there a consensus that America was—or should be—an example of Christian morality, and Christian leaders and theologians were engaged in sharp debates regarding the right response to these changes. Some of the perspectives articulated from those debates were in tension with the emerging discipline of public health, whose practitioners came to rely more on the social and health sciences than on a Christian moral vision; however, other perspectives within America's religious landscape were more closely aligned to public health research and practice.

"Difficulties Which Are Otherwise Inexplicable": American Protestantism and the Social Health of America in the Nineteenth Century

> Examining the social question in the highest light by which it can be viewed—that of Christianity—we find a solution of many difficulties which are otherwise inexplicable. . . . It shows that while none are so pure as to be exempted from suffering, such suffering is directly or indirectly attributable to an anterior departure from virtue; and that apart from death, and accident, and unavoidable disease, the wretchedness of humanity is resolvable to moral causes.[2]

New York City in the early decades of the nineteenth century was beset by innumerable social ills: regular outbreaks of disease, high levels of illiteracy, dangerous and poorly regulated working conditions in the factories of the rapidly expanding industrial base, and a burgeoning immigrant population mired in poverty. As the city inspector from 1842 to 1843 and the chief physician of the City Hospital from 1843 to 1870, John Griscom endeavored to address these circumstances. His efforts to address environmental conditions such as air quality, the social environment of immigrants living in tenements, and recurrent epidemics of contagions such as yellow fever spurred the emergence of some of the first formal public health programs in the United States. Such efforts were predicated on a distinction between medical care and public health, a distinction that Griscom was one of the first to describe:

> It is necessary to understand the distinction between *Public Health* and *Individual Health*. . . . The difference depends chiefly on the cause being *personal* or *general*. Thus an individual may be made sick by causes which affect no one else . . . and yet even these diseases, personal and peculiar as they seem to be, will sometimes be found [to be] dependent upon causes which affect large numbers at the same time. . . . In such cases, a well-directed inquiry into the condition in which people live, the position and arrangement of their working and lodging rooms, the character of their food, their habits of dress and cleanliness, the well or ill ventilated rooms they occupy by day and by night, would . . . fully account for the great and premature mortality of our citizens.[3]

A contemporary of Griscom's, Robert Milham Hartley, founded one of the first social service organizations in the United States, the New York Association for Improving the Condition of the Poor, in 1842. While Griscom endeavored to address the underlying causes of poor health among the citizens of New York as a physician, Hartley sought to address those broader societal factors through social services:

> The design of the Association was to advance the social, moral, and material interests of large masses of the community [to] provide for existing difficulties, avoid known evils, and secure beneficent results. . . . Moral means were to be employed, from the fact that no other would be adequate to produce the results, which the condition of the indigent required. It contemplated likewise preventive rather than remedial measures. It was primarily and directly to discountenance indiscriminate alms giving; to visit the poor at their homes, to give them counsel, to assist them when practicable in obtaining employment, to inspire them with self-respect and self-reliance, to inculcate

habits of economy, industry, and temperance, and whenever absolutely necessary to provide such relief as should be suited to their wants.[4]

John Griscom was a medical doctor and a devout Quaker. Robert Hartley
was a businessman and devout Presbyterian who ran a manufacturing trade
before founding the association. Both men were quintessential examples
of the de facto leaders of nineteenth-century America: white, male, devoutly Protestant, well educated, and well-to-do. From the perspective of
these leaders, the physical and social ills facing their city and nation were
the result of pauperism, a nineteenth-century notion of pervasive poverty
as rooted in individual moral weakness. Hartley, Griscom, and their peers
believed that moral force alone could overcome pauperism: "Official data
show, though imperfectly, how large a part of the pauperism of the City
and State is occasioned by indolence, intemperance, and other vices. . . .
To remove the evil we must remove the causes; and these being chiefly
moral—whatever subsidiary appliances may be used—they admit only
moral remedies."[5] These perspectives were universal among both religious
leaders and medical professionals in the early nineteenth century. For example, Griscom's father, a chemist who helped establish both the medical
school at Rutgers University and the American Bible Society, founded the
Society for the Prevention of Pauperism in 1817.[6] In writing the biography
of his father, the younger Griscom recounted the position of that society
that, while pauperism may consist of many causes, it arose chiefly from an
individual's moral weakness.[7]

The idea that the poor themselves bore the primary responsibility for
their condition was long lasting. Almost three-quarters of a century after
the founding of the Society for the Prevention of Pauperism, John Shaw
Billings, a well-respected surgeon and early leader of the nascent US
Public Health Service, echoed this perspective in a speech on public health
and municipal government: "Pauperism consists of a distinct class of
people who are structurally and almost necessarily idle, ignorant, intemperate, and more or less vicious, who are failures, or the descendants of
failures, and who for the most part belong to certain races."[8] For men such
as Billings, Hartley, and the elder and younger Griscoms, pauperism was
the source of the social ills that they hoped to remedy. Likewise, all of
these men believed that moral instruction rooted in Christianity was the
only efficacious response: "If there is one kind of effort more to be depre-
cated than another, it is that which attempts the reform of deep-seated
social evils, without the agency of the only power adequate to their
eradication—the moral spirit of Christianity."[9] Robert Hartley displayed

unerring faith in his moral vision of Christianity as a solution to the health and social ills facing his city. Two examples of Hartley's work highlight the certainty of that vision, and both anticipated the public health movement that would emerge in the United States decades later: his investigation into milk as a vector for disease transmission among the poor in New York City and his publication and distribution of missionary tracts.

In 1842, the same year that he founded the New York Association for Improving the Condition of the Poor, Robert Hartley argued that the sale of milk from sick cows was passing disease to poor citizens who purchased their milk from unregulated vendors. The book in which he published this argument, *An Historical, Scientific, and Practical Essay on Milk as an Article of Human Sustenance*, is a remarkable example of early public health writing; well over a century before the term "social determinants of health" was coined, Hartley examined the physical, social, and economic factors that contributed to the spread of disease through unsanitary cow's milk. He looked at the built environment of the city, including the pens where the cows were held, and argued that the architecture of both the cow stables and the tenements created ideal conditions for disease. He undertook an analysis of infant and childhood morbidity and mortality rates in New York in comparison to other large cities in the United States, cities in Europe, and rural areas where dairy production was part of large farms. He gathered testimony from those who had drunk cow's milk from the sources that he investigated and had subsequently fallen ill; he also included medical opinions from leading physicians in the city. Finally, he researched bovine physiology and examined the cows' diet in the unregulated dairies. He discovered that the cows' diet consisted primarily of distillery slop, "the refuse of grain diffused through water after it has undergone a chemical change, the alcohol and farina being extracted by the process of fermentation and distillation."[10]

Tying the social evil of pauperism to the production of alcohol, Hartley argued that this evil was leading to the poor health of the city's children, who were drinking contaminated milk coming from cows fed distillery slop. Further, he held the consumers both of liquor and of the tainted milk accountable:

It should not be forgotten that the consumer, whether of strong liquors or of milk produced from the dregs of whiskey is one . . . in this work of destruction. . . . He it is that kindles up the fires of the distillery, patronizes the rum-seller and the impure milk vender, and perpetuates the evils which flow from these occupations. For his own safety and for the benefit of his suffering fellow-creatures, he is in duty bound to abstain from all such use.[11]

In short, *An Essay on Milk* was a groundbreaking investigation into a public health problem undertaken not by a medical doctor or scientist but by a businessman interested in the health condition of his city.

In writing that investigation, Hartley invoked religion freely. The title page of the 1842 edition contains a short epigraph: "Μη των βοων μελει τω θεω. Δι ημασ γαρ εγγραφη. Paul."[12] This is the Greek translation of a verse from Saint Paul's first epistle to the church in Corinth: "Is it for oxen that God is concerned? Or does he not speak entirely for our sake?" (1 Corinthians 9: 9b–10).[13] The introduction and first four chapters of the book tie the topic of unsanitary milk to the providence of God, the proper relationship between human beings and animals according to biblical narratives, and the importance of pastoral life to the ancient Israelites. Among the list of proposed reforms to address the problem, Hartley calls for the suspension of milk sales on Sunday to avoid profaning the Sabbath. He closes the book with a concluding paragraph that links attention to public health to a particular vision of Christianity:

> Whilst the inquiry [into the sanitary conditions of milk], therefore, especially invites the attention of medical men, from whom, as the constituted guardians of public health, much is naturally expected, yet neither is our farther knowledge of the subject, nor the extirpation of the evils to which such knowledge refers, necessarily limited either to their investigations or exertions. . . . All indeed who desire and expect the ultimate removal of the woes which afflict and debase their world . . . will assuredly advance not only their own immediate good and that of the community around them, but happily become instrumental in preparing the way for the advent of that promised era of primeval purity and peace, so long foretold in prophecy, and invoked in sacred song."[14]

For Robert Hartley, that vision of Christianity "foretold in prophecy and invoked in sacred song" was the foundation for addressing the public health problem of tainted cows' milk. That same foundation also guided the second example of Hartley's influence on public health: his leadership of missionary tract societies.

Tract societies played a key role in spreading Hartley's Christian moral vision and connecting it to practical information to address the living and health conditions of the poor. England had been the home of the tract movement since the late eighteenth century. For a number of years, tracts provided fictional narratives of wayward souls finding salvation through God's miraculous Providence in Jesus Christ, but by the middle of the nineteenth century, the catalog of tract titles had grown to encompass social concerns such as pauperism, and the tract movement had spread around the world as a central program of British Protestant missionary movements.[15] By 1832, the American Tract Society, which was headquartered in Boston, was publishing close to seven hundred titles in six different languages with a total circulation of over fifteen million copies,[16] a truly astounding number when one considers that the population of the United States in the 1830 census was 12,858,670.[17]

Hartley was an important leader of the New York chapter of the American Tract Society, and he used the activities of the New York Association for the Improving the Condition of the Poor to spread the gospel contained in the tracts:

> The Association began the issuing of tracts, designed to inform the more unfortunate in the community what was expected of them, though they were poor; how to conduct themselves in their poverty; what to adopt, what to avoid; how to buy, cook, economize; in a word, how to live—live happily, live successfully. . . . We would merely mention some of the more prominent of these topics, that received consideration and were given to the public. Street Begging and Vagrancy; The Proper Subjects of Charity; Domestic Economy; Food and Drink, with the best Modes of Preparation; Plans for the Better Distribution of Medical Attendance and Medicines for the Indigent Sick, by the Public Dispensaries of the City; Sanitary Law; Truancy; Sewerage; Employment; Apprentices; Dwellings; Widows; Orphans; Tenements; Crowded Dwellings; Public Health; Reformatories, and numerous others.[18]

The tracts, in short, provided a way to communicate health messages in the context of a Christian moral frame. This message marrying Christianity and health was not unique to Hartley. John Ordronaux, a prominent New York surgeon, spoke about the key role of the American Tract Society in improving the health of the city in his 1866 keynote address to the New York Academy of Medicine:

> Let the poor be taught that there is religion in cleanliness, in ventilation, and in good food; let them but once be induced to put these lessons into practice, and we may rest assured their spiritual culture and moral elevation will be

rendered all the more easy and certain. Disease, like sin, is permitted to exist; but conscience and revelation on the one hand, and reason and science on the other, are the kindred means with which God has armed us against them.[19]

Christianity and public health education, then, were brought together in the distribution of Hartley's tracts. Tract societies had initially been developed as mechanisms for evangelism; now Hartley was using them to address social ills.

The staff of Hartley's association visited the tenements that were home to New York's poorest citizens, conducted assessments of the living conditions that they found, educated residents about various means to improve their living conditions, and offered time-limited financial support (under strict conditions so as not to encourage long-term reliance on charity).[20] In the 1840s and 1850s—over twenty years before coordinated public health responses were developed by medical organizations—Robert Hartley built "the most coherent and far-seeing public health program of any benevolent group while medical societies still concerned themselves marginally with such matters."[21]

As Robert Hartley worked to respond to social ills through his organizations, John Griscom sought to use the power of local government. Griscom conducted research into the links between fresh air and illness, hypothesizing that poor air circulation, common in New York tenements, made the poor more susceptible to illness.[22] He interviewed "tract missionaries" such as the staff of the Association for Improving the Condition of the Poor to gather data on the living conditions of poor New Yorkers. Those missionary interviews comprise almost one-fourth of Griscom's *The Sanitary Conditions of the Laboring Population of New York*, a landmark study of the social conditions that impact public health. In interviewing these missionaries, Griscom asked questions covering the full range of living conditions:

1st. To what extent does the congregation of different sexes, and various ages of the same family of the poor, in one apartment, influence their morals, and do they, or do they not, seem to place a lower estimate on moral character, (though free from actual vice,) than others, a grade above them in physical condition?

2d. Have you found physical distress to present a bar to your moral and religious instructions, and do you think relief from their bodily ailments would enable you to be of greater service to the poor in your calling?

3d. Have you observed that personal and domiciliary negligence and filthiness tend to depress still more the moral sensibility, and make the poor more reckless of character—and do you believe, that domiciliary and personal cleanliness, though combined with an equal degree of poverty, give to the individual or family, more self-respect, more aptitude to receive instruction, and more happiness?

4th. If constrained by law to keep themselves, their furniture, clothing and dwellings, more clean, by frequent use of water and lime, do you think there would be a greater inclination to improve their associations, and obtain a better state of moral and social feeling?

5th. In your opinion would regular domiciliary visits by an officer of health, empowered to enforce a law to promote the cleanliness of house and persons, have any influence in raising the tone of feeling among the poor, as well as relieving sickness and prolonging life?

6th. Are there not many who would be pleased to be aided and instructed in the best mode of improving the condition of their dwellings, and be glad to receive the visits of such an officer?[23]

One sees in these questions an implicit perspective different from that of Hartley and his fellows, a belief that social forces play a more central role than individual moral fabric in causing and sustaining pauperism and that interventions "by an officer of health" may help address those forces. At points in *The Sanitary Conditions of the Laboring Population of New York*, Griscom makes these implicit connections explicit:

Let us first cast the beam from our own eye. We are parties to their degradation, inasmuch as we permit the inhabitation of places, from which it is not possible improvement in condition or habits can come. We suffer the sublandlord to stow them, like cattle, in pens, and to compel them to swallow poison with every breath. They are allowed, may it not be said required, to live in dirt, when the reverse, rather, should be enforced.[24]

Griscom was prescient; his perspectives anticipated current initiatives to address the social determinants of health. His perspectives also anticipated a turn within both sociological analysis and theological reflection that saw disparities between classes, races, genders, or other social conditions arising not from the weak moral characters of people labeled as "paupers" but from social conditions that favored some at the expense of others:

Now where are the advantages of this study [of the sanitary living conditions of the working poor] most needed? among what classes of the community are its precepts and laws, its vital and saving influences, its checks and guards against disease and danger, most required? Is it among those who live in high-ceiled rooms, who have plenty of time and means to go abroad and seek fresh air in the country, who can afford to live on the choicest delicacies, and dress in the most comfortable manner, who have no fear of want, and are not compelled to study the most economical mode of living? or to seek out, from a very limited field, the best they can do for themselves? No! indeed, such need comparatively little aid. They may turn night into day, and dissipate their time and strength in debauchery and folly, but they are not compelled to reside in cellars, and chambers ill ventitilated [sic], or to associate with filth, in foul air. *They* are to be reached only by *moral* teaching.[25]

Pauperism, in Griscom's view, was not the effect of weak moral character but of inequitable social conditions. The question of moral conviction lay not in front of the pauper but before the well-to-do, for "they are to be reached only by the moral question." Griscom's views directly challenged those of his day, and his questions about social forces and social justice were met with resistance. Indeed, one of the tract missionaries interviewed by Griscom goes out of his way to reject the implications of his questions:

That the physical condition of an individual or a family, has a powerful and important bearing on the moral character, for weal or woe, needs no labor to prove; although neither of us has any idea of embracing [the teaching] that most of the ills of life, as now experienced in the world, flow not from the moral obliquity of human nature, but from the *wrong, civil, and physical* position of men.[26]

These tensions between moral responsibility and social forces would play out in the coming decades, within Christianity and in the broader society. As the modern American public health movement began to coalesce in the mid-nineteenth century, it was grounded in the Christian moral and social vision of religiously observant medical and social service leaders who believed that their religion provided the only legitimate and effective response to the social and physical ills facing the American populace. This unified vision would not last. New tensions would arise among various factions within Christianity and between some Christian religious leaders and researchers and practitioners in the medical and social sciences.

"The Gospel Remedy for Sin and Misery": Christianity's Relationship to Modern Society

> We must beware of expecting too much from any social or eco-
> nomic reform. . . . There is but one force that can save, can regener-
> ate humanity. Only one can give life. . . . When Christ himself was
> here, though surrounded by crying abuses, oppression, and tyranny,
> he attempted no civil reforms; nor has he left his Church any com-
> mission to purify the government of earth,—not because he was
> indifferent to the woes of humanity, but because the remedy was
> not to be found in any external conditions or any human means.[27]

In 1845, John Griscom and Robert Hartley were working to bring about an
American society grounded in a particular Christian moral vision, one in
which religious institutions and governmental organizations worked together to address the social problems that led to ill health among the nation's poorer citizens. By 1920, George Price, a Seventh-day Adventist
from Canada, warned against an overreliance on the institutions of modern
society to save humanity from illness and suffering, arguing that only faith
in Jesus could save human beings from sin. Any effort to examine the historical role of religion in the founding of the modern public health movement must take into account the changes in worldview that occurred in the
decades between the 1840s era of progressive optimism exemplified by
Griscom and Hartley and the 1920s era of suspicion demonstrated by
Price.

Progress or Salvation: The Purpose of Christian Faith in America

Hartley and Griscom endeavored to address pressing public health needs
by relying on a Christian moral vision made real in American society. This
theological vision understood salvation not so much as the rescue of an
individual soul from sin and hellfire but more as the dawn of God's kingdom on earth, ushered in through an American society that had overcome
its various social ills by turning toward the truths of Christianity. This theology had a profound impact on American Protestantism in the nineteenth
and early twentieth centuries, forming the foundation for a broad-based
social reform movement that came to be known as the social gospel. Walter
Rauschenbusch, an American Baptist theologian, was the primary spokes-
person for the movement. Rauschenbusch made a theological case for the
social gospel, arguing that it represented the continuation of the gospel

narratives of Jesus' work of healing and care for the poor. Writing fifty years after Griscom and Hartley, at a point at which some social reformers had begun to criticize the connection of social progressivism to Christianity, Rauschenbusch rearticulated the need for that connection:

> The majority of social-reform workers . . . fluctuates somewhere between contempt and avowed hostility toward the church and spiritual religion. We of "The Brotherhood of the Kingdom" believe that such a separation is unnecessary, unwise, and undesirable, detrimental to the full success of both parties concerned, and perilous to the future of humanity. . . . We must overhaul all the departments of our thought and work out that social Christianity which will be immeasurably more powerful and more valuable to the world than either an unsocial Christianity or an unchristian socialism. After the process of union is in a measure completed in ourselves, we can become mediators for others, breaking down the middle wall of partition between Christianity and the social movement, bringing them into their just and natural relation to each other, infusing the exalted fervor and power of religion into the social movement, and helping religion to find its ethical outcome in the transformation of social conditions.[28]

Just as growing numbers of those working for social reform expressed suspicion toward religion, not all Christians shared Rauschenbusch's vision of a Christianized social order. In fact, there had long been disputes among Christians as to the chief purpose of Christian faith. Many Christians grounded their belief in an experience of personal salvation from sin. Seen in this way, Christianity brought not a perfected social order or a civilizing influence upon the morally weak pauper but salvation from damnation for every sin-sick soul. Social problems such as the poor living conditions of tenement dwellers in New York City or the poor health of milk cows were of little concern in the face of the possibility of eternal damnation as the consequence of sin. The purpose of Christian faith for these believers was to regenerate a sinful soul through the exorbitant grace of God, not to Christianize the social order.

These two distinct theological perspectives can be traced across the history of American Protestantism into the present. Both of them have influenced the relationship between American Christianity and the public health movement for over 150 years. The social gospel perspective has supported an alignment between religion and public health, while the perspective focused on individual salvation has contributed to tensions between religion and public health. These alignments and tensions have taken on various forms at various times, but the fault lines between these two visions of Christianity were revealed in the early decades of the twentieth century, when the rise of the temperance movement and the controversies surrounding Charles Darwin's theory of evolution put those competing visions in stark relief.

Depravity or Disease: Alcohol, Religion, and Public Health

When the United States was founded in the late eighteenth century, drinking was commonplace: "Alcohol was pervasive in American society; it crossed regional, sexual, racial, and class lines. Americans drank at home and abroad, alone and together, at work and play, in fun and in earnest. They drank from the crack of dawn to the crack of dawn."[29] While drinking was commonplace, drunkenness was evidence not of the disease of alcoholism but of the moral failing of a weak free will bedeviled by vice. In 1754, Jonathan Edwards wrote on the nature of that will: "When a drunkard has his liquor before him, and he has to choose whether to drink or no. . . . If he wills to drink, then drinking is the proper object of the act of his Will; and drinking, on some account or other, now appears most agreeable to him, and suits him best."[30]

By the mid-nineteenth century, that religious framework had been supplemented by a medical one that spoke of drunkenness as a kind of disease. Benjamin Rush was a nephew of Samuel Finley, an evangelist, and an early president of Princeton University who was part of the eighteenth-century religious revival in the United States known as the Great Awakening. Rush was a prominent physician in the young country; to this day, his profile adorns the seal of the American Psychiatric Association.[31] In his tract *An Inquiry into the Effects of Ardent Spirits upon the Human Body and Mind*, Rush described intemperate drinking of distilled spirits as a "disease of the will."[32] Disease, the language of medicine, had joined depravity, the language of theology, to describe the causes of habitual drunkenness. Until the beginning of the twentieth century, all of the various temperance organizations formed in the United States in the early 1800s used some combination of religious and medical rhetoric to make their cases. In doing so, they reflected a common moral vision akin to that of Griscom and Hartley, one in which Christianity alone could provide the moral force to overcome this "disease of the will," though clinical intervention could support a cure. For example, Walter Rauschenbusch, the primary author of the social gospel, was a strong advocate not only of voluntary temperance pledges but also of legislated prohibition.[33] The act of will—the pledge of sobriety—should be supported by a societal intervention—the legal prohibition of the dangerous substance.

However, dissenting voices began to speak out, disturbed by the moralizing that they saw as characteristic of temperance proponents who were eager to legislate abstinence for all. One early group of dissenters was the Committee of Fifty for the Investigation of the Liquor Problem; the group, which included business leaders, social scientists, physicians, and clergy, described their efforts thus:

> Our members represent many different attitudes of mind toward practical methods of temperance reform. . . . The problem before such a committee was that of formulating the facts on which thoughtful students of various traditions and tendencies might agree. The series of special investigations are not missionary tracts or moral appeals, but scientific studies of physical and social facts.[34]

The committee's reports represented a shift in the understanding of the relationship between religious viewpoints and other sources of knowledge such as medicine or the social or natural sciences. No longer was there an assumption of a unified vision.

The recommendations of the committee had little impact on popular opinion or public policy at the time the report was published. In fact, fifteen years after the publication of the committee report, prohibition was enshrined into the US Constitution with ratification of the Eighteenth Amendment in 1920. Religious studies scholar Susan Harding nonetheless argues that the document marked an end to Protestant hegemony in the United States:

> The recommendations in the committee's volumes were largely ignored when they were published, a reflection of just how dominant the conservative Protestant "organized church forces" were at the time. But their formulation, and the coalition that came together to write them, points to the breakup of Protestant unity that was under way, even around the one issue [temperance] that had for so long brought all kinds of Protestants together.[35]

The repeal of Prohibition in 1933 marked the dissolution of a common moral vision of a Christianized social order.

The relationship between the kind of Protestantism that had given rise to such a vision and American society at large was being renegotiated: "Science, reason, an etiquette of civility, and ecumenism, in the sense of both diversity of religious perspectives and of forgoing claims of religious superiority, came together in the repeal effort as integral elements of the emerging normative religiosity and public morality, which we know retrospectively as modern secularity."[36] Of course, this was not the only vision that Protestantism birthed. A Protestant vision of individual salvation remained a dominant religious belief in America. Adherents to that vision were far less likely to arrive at some level of accommodation with a secular American society.

Protestant Fundamentalism's Relationship to Secular Society

Many analyses of American Protestant fundamentalism argue that the fundamentalist movement of the early twentieth century was antimodern, refusing to recognize the truth of evolutionary science in favor of clinging to superstition and simplistic, anachronistic readings of scripture. While it is true that American Protestant fundamentalism was (and is) concerned with salvation from sin, so are other Christian traditions that are not fundamentalist. To understand the motivations of American Protestant fundamentalism, that characteristic must be analyzed in conjunction with another: a suspicion or cynicism toward modern society. These two characteristics together functioned to protect fundamentalism's adherents from a dangerous, rapidly changing world, providing them with a clear, firm set of beliefs that offered a vision of eternal salvation and a structure from which to resist the dangers of a society gone astray.

In his analysis of William Jennings Bryan's closing argument in the Scopes Monkey Trial, Matthew Tontonoz demonstrates these dual characteristics of fundamentalism. Based on his analysis, Tontonoz, who is both a biologist and a social historian, argues that the lawyer was not so much a rigid biblical creationist as a devout but open-minded Christian who feared the social and political implications of Darwinian evolutionary theory.[37] For Tontonoz, Bryan's closing argument demonstrates that the lawyer rejected Darwinian evolutionary theory because it gave a stage to social and political views that he as a Christian could not abide, namely social Darwinism and eugenics. As a strong proponent of the social gospel and a staunch critic of unregulated capitalism, Bryan was disturbed by the use of Darwin's theory to construct harsh social theories that justified the dismantling of social support programs in the interest of allowing the "survival of the fittest."[38]

This concern for the dangers of an American society no longer grounded in Christian belief came to typify a key component of American fundamentalism. Bryan, then, found himself in allegiance with fundamentalism not so much because of his theological belief but because of a social and political belief that religion offered a necessary moral anchor for American society. In contrast, many in the field of public health had come to see religion as a neutral variable at best and as a social force inimical to scientific inquiry at worst. There was no longer an inherent, unexamined alignment between a certain kind of Christian moral vision and public health practice. In less than one hundred years, those alignments had ended or at least shifted.

The Relationship between Religion and Public Health in the Present and the Outlines of a (Possible) Future

In the first half of the nineteenth century, the connections between public health and religion—specifically Christianity—were just being forged. At that point, the social worldviews of religious leaders and of medical doctors were largely in lockstep: religion provided the necessary moral grounding for a godly, prosperous, productive, and upright society. That moral force could be used to address social ills such as squalid living conditions and entrenched poverty.

When Jim Curran and William Foege described the affinity between public health and religion, they were, in effect, describing a very specific form of American Christianity typified in the movement that Curran referenced: the social gospel. Today, American religion and public health are no longer in lockstep. Christian Protestantism itself has split. The movements within American mainline Protestantism that align most closely with public health research and practice in the early twenty-first century rely on a theological vision of social justice. But these movements are no longer the only (or even the predominant) Protestant movements today, either in the United States or internationally. And, of course, we have finally begun to realize that religion itself is much broader and more complex than the forms of American Protestantism that have figured so strongly in the history of American public health. Other forms of Christianity play key roles. Other religions play key roles. Although the relationships between the modern public health movement and these myriad religious forces are no longer singular or linear, this chapter closes by offering four brief descriptions of those relationships.

If American fundamentalism through the first decades of the twentieth century had been marked both by a strict theological system and by a refusal to engage with corrupt social and political organizations, the movement shifted perceptibly in the 1970s, toward an eagerness to work within social and political structures to push for an American society grounded in a Christian moral vision. This robust, politically engaged, conservative Protestantism offers the first example of the relationship between public health and contemporary religious movements. Susan Harding argues that the emergence of this religious movement in the late 1970s unsettled American civil society because it represented the return of a movement whose expulsion at the end of Prohibition had marked the beginnings of modern secularism in America: "This particular religious outsider—the white moralistic Protestant fundamentalist—was the one whose expulsion had defined the body politic as secular in the modern sense."[39] The relationship between defenders of programs in public health and this religious movement is often characterized by mutual suspicion and mistrust, most notably in contentious areas such as sexual and reproductive health. To the extent that this expression of Christianity remains active in American society, the relationship between it and public health will need to be explored; to date, however, there have been few contexts in which that is occurring.

In contrast, the second type of relationship, that between public health and the present-day descendants of the social gospel movement, is much clearer. In 1845, John Griscom presciently argued that scientific inquiry into the social factors that contributed to the growth of the New York tenements would also support a moral inquiry into the obligations of those who were not living in the slums to do something about them.[40] Griscom rejected the prevailing idea that the poor were poor as a result of their moral weakness; in short, he rejected the notion of pauperism. His perspective anticipates the perspectives of liberation theology, a theological tradition that refutes the notion that those who are poor are responsible for their poverty, arguing instead that God displays a "preferential option for the poor," who can offer testimony from their own lives to the revelation of God's love at work.[41] This shift from blaming the poor for their material condition to seeing them as offering revelation of God's work in the world has influenced public health practice in a variety of contexts, most notably through the work of Paul Farmer.[42]

Arguing that those who are poor do not bear primary responsibility for their plight has not always been popular. There is within both public health and religion an eagerness "to care for those in need," but, as feminist Christian ethicist Mary McClintock Fulkerson warns, "the impulse of care for the other is inevitably shaped by the impulse to control."[43] This impulse to control can be seen in blaming those who face the ill effects of social disparities for those effects—the pauper suffers from the moral weakness of pauperism.

Many forms of contemporary theological thought have developed strong traditions of internal critique in the wake of a long history of social control carried out in the name of God. Drawing on the work of scholars such as French philosopher and theologian Paul Ricœur, theologians have described the importance of an attitude of suspicion in relation to one's own thought.[44] In fact, the intention with which many theologians and religious studies scholars attend to their own social location and biases offers a well-developed practice of self-critique for public health researchers and practitioners. This practice represents the third kind of relationship between religion and public health; religious thought and practice that is informed by this attitude of suspicion can offer public health research and practice a method for self-critique in regard to its own impulse to control.[45]

The fourth and final relationship between religion and public health is to be found in the influences of religions other than Christianity. Christianity has dominated the history of the relationship between religion and the American public health movement; this is no longer the case, nor should it be. Those of us working in the intersection of religion and public health would do well to build the scholarship, research, and applied practice to help us understand more fully the influences of religion outside of Christianity.

The history of progressive modern Protestantism influenced the work of reformers such as John Griscom and Robert Hartley. This vision of American Christianity had strong historical connections to the modern public health movement; those connections can still be seen today, as Jim Curran's invocation of the social gospel demonstrates. Nonetheless, the relationship between public health and religion in these first years of the twenty-first century and beyond will not be so clear and singular. As interdisciplinary scholarship in the intersection of religion and public health continues to emerge, it will be important to identify theoretical frameworks and research methodologies to help us understand the complexities of that relationship.

Notes

1. William Foege, *House on Fire: The Fight to Eradicate Smallpox* (Berkeley: University of California Press, 2011).
2. Isaac S. Hartley, *Memorial of Robert Milham Hartley* (1882; repr. New York: Arno Press, 1976), 307.

3. John Hoskins Griscom, *The Sanitary Condition of the Laboring Population with Suggestions for Its Improvement* (New York: Harper, 1845), 3–4; emphasis in original.

4. Hartley, *Memorial*, 186–187.

5. Hartley, *Memorial*, 307–308.

6. Rossiter Johnson, *The Twentieth Century Biographical Dictionary of Notable Americans: Brief Biographies of Authors, Administrators, Clergymen, Commanders, Editors, Engineers, Jurists, Merchants, Officials, Philanthropists, Scientists, Statesmen, and Others Who Are Making American History*, Vol. 4, Ericsson-Gwin (Boston: Biographical Society, 1904), 448.

7. John Hoskins Griscom, *Memoir of John Griscom, LL.D., Late Professor of Chemistry and Natural Philosophy* (New York: Robert Carter and Brothers, 1859), 159.

8. John S. Billings, *Public Health and Municipal Government: An Address Delivered before the American Academy of Political and Social Science at the Art Club, Philadelphia, Jan. 14, 1891* (Philadelphia: American Academy of Political and Social Science, 1891), 6.

9. Hartley, *Memorial*, 309.

10. Robert M. Hartley, *An Historical, Scientific, and Practical Essay on Milk, as an Article of Human Sustenance; with a Consideration of the Effects Consequent upon the Present Unnatural Methods for Producing It for the Supply of Large Cities* (1842; repr. New York: Arno Press, 1977), 10.

11. Hartley, *An Historical, Scientific, and Practical Essay on Milk*, 346.

12. Hartley, *An Historical, Scientific, and Practical Essay on Milk*, title page.

13. All biblical references in this chapter follow the New Revised Standard Version.

14. Hartley, *An Historical, Scientific, and Practical Essay on Milk*, 350.

15. Samuel Gosnell Green, *The Story of the Religious Tract Society for One Hundred Years* (London: Religious Tract Society, 1899).

16. American Tract Society, *Nineteenth Annual Report of the American Tract Society* (Boston: Perkins & Marvin, 1833).

17. US House of Representatives, *Abstract of the Returns of the Fifth Census, Showing the Number of Free People, the Number of Slaves, the Federal or Representative Numbers, and the Aggregate of Each County of Each State of the United States* (Washington, DC: Dugg Green, 1832). Available online at http://www2.census.gov/prod2/decennial/documents/1830a-01.pdf.

18. Hartley, *Memorial*, 197, 200.

19. Quoted in Charles E. Rosenberg and Carroll S. Rosenberg, "Pietism and the Origins of the American Public Health Movement: A Note on John H. Griscom and Robert M. Hartley," *Journal of the History of Medicine and Allied Sciences* 23, no. 1 (January 1968): 26–27.

20. Hartley, *Memorial*, 184–203.

21. Rosenberg and Rosenberg, "Pietism and the Origins of the American Public Health Movement," 31.

22. John Hoskins Griscom, *The Uses and Abuses of Air: Showing Its Influence in Sustaining Life, and Producing Disease; With Remarks on the Ventilations of House, and the Best Methods of Securing a Pure and Wholesome Atmosphere Inside of Dwellings, Churches, Court-Rooms, Workshops, and Buildings of All Kinds* (New York: Redfield, 1854).

23. Griscom, *The Sanitary Condition of the Laboring Population*, 25.

24. Griscom, *The Sanitary Condition of the Laboring Population*, 23. Italics are original.

25. Griscom, *The Sanitary Condition of the Laboring Population*, 57; emphasis in original.

26. Griscom, *The Sanitary Condition of the Laboring Population*, 28, quoting Samuel Russell Jr., missionary of the Eighth Ward; emphasis in original.

27. George McReady Price, *Back to the Bible or the New Protestantism* (1916; repr. Washington, DC: Review and Herald Publishing Association, 1920), 217–218.

28. Walter Rauschenbusch, "The Ideals of Social Reformers," *American Journal of Sociology* 2, no. 2 (September 1896): 202–203.

29. W. J. Rorabaugh, *The Alcoholic Republic: An American Tradition* (New York: Oxford University Press, 1979), 20–22.

30. Jonathan Edwards, *Freedom of the Will, Which Is Supposed to be Essential to Moral Agency, Virtue and Vice, Reward and Punishment, Praise and Blame* (1754; repr. London: Hamilton, Adams, 1860), 8.

31. The seal can be seen on the homepage of the American Psychiatric Association's website, http://www.psych.org.

32. Benjamin Rush, *An Inquiry into the Effects of Ardent Spirits upon the Human Body and Mind with an Account of the Means of Preventing and of the Remedy for Curing Them* (1758; repr. Boston: James Loring, 1823). Interestingly, Rush rejected the notion that beer, wine, or fermented cider could lead to drunkenness. The only danger he saw came from distilled liquors.

33. Susan Harding, "American Protestant Moralism and the Secular Imagination: From Temperance to the Moral Majority," *Social Research* 76, no. 4 (Winter 2009): 1294.

34. Francis G. Peabody, "Introduction," in *The Liquor Problem: A Summary of Investigations Conducted by the Committee of Fifty* (New York: Houghton Mifflin, 1905), 7–8.

35. Harding, "American Protestan Moralism," 1297.

36. Harding, "American Protestan Moralism," 1302.

37. Matthew Tontonoz, "The Scopes Monkey Trial Revisited: Social Darwinism Versus Social Gospel," *Science as Culture* 17, no. 2 (2008): 121–143. Bryan's closing argument was never read at the trial. Clarence Darrow, wary of Bryan's rhetorical skill, did not offer a closing argument; as a result, Bryan was not permitted to offer one either. He intended to offer it as a public speech following the trial, but he died immediately afterward. The text of his argument was published in the *New York Times* on July 29, 1925.

38. Tontonoz, "The Scopes Monkey Trial Revisited," 127–129, 135–136. Tontonoz's argument echoes that more fully developed by Michael Kazin in *A Godly Hero: The Life of William Jennings Bryan* (New York: Anchor Books, 2006).

39. Harding, "American Protestan Moralism," 1303.

40. See Griscom, *Sanitary Condition*, 57.

41. See Gustavo Gutierrez, *A Theology of Liberation* (Maryknoll, NY: Orbis Books, 1973).

42. See, for example, Tracy Kidder, *Mountains Beyond Mountains: The Quest of Dr. Paul Farmer, a Man Who Would Cure the World* (New York: Random House, 2009). Farmer and the liberation theologian Gustavo Gutierrez were the featured speakers

in a forum at Notre Dame on global health and liberation theology on October 24, 2011, convened to examine the connections between liberation theology and the public health work of Farmer's group Partners in Health. For a video of that discussion, see http://www.pih.org/blog/video-dr-paul-farmer-and-rev-gustavo-gutierrez.

43. Mary McClintock Fulkerson, *Changing the Subject: Women's Discourses and Feminist Theology* (Minneapolis: Fortress Press, 1994), 383.

44. Paul Ricœur, *Freud and Philosophy: An Essay on Interpretation* (New Haven, CT: Yale University Press, 1970), 27. This attitude of self-critique is often described as a hermeneutic of suspicion.

45. For a sustained description of the ways in which progressive Protestantism engaged in this type of critique long before Western medicine did, see Pamela E. Klassen, *Spirits of Protestantism: Medicine, Healing, and Liberal Christianity* (Berkeley: University of California Press, 2011).

16 | Anthony Comstock: A Religious Fundamentalist's Negative Impact on Reproductive Health

LYNN HOGUE AND CAROL HOGUE

RELIGION'S ROLE AS A SOCIAL determinant of health is a central thesis of this book; that role can be positive, negative, or mixed. This chapter explores a darker side of religion's role, tracing the long shadow cast by religious fundamentalism on US laws regarding contraception and abortion. In the late nineteenth century, one man—Anthony Comstock—managed to imbue state and federal law with his religiously fundamentalist views on sexual morality so deeply that his effect is still felt today, though Comstock died in 1915 and the legal structures that he championed have been largely disassembled. The story of the Comstock laws is an illustration of the destructive effects of religious fundamentalism harnessed to the coercive power of the state.

Fundamentalism takes various forms, including the one associated with North American Protestantism, from which Comstock's crusade sprang. Protestant fundamentalism is an intellectually reactionary response to American Protestantism's "seeking ways to adapt traditional beliefs to the realities of 'modern' scholarship and sensibilities."[1] Of the central features of this particular version of fundamentalism, notably evangelism, biblical inerrancy, premillennialism, and separatism, the concepts of scriptural inerrancy and biblical infallibility have had the greatest impact on science and health by promoting an anti-science bias.[2]

Fundamentalism should be thought of in a larger sense, which is captured by Martin Marty and Scott Appleby in the concluding chapter of *Fundamentalisms Observed*, the first volume of the Fundamentalisms Project:

Our own caution about applying the term "fundamentalism" beyond its original historical context would be supplanted by reluctance were we to allow the Protestant Christian case, for which the term was coined, to dictate the content of the term. Instead . . . , we have begun by emptying the term of its culture-specific and tradition-specific content and context before examining cases across the board to see if there are in fact "family resemblances" among movements commonly perceived as "fundamentalist."[3]

In the introduction to *Fundamentalisms Observed*, Marty and Appleby provide a distillation of fundamentalism that is characterized by militancy: fundamentalists *fight back* ("Fundamentalists begin as traditionalists who perceive some challenge or threat to their core identity, both social and personal."). They *fight for* a worldview governing such matters as the family, particularly "certain understandings of gender, sex roles, the nurturing and educating of children." Particularly relevant for this analysis, "they will fight for their conceptions of what ought to go on in matters of life and health, in the world of the clinic and the laboratory." They *fight with* resources drawn from "real or presumed pasts, to actual or imagined ideal original conditions and concepts . . . regarded as fundamental." Finally,

Fundamentalists also *fight against* others. These may be generalized or specific enemies, but in all cases, whether they come from without or within the group, they are the agents of assault on all that is held dear. The outsider may be the infidel, the agent of antithetical sacred powers, the modernizer, but he or she may also be the friendly messenger who seeks compromise, middle ground, or a civil "agreement to disagree." The insider as threat is likely to be someone who would be moderate, would negotiate with modernity, would adapt the movement.[4]

As so defined, fundamentalists can be found in many religious traditions: Roman Catholic, Jewish, Islamic, and Hindu as well as Buddhist, Confucian, and Shintoist, to name but some of those surveyed by the Fundamentalisms Project.

At bottom, for the purposes of this chapter, fundamentalism can be defined as an unyielding "attachment to a set of irreducible beliefs . . . that forestalls further questions," that is, "anachronistic, anti-intellectual," and antiscientific.[5] This definition clearly fits Anthony Comstock. His nineteenth-century anti-vice crusade ignored the emerging science of human biology on which reproductive rights and liberties are based in favor of a naïve view constructed from religious and moral preconceptions and presuppositions.

The Origins of Comstockery

Anthony Comstock was born March 7, 1844, in New Canaan, Connecticut, the fourth of ten children. His father, for whom he was named, was initially a subsistence farmer but eventually became the prosperous owner of a 160-acre farm and two sawmills.[6] The Comstocks were Congregationalists, and it was from his parents that Anthony acquired the religious disciplines of daily prayer, hard work, regular attendance at church, and virtuous living as measured by biblical norms. From his mother, Polly, he learned the lessons of God's protection of the moral heroes of Old Testament; from his Congregationalist ministers, he learned "that the devil inhabited the human mind and tempted the body at every opportunity."[7] Corporal punishment was an important part of Anthony's upbringing and shaped his adult views of guilt and punishment.[8]

Anthony's experience in the Union Army during the Civil War served primarily to reinforce and amplify his religious self-righteousness. Diary entries reflect his revulsion at the drinking, smoking, and profanity of his comrades and record his retreats into pietistic reflection.[9] Following the war, he returned to his home in New Canaan, only to discover that economic hardship had struck his family and the farm was lost.

He eventually found his way to New York City, where he worked as a clerk for some time. City life was a shock. "Temptations to immoral activity seemed abundant around him. [He was surrounded by] billiard saloons, theaters, gambling establishments, and houses of prostitution," all of which profoundly offended his religious sensibilities.[10] Comstock eventually bought a small home in Brooklyn and in 1871 married Margaret Hamilton, ten years his senior and the daughter of a Presbyterian elder. They had a daughter, Lillie, who failed to thrive and died on June 28, 1872, "a day Comstock strangely spent in court pursuing a pornographer," according to his biographer, Anna Louise Bates.[11]

Comstock is important to our understanding of religion as a social determinant of health because his religious crusade against his definition of vice, ostensibly to protect children, has had a profound impact on sexual and reproductive health in the United States into the present. As Bates notes, "Comstock believed obscene pictures and writing tempted children to indulge in unhealthy practices. Even educational literature about human anatomy was suspect, for it provided children with knowledge about their sex organs. Without such knowledge reasoned Comstock, children would not be tempted to vice."[12] Comstock saw vice as a continuous path beginning with knowledge gained from literature and pictures in one's youth progressing to masturbation and then on to promiscuous nonmarital sex, some with prostitutes facilitated by the use of contraceptives to avoid pregnancy and sexually transmitted diseases, and ultimately to out-of-wedlock pregnancy, which led either to abortion or to the "burden" of children and social opprobrium. All of the steps along this path were for Comstock inextricably linked; they were all part of an arc of evil that it was his duty to extirpate. Later in his career Comstock explained his moral vision as follows:

> In the heart of every child there is a chamber of imagery, memory's store-house, the commissary department in which is received, stored up and held in reserve every good or evil influence for future requisition. If you allow the Devil to decorate the Chamber of Imagery in your heart with licentious and sensual things, you will find that he has practically thrown a noose about your neck and will forever after exert himself to draw you away from the Lamb of God which taketh away the sins of the world.[13]

Efforts to explain Comstock's motivations during his lifetime and shortly after his death sought answers in Freudian psychology[14] or attributed his actions to his conservative Protestant religious faith. However, more thorough, balanced, and recent biographical work finds Comstock to have had a conventional, apparently normal sexual and family life and to have possessed religious beliefs generally shared by his white, Anglo-Saxon, Protestant contemporaries.[15] It is precisely because his view was reflective of mainstream fundamentalism that his story is a useful case study of the negative impact of religious fundamentalism on health.

The Rise of Comstockery

In 1866, Comstock joined the Young Men's Christian Association (YMCA), an organization that offered "wholesome, Christian alternatives to the vices characteristic of city life" solely to "young Christian men in good standing in evangelical churches." The YMCA opposed vices such as gambling, alcohol, prostitution and "licentious literature,"[16] which threatened the morals of young men flocking to burgeoning cities like New York. It was through the YMCA that Comstock heard a lecture on the dangers of lurid and sexually stimulating literature, and he resolved to make fighting vice, particularly sexual immorality and its stimulants, his life's work. He began with part-time efforts against those whom he considered smut sellers and gradually gained in both confidence and belligerence as his efforts met with support from the police and courts. Based on his demonstrated success in targeting for harassment printers and retailers who produced and sold pornographic literature, Comstock gradually ingratiated himself with leaders and wealthy supporters of the YMCA, including businessmen such as J. Pierpont Morgan and Samuel Colgate.[17] At the same time, his concept of licentious literature expanded to include not only sexually explicit stories and pictures but also newspaper advertisements for birth control devices and abortions and eventually even news stories that challenged prevailing Victorian norms of love and marriage in ways he believed were harmful.[18] His goal was to serve as a moral censor to enforce his own religiously based, fundamentalist views of social propriety.

The enactment of the federal Comstock laws that proved central to Comstock's anti-vice enterprise grew out of his disappointment with the outcome of federal prosecutions under an 1872 anti-obscenity law, particularly the unsuccessful prosecution of sisters Victoria Woodhull and Tennessee Claflin, who published *The Woodhull and Claflin Weekly*. The women scandalized Comstock with their advocacy of "free love, short skirts, birth control" and other ideas that offended his notions of propriety.[19] They were arrested in 1872 for publishing two articles, one about a purported sex scandal involving the Reverend Henry Ward Beecher and the other about a stockbroker whom they accused of seducing a 15-year-old girl after taking her to a brothel. The prosecution ultimately failed when the judge "charged the jury not to convict, explaining that 'under the [obscenity] act of 1872, newspapers were not included . . . and . . . therefore there was no evidence to sustain the prosecution.'"[20]

YMCA directors were initially cool to Comstock's proposal of a new law that would remedy the shortcomings of existing federal law. They expressed concerns about the impracticality of pursuing new legislation late in the congressional session and feared the impact of unwanted publicity on contributions to the organization. However, with the support of YMCA president Morris Jesup, Comstock's effort to secure a new federal statute went forward.[21] The YMCA initially created and secretly funded a Committee for the Suppression of Vice, so that Comstock could pursue his anti-vice crusade without the organization's overt involvement, although later Comstock's activities were quite open.[22] Also through his contacts at the YMCA, Comstock forged an alliance with New York Congressman Clinton L. Merriam who shared Comstock's detestation of sexual vice and who had supported the federal law that was unsuccessfully used in the attempt to prosecute Woodhull and Claflin. Merriam was instrumental in helping Comstock steer the new legislation through Congress.

The history of federal efforts to regulate morality is brief. Federal regulation began in 1842, when Congress outlawed the importation of obscene material. In 1865, apparently concerned about obscene material mailed to Union troops, Congress banned from the mail "obscene book[s], pamphlet[s], picture[s], print[s], or other publication[s] of vulgar and indecent character." That provision was broadened slightly in 1872 with Congressman Merriam's support.[23] There were sound reasons for Congress's tepid approach to the regulation of morals. American courts and, until fairly recently, Americans in general have taken a cautious view toward the federalization of crimes. Crimes fall under the "police power" or the power to regulate matters of health, welfare, safety, and morals, which was left to the states under the federal system. The federal government had to rely largely on express powers allocated to it, principally those enumerated in Article I, §8 of the Constitution. As early as 1836, Congress had deliberated its power under the Postal Clause ("Congress shall have Power To establish Post Offices and post Roads") to exclude material from the mail. The debate then focused on anti-slavery materials viewed as "incendiary" by southern states. A committee chaired by Senator John C. Calhoun of South Carolina decided that while "Congress could not prohibit the transmission of the incendiary documents through the mails," it could cooperate with the states and "prevent their delivery by the postmasters in the States where their circulation was forbidden."[24] By the 1870s, Congress was open to a more robust application of its power to regulate the mail.

What Comstock achieved with the Comstock Law, as it came to be known, was the first comprehensive, federal, anti-obscenity law. The enactment of the 1873 Comstock Act marked an important turning point in morals regulation by "making a federal case" out of what had previously been controlled locally. The 1873 Comstock Law declared that "no obscene, lewd or lascivious book . . . , picture . . . , or other publication of an indecent character, or any article . . . intended for the prevention of contraception [sic] or procuring of abortion . . . shall be carried in the mail." This law effectively banned only materials concerning contraception and abortion; a subsequent amendment, enacted in 1876, was necessary to ban obscene and indecent materials generally. Violators were subject to a fine and imprisonment.[25]

A key to the Comstock laws was the linkage of sex and obscenity. Justice Marshall once put it aptly when he pointed out that the "driving force" behind the 1873 law was Anthony Comstock's belief that "anything remotely touching upon sex was . . . obscene."[26] The new law was so broadly written that it embraced not only literary and pictorial depictions of sex, the "smut" that Comstock abhorred but also information and advertisements about family planning as well as medical and scientific information about human sexuality important to reproductive health and essential to avoiding unwanted pregnancy. Of course it also affected newspapers sent through the mail, both their articles and advertisements, and it also prevented the sale and distribution of contraceptives and abortifacients through the mail. Once states followed suit with local bans on the retail sale of similar papers, pamphlets, and books as well as birth control devices such as condoms, the chokehold on family planning was complete.

In what was to mark an important enhancement of his vice-fighting abilities, Comstock also procured an appointment as a special agent of the Post Office Department with arrest powers and the right to carry a weapon. (In fact, Comstock had carried a pistol for self-protection and the intimidation of others since his early days as an amateur vice fighter.) This empowered him to enforce the newly expanded federal law, if necessary, with a national scope. Eventually, he was successful in persuading several states to enact state versions of the federal law, ultimately acquiring state law enforcement powers in his home state of New York.

Comstockery and Reproductive Rights

This consolidation of governmental power to suppress information about contraception as well as medical means to control family size, all in the name of morality, had profound implications for human reproduction and reproductive health in the United States. There are three necessary conditions for effective family planning: the will to control fertility, appropriate contraceptive technology to avoid conception, and information about how to access and use that technology. The nineteenth century saw the advent of all three of these conditions on a broad scale for the first time in human history.[27] Francis Place in England and Charles Knowlton in the United States popularized the desirability of birth control by emphasizing the desirability of smaller families; they also published information on how to limit births, although that information was suppressed in the United States. At the same time, technology brought about through advances in the vulcanization of rubber made condoms widely available.

Anthony Comstock's crusade was designed to deny access to information about fertility control. With the passage of the Comstock Law, women and their partners lost the ability to control family size and to avoid unwanted pregnancy through the use of birth control and, as a last resort, therapeutic abortion, as contraception and abortion were driven underground. As a result, private and public health suffered. Information about human reproduction dried up, condemned as obscene. Even medical texts detailing human reproduction could not be mailed. What little information was available for lay consumption was suppressed by Comstock's relentless pursuit of the "lewd and obscene." The same was true of contraceptives. Comstock's ruthless campaign focused in major metropolitan areas, principally New York, had a nationwide impact. "Comstockery," as it became known, became a nationally recognized phenomenon.

As part of the national Comstock movement, many states enacted their own laws to regulate sex and matters relating to sex, including contraception and birth control. Early in the twentieth century, a New York court upheld a state Comstock statute, enacted in 1887, that made it illegal to sell or give away information or devices for the prevention of conception.[28] The subject of the law, information about contraception and technology intended to facilitate it, was properly within the state's police powers, the court asserted, and the state legislature could decide that disseminating information about contraceptives and selling or distributing them was contrary to public morals and welfare. A major justification for the law was the danger that without the threat of pregnancy, which represented a potent deterrent to the unrestrained expression of sexual passion, adultery and fornication would increase.

The direct regulation of contraceptives, particularly those distributed through nonmedical sources, was an important weapon in a state's arsenal against the availability of information and technology. For example, the Massachusetts case of *Commonwealth v. Goldberg* involved a prosecution for violation of a law enacted in 1879 that criminalized the advertising of "any drug, medicine, instrument or article whatever for the prevention of conception." The defendant sold condoms at his novelty shop, where they were advertised on cards and pamphlets available over the counter. In upholding the conviction, the court noted that all of the advertising "bore stories or anecdotes of a vulgar nature, three of which referred to sexual intercourse and of the three one referred to the birth of a child as the result of such intercourse. . . . [The condoms were advertised] to insure safety in sexual intercourse, not only from disease but also from the normal result of such intercourse—conception."[29]

The effect of nineteenth-century laws like these was to foreclose retail access to information and effectively keep sex in the dark. Laws with criminal penalties attached to them limited the advertising and display of condoms even in drug stores and provided that only licensed pharmacists could dispense them. Similar laws precluded the ready availability of condoms by forbidding their sale through vending machines in locations like service stations and taverns. This allowed religiously motivated fundamentalist moralists who objected to the practice of contraception to force their values onto others through law.[30]

The examples from New York and Massachusetts are cases of "little Comstock laws" adopted by states following the model of Comstock's 1873 law. Some states had adopted limitations on obscene material well in advance of Comstock's movement. For example, Vermont adopted a law in 1821 prohibiting "the publication or sale of 'lewd or obscene' material." After the passage of the federal Comstock Law, such obscenity legislation became almost commonplace. By the end of the nineteenth century, some thirty states had followed suit.

Undoing Comstockery

Deconstruction of the legal framework supporting Comstock's moral and religious enterprise with its far-reaching negative health consequences was ultimately accomplished by a difficult, slow-moving, piecemeal process that unfolded over many decades. That process largely took place through cases decided by the US Supreme Court. Two independent legal developments eventually ended the Comstock era. One was the emergence of a robust doctrine of privacy that effectively nullified Comstock laws and led to greater availability of the information and technology to facilitate effective control of human reproduction. Access to contraception and even abortion would eventually receive constitutional protection. A second development was the creation of a First Amendment doctrine that protected information about sex and human reproduction, tightening the definition of obscenity so that literature that included information about sex and contraception could no longer be banned. First Amendment protection was extended to advertising as well, so that consumers could learn about the utility and availability of contraceptives and abortion services.

Early attacks on the Comstock laws were largely unsuccessful. The facts of the *Byrne* case in New York, decided in 1917, demonstrate how little had changed legally since the nineteenth century. Ethel Byrne was convicted under New York's Comstock law, passed in 1887, of selling a contraceptive and information about human reproduction. The language of Judge Cropsey captures the uphill battle faced by birth control proponents during the Comstock era:

> The information would make people generally believe that by using the means suggested the act of intercourse could be had without the fear of resulting pregnancy. While there are other reasons that keep unmarried people from indulging their passions, the fear that pregnancy will result is one of the potent ones. To remove that fear would unquestionably result in an increase of immorality.[31]

Margaret Sanger, the mother of modern-day family planning, often ran afoul of Comstock laws as she struggled to disseminate information about birth control technology through magazine articles and books.[32] Although she was successful in attracting media attention to the birth control cause, the results of her legal battle were mixed. In the *Sanger* case,[33] she conceded the constitutionality of the Comstock laws as applied to unmarried persons but argued that the law was unreasonable as applied to married couples insofar as a medical necessity for contraceptives and contraceptive information was concerned. The court accepted this argument, thereby creating a medical exception to the Comstock laws that gradually opened the way for population control measures to be distributed through birth control clinics. The idea of a medical exception comes from the *Byrne* decision, in which the judge conceded that under the New York law "a physician would be justified in prescribing the prohibited articles or drugs, if in his opinion the health or condition of the patient required it."[34] This idea, that a woman's health interest would limit the government's ability to interfere with medical decisions affecting her, would later resonate in many of the important abortion decisions, including *Roe v. Wade*,[35] *Planned Parenthood of Southeastern Pennsylvania v. Casey*,[36] and the controversial "partial-birth abortion" case *Stenberg v. Carhart*.[37]

Federal Courts to the Rescue

Gradual social, political, and religious changes dissolved the consensus supporting Comstockery as a legal regime. The concomitant process of deconstruction by the courts was in many respects more complicated and disjointed than the process that brought about Comstockery in the first place. It effectively began with the decision in the *Griswold* case in 1965.[38]

Connecticut's state Comstock law criminalized the *use* of contraceptives as well as the provision of assistance or advice about contraception. In that respect, Connecticut's law was both harsher and more intrusive than other state and federal laws,[39] but its approach had been acknowledged to be constitutional in the *Byrne* case.

Connecticut's ban on the use of contraceptives and on sharing information about them was struck down in the *Griswold* case as a violation of the right of privacy derived from the constitutional protections identified in the Bill of Rights. Although the justices could not precisely describe the sources of this right of privacy, a majority of them nevertheless agreed that it existed with sufficient robustness to invalidate Connecticut's law. This chink in the armor of Comstockery would lead to its eventual destruction.

Because the case dealt with a challenge to the law by married couples and physicians who counseled them, *Griswold* appeared at first to be limited to state laws that interfered with marital privacy, but it quickly became apparent that the right of privacy was far more sweeping in its reach. In 1972, in *Eisenstadt v. Baird*, the Supreme Court struck down the Massachusetts Comstock law based on a much-expanded view of Griswold's privacy right: "If the right of privacy means anything, it is the right of the *individual*, married or single, to be free from unwarranted governmental intrusion into matters so fundamentally affecting a person as the decision whether to bear or beget a child."[40] Gone from this viewpoint was the idea that states could use their police power to enforce moral reservations about birth control practices or even sexual relations by unmarried persons.[41]

Five years later, the Supreme Court took another major step in ending the Comstock era when it struck down a New York prohibition on the sale or distribution of contraceptives to minors under 16 years of age. In *Carey v. Population Services International*, the high court was divided on the theory underlying the result; only four justices were willing to see the result as based on the privacy doctrine that had emerged from *Griswold* and *Eisenstadt*, but seven of nine justices saw the law as unconstitutional.[42]

The Comstock Laws (Finally) Take a Direct Hit

In 1983, the US Supreme Court directly ruled on a modern version of the Comstock laws in *Bolger v. Young's Drug Products Corporation*.[43] *Bolger* concerned a challenge by a manufacturer and distributor of contraceptives to a federal statute prohibiting unsolicited mailing of contraceptive advertisements. The statute was struck down as an unconstitutional restriction on commercial speech. This ruling was probably the final direct blow to the Comstock laws delivered by the Supreme Court.[44] A foundational case for the decision in *Bolger, Bigelow v. Virginia* (1975) held that the advertising of abortion services was protected as commercial speech within the First Amendment. Prior to *Bigelow*, commercial speech had not been held to be protected by the First Amendment. *Bigelow*'s rationale was that since abortion was legal under *Roe v. Wade* (1973), advertising it could not be prohibited.[45]

Restraint on information had historically been one of the props upon which Comstockery depended. As direct advertising bans began to fall, the linkage between contraceptive and birth control information also began to crumble, and the Supreme Court began to tackle obscenity as a classification.

Obscenity Revisited

Initially, information about sex and contraception was treated as obscenity whose dissemination could be criminalized. Contemporaneously with the emergence of a privacy doctrine in cases like *Griswold, Eisenstadt,* and even *Carey* and despite the lack of consensus on the privacy point, the Supreme Court undertook a reexamination of the protection accorded sexually explicit speech and writing under the First Amendment. Historically, the definition of obscenity had a broad reach that included virtually anything having to do with human sexuality. Obscenity and the First Amendment were complete strangers to one another. A weak and largely undeveloped First Amendment provided no protection because of court-imposed limits on it.

Gradually, however, the value of obscenity law as a blunt instrument for suppressing information about birth control and abortion was limited through a series of cases that began with *Roth v. United States* in 1957.[46] *Roth* found that sex and obscenity were "not synonymous." Obscenity required a prurient portrayal of sex, one that appealed to a person's baser instincts or a morbid, lascivious, or lewd interest in sex. Presentations of sex or sexual information that did not cross into this forbidden area would not be considered obscene. Even the private possession of obscenity was held protected in *Stanley v. Georgia* (1969), a case involving the "mere possession" of ordinary obscene materials. Throughout all of these legal developments, obscenity remained a viable legal concept even for constitutional purposes; that was the outcome of the seminal case of *Miller v. California* (1973), a case that coalesced the touchstones of obscenity into three elements. Those elements are "whether 'the average person, applying contemporary community standards' would find that the work taken as a whole, appeals to the prurient interest [borrowing from *Roth*]; whether the work depicts or describes, in a patently offensive way, sexual conduct specifically defined by the applicable state law, and whether the work, taken as a whole, lacks serious literary, artistic, political, or scientific value." By these standards, of course, information about sex and the means to limit human reproduction enjoy First Amendment protection.[47]

Visual depictions that had earlier been a vexation for those seeking to inform about sex and the human body also came to enjoy protection in this period. As the court summarily stated in the 1981 case *Schad v. Mount Ephraim*, "'Nudity alone' does not place otherwise protected material outside the mantle of the First Amendment."[48] Comstockery's use of obscenity laws to restrict information about sex and human reproduction was effectively nullified.[49]

Abortion

Information about sex and contraception could no longer be restricted. Three other cases dealt with another demon of Comstockery: abortion. The nation as a whole remains conflicted on the subject of abortion. Of course, no polling data exist for the nineteenth century when the Comstock laws were enacted to tell us what the popular opinion was about abortion. Studies of abortion note that the demand for abortion services, as reflected by the practice of abortion, is—like the demand for sex—inelastic. Abortion occurs at roughly the same rate regardless of whether it is legal. The idea that abortion should be safe, legal, and rare is supported by contemporary polling data and probably reflects what even nineteenth-century folk would have thought about it, taking behavior as a reflection of attitudes.[50]

There is no controversy about the terrible toll on women's lives exacted by illegal and unsafe abortion. In the United States, it was estimated that one in five pregnancies were terminated by illegal abortion in 1960, resulting in as many as five thousand women's deaths per year.[51] By the late 1960s, legal abortion was safer for women than carrying the pregnancy to term and risking death from childbirth. The relative safety of abortion for women underlay the Supreme Court's decision in *Roe v. Wade*.[52] Moreover, legalizing abortion did not increase the number of abortions—rather, it substituted safe for unsafe abortions. The number of women's deaths attributed to abortion plummeted; only twelve such deaths were reported in 2008.[53] This represents a mortality rate of less than one per 100,000 legal abortions (compared to a maternal mortality in excess of fifteen per 100,000 live births).[54]

The right to privacy received perhaps its greatest extension in 1973 in the landmark case of *Roe v. Wade*, in which the Supreme Court recognized a "right of personal privacy" so potent as to restrict the ability of government to deny a woman the right to have an abortion when a pregnancy threatened her health and well-being or her life. This formula—essentially that laws enacted under the police power cannot block health-saving or life-saving medical services, a theme evident as early as 1917, in the New York *Byrne* case—is a persistent one. The *Casey* decision, nineteen years later, retained the "essential holding" of *Roe* that the right to an abortion was constitutionally protected from the imposition of "undue burdens" that restricted abortion.[55] After *Casey*, however, states were free to make decisions that had the effect of limiting the availability of the procedure, such as prohibiting licensed physicians' assistants from performing abortions, and those steps were not considered to impose an undue burden.[56]

Taken together, these cases have removed another support from the underpinnings of Comstockery. Abortion is the only alternative for women who have become pregnant and who do not desire to undergo the very real risks of pregnancy or wish to accept the burden of unwanted offspring. In the nineteenth century, adherents of a pronatalist philosophy and followers of a harsh, moralistic philosophy like that reflected in Comstock's fundamentalist religious view saw pregnancy and venereal disease as punishment for sin. Sin codified as crime could justify bans on abortion and information about abortion; that would be natural and logical. The emergence of a robust constitutional doctrine of personal privacy grounded in the liberty of women as well as men to control their reproductive destinies has changed the legal and constitutional terrain so that flat bans on abortion and accurate information about it are no longer legally tolerable.

New Word from Congress

Around the same time that the courts were dismantling Comstockery, public support for family planning translated into legislation, culminating in the passage of Title X of the Public Health Service Act in 1970. Enactment of Title X can be seen as a congressional repudiation of the approach to contraception and human reproduction implicit in the Comstock laws. The overall goal of Title X was "to assist in making comprehensive voluntary family planning services available to all persons desiring such services."[57] Specific funding was provided for family-planning services to low-income women and also to support population research. As we write, the Affordable Care Act of 2010 has begun to require insurance coverage without copayment for FDA-approved prescription contraceptives for women.

Comstock's ghost still haunts women, however. Attacks on the Affordable Care Act's contraceptive coverage provisions, irrespective of their underlying legal or constitutional theory, have as their goal the use of governmental power to deny women the ability to avoid unwanted pregnancy with its attendant dangers. By so doing, backers of these legal attacks seek to impose their fundamentalist moral or religious beliefs on women who bear the consequences of restricted access to the most effective contraceptives and safe, legal abortion when all else fails.

The Public Health Impact of Comstockery

For nearly a century, public health investigators have known that maternal and infant mortality is higher when childbearing begins at too early an age or continues when the mother is older or physically impaired. For even the healthiest women, pregnancies occurring in rapid succession are more likely to end poorly for the mother and baby than are pregnancies spaced two to three years apart. Family planning, then, has a tremendous positive impact on individual and public health. It is also an economic good that is positively correlated with per capita GDP while reducing demand on food, space, and other resources. It contributes to the empowerment of women through increased educational attainment and employment. It also saves lives—an estimated 1.2 million infant deaths a year avoided.[58]

Given this knowledge, it may never be possible to estimate the number of women's and children's lives lost or ruined as a result of the Comstock laws. However, two "natural experiments" have allowed estimates of the impacts of Comstockery. The first involved the work of Charles Knowlton (1800–1850), the American physician who first suggested a health basis for birth control use. His book *Fruits of Philosophy or the Private Companion of Young Married People* (1832) was the first comprehensive text on birth control for laypersons published in the United States. Knowlton was involved in three trials and subjected to a fine and three months in jail, but—unlike Margaret Sanger—his problems attracted little publicity, and his book, which was suppressed, had virtually no impact in the United States. However, forty years later, two other free-thought advocates, Charles Bradlaugh and Annie Besant, republished the book in the United Kingdom. Their subsequent trial gained much notoriety. Newspapers reported the arguments in favor of family limitation and open discussion of contraception. The defendants prevailed in 1879, the same year that Annie Besant published her book *The Law of Population*.[59] In the ensuing years, British birth rates dropped almost 50 percent, from a high of 36.3 per 1,000 people in 1876 to 16.7 per 1,000 in 1927, most likely due to increased contraceptive use, according to Norman Himes, who published a study of the demographic shift in the *New England Journal of Medicine* in 1928.[60] Estimated declines in US fertility over the same period were much less steep.

Later in the twentieth century, just as state Comstock laws were beginning to be overthrown, economist Martha J. Bailey utilized another "natural experiment" to estimate the impact of Comstockery on the use of oral contraceptives. She analyzed nationally representative surveys of reproduction and contraception among married women conducted in 1955, 1965, and 1970, just before and shortly after the introduction of the birth control pill in 1957 (first as a medication for menstrual problems and then in 1960 as a means of contraception).[61] Bailey found that women in states with Comstock laws were substantially less likely to have used the pill by 1965, when *Griswold* was decided. However, once the information bans were lifted, pill use expanded to all states, and by 1970 there was no significant difference in use across the United States. She estimates that hundreds of thousands of births—124,000 in 1965 alone—would have been prevented had there been no Comstock laws in place in 1957.

The impact of the Comstock laws on population control was direct and significant, but other public health issues were also affected. For example, an Oregon law enacted in 1909 that criminalized "the advertising of treatment or cure of venereal or other diseases" was upheld on the Comstockian theory that the personal and public health benefits of preventing communication of sexually transmitted diseases should be subordinated to the need to deter or punish those who chose to engage in illegal and immoral behavior.[62] Pregnancy and infection, the thinking ran, would be their just punishments.

Conclusion

Increasingly, health and health care—that is, the means of securing health—are recognized as basic human rights. Numerous international conventions, among them the Universal Declaration of Human Rights; the International Covenant on Economic, Social and Cultural Rights; and the UN Convention on the Rights of the Child, accept as a given that there is a right to health and the means to secure it. An "overwhelming number of Americans [consistently support] the idea that health care should be a right."[63] In the 1941 State of the Union Address in which he delineated the four freedoms (freedom of speech and expression; freedom of worship; freedom from want; and freedom from fear), President Franklin D. Roosevelt identified freedom from want as encompassing "economic understandings which will secure to every nation a healthy peacetime life for its inhabitants everywhere in the world." He later linked the realization of a healthy life "to adequate medical care and the opportunity to achieve and enjoy good health."[64]

Because it profoundly affects the health of women and children as well as that of families and communities, the ability to control fertility is inextricably linked with the right to health. Anthony Comstock's crusade was designed to deny access to information about fertility control, using state and federal law to enforce a fundamentalist, religiously based moral view toward contraception, abortion, and obscenity, among other things. The effort to extirpate Comstockery's legacy from the United States is not entirely over. As this book goes to press, an important decision by Federal District Judge Korman will go into effect.[65] Judge Korman's order requires that the Food and Drug Administration (FDA) certify Plan B One-Step as a nonprescription morning-after contraceptive pill available to all women and girls without age restriction. During the administration of George W. Bush, neo-Comstockians in the FDA had sought to limit access to Plan B, a safe and effective contraceptive pill that prevents conception if taken within seventy-two hours after sexual intercourse, by requiring young teens to obtain a prescription for it. Judge Korman concluded that the FDA had acted in bad faith.[66] The Obama administration's Justice Department initially followed the Bush administration's Comstockian playbook, citing the dangers of sex to the young. However, the administration recently announced that it would acquiesce to Judge Korman's order. It is difficult to imagine that Comstockian evils are at an end, even in the United States, but recent developments portend a steady if bitterly contested progress in gaining basic human rights to privacy and autonomy.

There are important lessons to be learned from this ongoing struggle about the need to confront fundamentalism and the dangers inherent in the alliance between religious fundamentalism and governmental power. Comstockery is one example of the potential for religion to be a potent, negative social determinant of health. The story of Anthony Comstock and his followers yields some major lessons related to the suppression of information about contraception and family planning. First, viewing sex exclusively through the lens of fundamentalist religious presuppositions divorces human reproduction from science. Second, ignoring science increases human suffering as people are forced to endure the consequences of unwanted pregnancy. Third, private fundamentalist religious views are most toxic when harnessed with the coercive power of law and state enforcement. Although Comstock laws are no longer valid, they have had a long-lasting negative effect on public health. Comstockians in the United States whose efforts restricted the availability of the information and technology to place control of human reproduction in the hands of individuals gave us not only abortions and unwanted offspring, but families who struggle at the economic and social margins. In today's global village, 220 million women seek contraceptive services that they cannot obtain due in large measure to the ongoing, corrosive influence of religious fundamentalism forced on unwilling nonadherents through state coercion.

Notes

1. Nancy T. Ammerman, "North American Protestant Fundamentalism," in *Fundamentalisms Observed*, eds. Martin E. Marty and R. Scott Appleby (Chicago: University of Chicago Press, 1991), 4–8.
2. Mark A. Noll, *The Scandal of the Evangelical Mind* (Grand Rapids, MI: Eerdmans, 1994), 187–188.
3. Martin E. Marty and R. Scott Appleby, "Conclusion: An Interim Report on a Hypothetical Family," in Marty and Appleby, *Fundamentalisms Observed*, 816.
4. Martin E. Marty and R. Scott Appleby, "Introduction: The Fundamentalism Project: A User's Guide," in Marty and Appleby, *Fundamentalisms Observed*, ix–x.
5. We are indebted to the anthropologist Judith Nagata for the phrasing of the definition posited here, although the definition itself is not hers.
6. Anna Louise Bates, *Weeder in the Garden: Anthony Comstock's Life and Career* (Lanham, MD: University Press of America, 1995), 29–30. Many of the details of Comstock's biography discussed in this chapter are drawn from Bates's excellent study.
7. Bates, *Weeder in the Garden*, 32.
8. Bates, *Weeder in the Garden*, 36.
9. Bates, *Weeder in the Garden*, 40–42.
10. Bates, *Weeder in the Garden*, 51.
11. Bates, *Weeder in the Garden*, 56.
12. Bates, *Weeder in the Garden*, 15.
13. Bates, *Weeder in the Garden*, 36–37, quoted from *Harper's Weekly*, May 22, 1915.
14. One of the most flagrantly Freudian accounts of Comstock's life and activities is Heywood Broun and Margaret Leech, *Anthony Comstock: Roundsman of the Lord* (New York: Albert & Charles Boni, 1927); these quotations are representative of the Leeches' approach: "Psychically Comstock was certainly sick through the greater part of his year's enlistment" (51). "Here, again, the consulting Freudian might con-

tend that the weakness which tantalized and sometimes conquered Tony were the same 'lines of temptation' of which he spoke to Trumbull [Comstock's biographer] when he told him of the fierce trials to which the Devil made him submit while he was still a boy on the farm" (56).

15. See Bates, *Weeder in the Garden.*
16. Bates, *Weeder in the Garden*, 51–52.
17. Bates, *Weeder in the Garden*, 52.
18. Nicola Kay Beisel, *Imperiled Innocents: Anthony Comstock and Family Reproduction in Victorian America* (Princeton, NJ: Princeton University Press, 1997), 97.
19. Bates, *Weeder in the Garden*, 71.
20. Beisel, *Imperiled Innocents*, 8 and n. 12.
21. Bates, *Weeder in the Garden*, 80.
22. Broun and Leech, *Roundsman*, 84–85.
23. On the early history of obscenity regulation, see Justice Brennan's dissent in *Paris Adult Theatre I v. Slaton*, 413 U.S. 49, 104–105 (1973).
24. *Ex parte Jackson*, 96 U.S. 727, 734–735 (1877).
25. On the background of the Comstock Act generally see Margaret A. Blanchard, "The American Urge to Censor: Freedom of Expression Versus the Desire to Sanitize Society—From Anthony Comstock to 2 Live Crew," *William & Mary Law Review* 33, no. 741 (1992).
26. For Justice Marshall's description of Comstock, see *Bolger v. Young's Drug Products Corp.*, 463 U.S. 60, 70 n.19 (1983).
27. For a brief history of birth control advocacy in the nineteenth century, see Abdel R. Omran, *The Health Theme in Family Planning* (Chapel Hill, NC: Carolina Population Center, 1971).
28. On New York's regulation of information about contraception and contraceptives, see *People v. Byrne*, 99 Misc. 1, 163 NYS 682 (1917).
29. *Commonwealth v. Goldberg*, 316 Mass. 563, 55 N.E. 2d 951 (1944).
30. On the limitation of condom dispensing to licensed pharmacists see *People v. Pennock*, 294 Mich. 578, 293 N.W. 759 (1940) and *Sanitary Vendors, Inc. v. Byrne*, 40 N.J. 157, 190 A.2d 876 (1963), which barred the sale of packaged condoms in vending machines. Some states also used their authority to control liquor sales to suppress the use of condom vending machines; see *Howell v. Bryant*, 99 Ohio App. 49, 130 N.E. 2d 837, appeal dismissed, 162 Ohio 445, 123 N.E. 2d 407 (1954); *State v. Arnold*, 217 Wis. 340, 258 N.W. 843 (1935). On the judicial response to the Comstock laws, see C. Thomas Dienes, *Law, Politics, and Birth Control* (Champaign: University of Illinois Press, 1972), 49–74; see also *People v. Byrne.*
31. On the judicial response to the Comstock laws see Dienes, *Law Politics and Birth Control*, 49–74; see also *People v. Byrne*, 99 Misc. 1, 35 N.Y.Crim.R. 406, 163 N.Y.S. 682 (1917).
32. For Margaret Sanger's story, see Dienes, *Law, Politics and Birth Control*, 78–88.
33. *People v. Sanger*, 222 N.Y. 192, 118 N.E. 637 (1918).
34. *People v. Byrne.*
35. 410 U.S. 113 (1973).
36. 505 U.S. 833 (1992).
37. 530 U.S. 914 (2000).

38. *Griswold v. Connecticut*, 381 U.S. 479 (1965).

39. For a discussion of the background of the *Griswold* case from a skeptical perspective, see Robert H. Bork, *The Tempting of America: The Political Seduction of the Law* (New York: Free Press, 1990), 95–100.

40. *Eisenstadt v. Baird*, 405 U.S. 438 (1972).

41. For the evolution of the privacy doctrine, see *Eisenstadt v. Baird*, and *Carey v. Population Services International*, 431 U.S. 678 (1977). Recent cases, particularly *Lawrence v. Texas*, 539 U.S. 558 (2003), which struck down a Texas sodomy law, call into question the constitutional validity of other morality-based restrictions on sex, such as laws on fornication or sex between unmarried persons. This is explored, albeit briefly, in L. Lynn Hogue, "Romer Revisited or 'The Devil in the Details': Is Georgia's Marriage Amendment Constitutionally Defective," *Florida Coastal Law Review* 7 (2005): 255, 260, and note 48 (questioning whether there is such a thing as a "right to sexual intercourse"). However, state authority over marriage preserved to the states under federalism may preserve the power to regulate adultery, bigamy, and polygamy; see L. Lynn Hogue, "Examining a Strand of the Public Policy Exception with Constitutional Underpinnings: How the 'Foreign Marriage Recognition Exception' Affects the Interjurisdictional Recognition of Same-Sex 'Marriage,'" *Creighton Law Review* 38, no. 449 (2005): 451–464.

42. Carey v. Population Services International.

43. 463 U.S. 60 (1983).

44. *Bolger v. Young's Drug Products Corp.*, 463 U.S. 60 (1983). For the origin of the law invalidated in *Bolger*, see 463 U.S. 60 at 70.

45. *Bigelow v. Virginia*, 421 U.S. 809 (1975).

46. 354 U.S. 476 (1957).

47. For the evolution of the obscenity doctrine see *Roth v. United States*, 354 U.S. 476 (1957); *Kingsley Int'l Pictures Corp. v. Regents*, 360 U.S. 684 (1959) ("Lady Chatterley's Lover"); and *Stanley v. Georgia*, 394 U.S. 557 (1969). Stanley's principle has been limited in the special instance of child pornography in *New York v. Ferber*, 458 U.S. 747 (1982), which points to a number of special harms peculiarly related to child pornography. The child pornography covered by the New York law in Ferber was not required to be obscene, although the films at issue, which showed young boys masturbating, probably were obscene under the Miller standards; *Miller v. California*, 413 U.S. 15 (1973).

48. *Schad v. Mount Ephraim*, 452 U.S. 61 (1981).

49. On the protection of nudity, see *Jenkins v. Georgia*, 418 U.S. 153 (1974) ("Carnal Knowledge"); *Erznoznik v. Jacksonville*, 422 U.S. 205 (1975) (nude scenes on drive-in movie screens); *Southeastern Promotions, Ltd. v. Conrad*, 420 U.S. 546 (1975) (nude rock musical *Hair*); *Schad v. Mount Ephraim*, 452 U.S. 61 (1981).

50. On the disparity between abortion rhetoric and practice, see the extensive and well-documented discussion of "the looking–glass world of abortion advocacy" in Mark A. Graber, *Rethinking Abortion: Equal Choice, The Constitution and Reproductive Politics* (Princeton, NJ: Princeton University Press 1996).

51. J. M. Kummer and Z. Leavy, "Criminal Abortion: A Consideration of Ways to Reduce Incidence," *California Medicine* 95(1961): 170–175.

52. *Roe v. Wade*, 410 U.S. 179 (1973).

53. K. Pazol, A. A. Creanga, S. B. Zane, K. D. Burley, and D. J. Jamieson, "Abortion Surveillance—United States, 2009," *MMWR Surveillance Summarie*, 61, no. 8 (November 23, 2012): 1–44.

54. A. P. MacKay, C. J. Berg, X. Liu, C. Duran, and D. L. Hoyart, "Changes in Pregnancy Mortality Ascertainment, United States, 1999–2005," *Obstetrics and Gynecology* 118(2011): 104–110.

55. *Planned Parenthood of Southeastern Pennsylvania v. Casey*, 505 U.S. 833 (1992).

56. Space does not allow a full account of recent Supreme Court decisions on abortion or the legal prospects for recent, primarily state, efforts to impose restrictions on abortion through such mechanisms as setting a limit on the time within which abortion must be sought or basing the law on factors unrelated to a woman's health such as supposed fetal pain in an abortion procedure.

57. On Title X, see Deborah R. McFarlane and Kenneth J. Meier, *The Politics of Fertility Control: Family Planning and Abortion Policies in the American States* (New York: Seven Bridges Press, 2001), 42–55.

58. W. Cates Jr., "Family Planning: The Essential Link to Achieving All Eight Millennium Development Goals," *Contraception* 81(2010): 460–461.

59. Annie Wood Besant, *The Law of Population: Its Consequences and Its Bearing upon Human Conduct and Morals* (New York: Asa K. Butts, 1878).

60. Norman Himes, "Charles Knowlton's Revolutionary Influence on the English Birth–Rate," *New England Journal of Medicine* 199(1928): 461–465. For more details on this history, see Omran, *The Health Theme in Family Planning*, note 27.

61. M. J. Bailey, *"Momma's Got the Pill": How Anthony Comstock and* Griswold v. Connecticut *Shaped U.S. Childbearing*, National Bureau of Economic Research, Working Paper 14675, January 2009, http://www.nber.org/papers/w14675.

62. *State v. Hollinshead*, 77 Or. 473, 151 P. 710 (1915).

63. Quoted in Jonathan Todres, "The Right to Health Under the U.N. Convention on the Rights of the Child" in *The U.N. Convention on the Rights of the Child: An Analysis of Treaty Provisions and Implications of U.S. Ratification*, eds. Jonathan Todres, Mark Wojcik and Cris Revaz (New York: United Nations, 2006), 234.

64. Quoted in Steven D. Jamar, "The International Human Right to Health," 22 S.U.L. Rev. 1, 2 (1994).

65. *Tummino v. Hamburg*, F. Supp.2d, 2013 WL 865,851 (E.D.N.Y. 2013).

66. *Tummino v. Torti*, 603 F.Supp.2d 519 (E.D.N.Y. 2009).

Religion and Public Health across the Life Course

Part III of this volume examines the scientific research on religion as a social determinant of physical and mental health. Building on the theoretical framework laid out in chapter 1 and the lifecycle structure of the religious practices described in Part I, we organize the research literature on religion and health from a population and life course perspective. The overall conclusion is that religion has a profound effect on physical and mental health, one that is measurable and usually, although certainly not always, positive. Thousands of studies of religion and its impact on health have been conducted, and many reviews of this literature have been published, but the life course perspective is a new way to think about their relationship; Vernon Reynolds and Ralph Tanner offer the only other similar approach.[1]

Religions have a fundamental interest in perpetuating themselves. All social groups, religious groups among them, want to survive and thrive, and they do that by increasing their numbers and supporting the longevity and well-being of individual members. A social group that grows and increases its strength and resources—among them the mental and physical health of its members—is flourishing. The flourishing of one group, however, may be a source of conflict or struggle with other groups, creating a real potential for harm to others. Moreover, even individuals who are members of the group may not see their own interests as being in line with the teachings of their faith, and, here again, the consequences of the group's imperative to pursue what is best for the group may result in harm to individuals. This is a functional perspective, to be sure, but it is a useful one. In this section, we examine the sometimes intentional, sometimes inadvertent ways in which religions promote their own existence by shaping the conditions of existence for their members.

In chapter 17, Laura Gaydos and Patricia Page begin at the beginning, with religion's role in reproductive health. As religions have a natural interest in increasing their numbers, they take a special interest in sexuality, conception, childbearing, and infant care—and the related practices of contraception, abortion, and fertility treatment. Gaydos and Page document the widely varying teachings with regard to contraception and reproductive health of the major religious traditions in the United States as well as the research on the extent to which dogma matches actual practice among laypersons. In chapter 18, Ellen Idler reviews the epidemiological evidence for religion as a social determinant of health, with a focus on mortality in populations as the primary indicator, linking the varying cycles of religious practice illustrated in Part I to the scientific research on religious practice and religious institutions as determinants of health from childhood through old age. Finally, in chapter 19, Brendan Ozawa-de Silva considers the relationship of religious and spiritual practice to mental health. His view, which is holistic and integrative, emphasizes the potential of religion to both help and harm.

One theme that emerges from these three chapters is the importance of religious teachings and the rules for living that they espouse. The chapters in Part III all note various injunctions of religious traditions, many of which have known health consequences. Religious teachings prohibiting abortion or contraception (noted in chapter 17); banning smoking, alcohol use, or the eating of meat (chapter 18); or upholding an ethic of care and protection (chapter 19) mark out boundaries of behavior for members of a faith tradition. They define what it means to be an observant member. Individuals who do not conform may be sanctioned or, more seriously, shunned or excommunicated. In the theoretical framework of chapter 1, these rules and sanctions are examples of the social control that religious institutions exert over their members—the "sticks" that regulate behavior and enforce the norms that guide it. For religious group members, such rules are part of the texture of everyday life and, for many, a key aspect of identity.

In each of the three chapters in Part III, we see the potential that religion carries for harming health as well as promoting it. These threats underscore the impact of religious practices on whole communities, not just on the individuals who are members. Religious beliefs against immunization can lead to the transmission of potentially deadly childhood illnesses to those outside the nonvaccinating religious group who are simply too young to have been vaccinated. Religious influence on policies banning abortion and contraception is not just an issue of the past (as we saw in a previous chapter); it contributes to the spread of HIV/AIDS and to the proliferation of sexually transmitted diseases. The moral injunctions to protect from harm and provide care for those in need is common to all religions, as

Brendan Ozawa-de Silva points out in chapter 19, but there are too many times and places where acts of harm are carried out in the name of religion—against those of another religion, ethnicity, or race or against insiders who violate the religion's teachings. Religion is a social determinant of health in these instances, just as much as when it provides the health-promoting forces of social support, social control, and social capital.

The scientific research on religion and health provides a way to calibrate the balance of these positive and negative influences. In the literature reviewed in chapter 18, we see evidence of a robust statistical association of religious involvement—usually measured as participation in religious services or as membership in specific religious groups—with lower rates of death. We review only the most methodologically rigorous studies, those that compare entire populations or follow representative samples over time and carefully adjust for health differences and social advantages or disadvantages so that the role of religious involvement is well defined. These studies show, on balance, that religious participation protects adults from mortality, often by several years.

Moreover, the studies demonstrate a number of plausible explanatory mechanisms for the association. People who attend religious services more often are less likely to smoke cigarettes, drink heavily, have multiple sexual partners, use illegal drugs, get divorced, or feel lonely. At the same time, they are more likely to wear seat belts, get health screenings, get married, have children, and belong to other community and voluntary associations. These social, psychological, and behavioral advantages are linked to better health; they are also characteristically clustered among those connected to religious groups. Thus, religion influences health in both direct and indirect ways, and the studies that we review demonstrate the multiple streambeds through which this influence flows.

The life course perspective, with its recognition of the milestones in an individual's life and the close relationship of health with aging, brings an important dimension of change and transition to our consideration of religion as a social determinant of health. It requires that we consider the selection of individuals into and out of religious contexts as they move through their life course. In some countries, individuals freely choose religious beliefs and affiliations, participating voluntarily in the practices and obligations of their faith. They can select themselves out of one religious context and into another one or into a completely secular set of social circles. In other societies—and for the majority of people on earth—there is considerably less choice and strong social pressure to conform. Only a life course perspective allows us to think about research on religion and health in adulthood and old age as the product of social forces and individual choices that have taken place in prior decades of life. Also, only a life course perspective allows us to see the accumulation of social and health advantage and disadvantage.

Our Part III authors share their perspectives on religion and health through the life course from the disciplines of public health, medicine, sociology, philosophy, and religious studies. Their own religious backgrounds are equally diverse. What we hope to bring to this discussion of religion and mental and physical health is a glimpse of the complex reality of religious experience, the substantive content of embodied religious experience that has been lacking in much of the epidemiological and social scientific research on religion and health. By linking health to the religious practices of the life course, we hope to give public health researchers a better understanding of what religions are and do. Above all, we want to underscore the fact that however much religious groups may have a natural interest in the physical and mental health of their members, it is spiritual well-being and a life lived according to the tenets and practices of their faith that is most important. Our perspective on public health research should not obscure this important fact.

Note

1. Vernon Reynolds and Ralph Tanner, *The Social Ecology of Religion* (Oxford: Oxford University Press, 1995). This work of anthropology, originally published in 1983, predates most of the contemporary scientific research on religion and health, but it did not get the attention that it deserved from researchers. The authors argue that "religions have down-to-earth functions in the control and management of the main events of the human life cycle—birth, marriage, death, and the events in between" (back cover). We thank our editor, Cynthia Read, for bringing this important work to our attention and Vernon Reynolds for his encouragement of our project.

17 | Religion and Reproductive Health

LAURA M. GAYDOS AND PATRICIA Z. PAGE

The Old Testament commands "be fruitful and multiply."

The aims of Hindu marriage are said to be dharma (cosmic order), praja (progeny) and rati (pleasure), with a notable focus on childbearing.

In Islam, the prophet (pubh) is reported to have said: "Marry the one who is loving and fertile, for I will be proud of your great numbers before the nations [on the Day of Resurrection]."[1]

ALL RELIGIOUS TRADITIONS HAVE A natural interest in reproductive processes and the health of mothers and children, though this interest is addressed more avidly by some traditions and belief systems than others. In this chapter, we focus on the role of religion in reproductive health decision-making and behaviors for women, their partners, and their families in the United States. We recognize that many of these issues have implications globally; the scope of this topic is so broad that we will begin our discussion here, recognizing that the issues become increasingly broad and complex across the world. Our discussion, beginning in the United States, offers a stepping-stone to this broader discourse.

Organized religions may have a two-pronged impact on reproductive health. For individuals, literature suggests that religious affiliation may influence timing of marriage, beliefs about sex outside of marriage, ideas regarding childbearing, desired family size,[2] contraceptives, and a myriad of other routine health decisions.[3] At the community level, faith institutions (churches, synagogues, mosques, temples) can shape community norms, whether through spoken values declared from the pulpit and in education classes or through unspoken values shared among a religious community. Religious institutions may also influence reproductive health directly by providing services, as in the case of hospital ownership, prescribing explicit rules about use of reproductive healthcare services, engaging in political action aimed at reproductive healthcare services, and framing public policies that fall in line with moral teachings. In all of these ways, faith institutions are instrumental, intentionally or unintentionally, in the establishment of community mores,[4] which significantly influence reproductive health.

As religion plays an influential role in childbearing and childrearing, it exemplifies one of the characteristics of the social determinants perspective: the profound effects of early life influences on health throughout the life course. Yet, as important as religion is, religious groups and practices do not exist in a vacuum. Many social, cultural, and economic factors are closely tied to religion, making it difficult to disentangle the nature of the relationships. For example, in the southeastern United States, African American women face significantly higher rates of unintended pregnancy and poor birth outcomes than either their Caucasian counterparts or African American women in other regions.[5] A large percentage of African American women in this region belong to historically black Protestant evangelical denominations, many of which have strong teachings against family planning, contraception, and abortion. Does that mean that religion drives the racial disparity in pregnancy outcomes in the Southeast? No. But religion is a factor that may be significant in understanding the decision-making processes and social determinants for this population.

In this chapter, we describe some of the ways in which religion is a social determinant of reproductive health. We note the influence of religious teachings and beliefs as well as the structural impact of religious institutions. But understanding this relationship is messy. Religion matters for understanding reproductive health, but many of the pathways and guideposts for this relationship are intertwined with other sociocultural factors and other determinants of health. In an effort to begin to understand these relationships, we discuss the available data on religious institutional policies and the practices of religious Americans.

Contraception and Family Planning

For most of history, women and couples have not had a reliable means to control fertility and plan their families according to their wishes and beliefs. While there have been reports of contraceptive use as far back as ancient Egypt and Mesopotamia, reliable means of family planning were not widely available until the mid-twentieth century. Since then, developed nations have seen a steady decline in birth rates. The ability to control fertility is widely recognized as important for the health of women and their families. Having children more than five years or less than two years apart can have significant detrimental effects on the health of both mother and child, including increased risks of anemia and third trimester bleeding during pregnancy[6] and increased risk of preterm birth and low birth weight as well as fetal/infant and maternal mortality.[7]

Use of contraception and family-planning methods is also closely tied to prevention of sexually transmitted infections, including HIV/AIDS. One of the most accessible and widely used forms of contraception in the United States is the male condom, which is also a critical tool in preventing the transmission of HIV. Religious traditions, beliefs, or mores related to condom use as well as beliefs about sexual initiation, sex outside of marriage, sex education, and a variety of other factors may increase or decrease risk for these sexually transmitted infections in a given population.

Beyond the health consequences, there are also economic ramifications for families unable to space children. The economic costs of pregnancy, childbirth, and raising additional children are significant and may create hardship for families with limited resources. As is widely discussed elsewhere in this volume, poverty and income are strongly related to health outcomes.

Religious Institutional Policies

In light of the recognized health benefits of family planning and contraception and the natural interest of religious groups in promoting healthy procreation, how do religions approach issues of family planning? There is no single answer to this question. Some religions support contraceptive use; others forbid it, and a myriad of policies exist in the middle ground (Table 17.1).

Perhaps the most varied policies on contraception are seen within Christian denominations. While Christian faiths typically forbade contraception prior to the twentieth century, there is now wide variation in the tenets and teachings on the topic. Most familiar to the majority of Americans is the strict stance of the Roman Catholic Church against any means of artificial contraception. In 1968, Pope Paul VI issued his landmark encyclical letter *Humanae Vitae* ("Human Life"), which reemphasized the

TABLE 17.1 Religious institutional policies on contraception use

	DENOMINATION/SECT	STANCE ON CONTRACEPTION
Christianity	American Baptist Church	Supports full range of contraceptive options.
	Assemblies of God	No official stance on the use of contraceptive options; deems contraception a "matter of personal conscience" between husband and wife and God.
	Church of Jesus Christ of Latter-day Saints[a]	No official stance on the use of contraceptive options; deems contraception a private matter between husband and wife.
	Southern Baptist Church	Supports the use of some forms of contraceptive options by married couples as long as they prevent conception from taking place (rather than destroying a fertilized egg or preventing implantation).
	Episcopal Church	Supports full range of contraceptive options.
	Evangelical Lutheran Church in America	Supports full range of contraceptive options.
	Greek Orthodox Archdiocese of America	Defines abstinence as only acceptable method of contraception.
	Presbyterian Church	Supports full range of contraceptive options.
	Roman Catholic	Forbids all artificial means of contraception.
	Seventh-day Adventist	Supports full range of contraceptive options.
	United Church of Christ	Supports full range of contraceptive options.
	United Methodist Church	Supports full range of contraceptive options.
	Unitarian Universalist Association of Congregations	Supports full range of contraceptive options.
Judaism	Reform/Constructionist Judaism	Supports full range of contraceptive options.
	Conservative Judaism	Supports full range of contraceptive options.
	Orthodox/Hasidic Judaism	Permits contraceptive use only to protect the woman's health or the health of existing children who are being nursed. Oral contraceptives are most widely accepted.
Islam		Support for contraceptive options varies, with nonhormonal/barrier methods most widely accepted. Sterilization is generally considered unacceptable and is illegal in some Islamic countries.

continued

TABLE 17.1 *continued*

	DENOMINATION/SECT	STANCE ON CONTRACEPTION
Hinduism		Support for contraceptive options remains varied. No evidence of public opposition to contraception in general.
Buddhism		Supports full range of contraceptive options that do not destroy life.
Chinese Religions	Includes Taoism, Confucianism, and Chinese Folk Religion	Supports full range of contraceptive options. Preference is given to natural methods/ remedies.
Native Religions		Supports full range of contraceptive options. Preference is given to natural methods/ remedies.

[a] There is debate whether the Church of Jesus Christ of Latter-day Saints should be considered a Christian denomination. Because Mormons self-describe as Christians, we include Mormonism under the Christian heading. SOURCES: Daniel C. Maguire, *Sacred Choices: The Right to Contraception and Abortion in Ten World Religions* (Minneapolis: Fortress Press, 2001) and *Sacred Rights: The Case for Contraception and Abortion in World Religions* (New York: Oxford University Press, 2003); P. Feldman, "Sexuality, Birth Control and Childbirth in Orthodox Jewish Tradition," *CMAJ* 146, no. 1 (1992): 29–33; "The DCR Report," The National Campaign to Prevent Teen and Unplanned Pregnancies, http://thenationalcampaign.org/resource/dcr-report—full-report; A. Srikanthan and R. L. Reid, "Religious and Cultural Influences on Contraception," *Journal of Obstetrics and Gynaecologly Canada* 30, no. 2 (2008): 129–137.

Church's teaching that it is always intrinsically wrong to use contraception to prevent new human beings from coming into existence. As defined in the *Humanae Vitae*, contraception is "any action which, either in anticipation of the conjugal act [sexual intercourse], or in its accomplishment, or in the development of its natural consequences, proposes, whether as an end or as a means, to render procreation impossible."[8] This includes sterilization, condoms and other barrier methods, spermicides, *coitus interruptus*, and all hormonal methods.

Few people realize that until 1930, all Protestant denominations agreed with the Catholic Church's teaching on contraception. The Anglican Church led the way in changing this trend, announcing at its 1930 Lambeth Conference that contraception was allowed in some circumstances and soon after allowing contraception across the board. Most other denominations have since followed suit, although there remain exceptions. For example, while most evangelical clergy (as many as 90 percent) support contraception,[9] there is ongoing opposition to contraception use in some evangelical communities[10] and the Amish continue to forbid artificial contraception, although they allow natural family planning.[11]

While there is no official Buddhist doctrine on birth control, Buddhist teachings about contraception are typically based on the idea that it is wrong to kill for any reason and generally favor fertility over birth control. However, in light of the nonspecific teachings, a Buddhist may accept all contraceptive methods, but with different degrees of hesitation. Abortion is likely to be perceived as the "the worst" method because it is equated with "killing a human-to-be." Therefore, Buddhist believers typically support contraceptive methods that prevent conception but not those perceived to destroy life or stop development of a fertilized ovum.[12]

Similarly, there is wide variation in beliefs about family planning within Hinduism and Islam and corresponding variation in clerical support or rejection of contraception. In general, Hinduism supports the idea of large families, but there is also support for the development of social conscience, which may lead to smaller family sizes. The Dharma (religious and moral codes of Hinduism) emphasizes the need to act for the good of the world. Some Hindus believe that producing more children than one's family or environment can support goes against this code. Conceiving more children than the family can support may also be seen as a violation of the Ahimsa (the nonviolent rule of conduct).[13]

In Islam, as in all religions, fertility is highly prized and children are seen as a gift of God to bring "joy to our eyes" (Qur'an 25:74). Muslim scholars agree that permanent methods of contraception (that is, sterilization) are not permitted. Conservatives argue that any family planning is an expression of a lack of trust in the sustaining God. Yet, contraception has a long history in Islam. Contraceptive medicine was actually developed in Islamic countries; Avicenna, the Muslim physician, discusses twenty different substances used for birth control in his book *The Canon of Medicine*.[14] The most common form of birth control when Islam began was called *azl*, also known as withdrawal or coitus interruptus. The five major schools of law in Islam all permit the practice of azl.

There is another important principle in Islamic teachings, *ijithad*, which means to analyze the unique data of a current moral problem and argue from Qur'anic principles, using analogy and logic to come to the best and most reasonable solution.[15] To this end, the Arab Republic of Egypt published a booklet called "Islam's Attitude towards Family Planning." In the introduction to the booklet, the authors state that research for the book included broad consultation with the most authoritative sources in Islam. After noting that azl is permitted, they argue that any method that has the same purpose as azl and does not induce permanent sterility is acceptable. They then go on to list such methods, including the cervical cap, the condom, contraceptive pills, injections to produce temporary sterility, and the "loop device" placed in the uterus to prevent implantation of a fertilized egg.

Traditional Jewish law regarding procreation focuses on two basic principles: (i) it is a mitzvah (good deed) to marry, procreate, and have children ("Be fruitful and multiply" [Genesis 1:28]); and (ii) it is forbidden to "waste seed" (that is, emit semen without purpose). This prohibition is often referred to as onanism, a term derived from the biblical narrative of Onan (Genesis 38:7–10), who, when forced by his father to marry his brother's widow, resisted his fraternal duty by refusing to consummate the marriage, instead letting the semen go to waste whenever he had relations with the woman (presumably by coitus interruptus, although the term onanism is actually also applied to masturbation). A passage in the Talmud called "The Beraita of Three Women" is another basis for much of Jewish teaching regarding contraception. It states that a woman may use a moch (contraceptive method) in any of three circumstances where a pregnancy would cause harm: the woman is underage, pregnant, or breastfeeding. Other passages of the Talmud also permit women to drink potions that make them infertile. These doctrines form the basis for Jewish acceptance of birth control.

In general, modern Judaism is permissive of contraceptive use, although there are variations by sect. Orthodox Jews are the most restrictive, generally permitting only contraceptive methods that do not destroy the sperm or prevent it from reaching its intended destination (such as the IUD and the oral contraceptive pill) and only under limited circumstances, including to prevent a pregnancy that might harm the mother, to limit the number of children when additional children might harm the welfare of the family, or to delay or space births. Contraception for the "selfish" purpose of preventing procreation is prohibited. Male birth control methods (particularly condoms[16] and vasectomy) are generally frowned upon, as they "waste seed," and the commandment to have children is historically directed at men. In contrast to Orthodox Jews, Reform, Conservative, and Reconstructionist Jews in the United States are widely accepting of the full spectrum of contraceptive methods. Many modern Jews feel that the benefits of contraception—be they the improvement of the woman's health, family stability, or disease prevention—are much more in keeping with the commandment to "choose life" than they are in violation of the commandment to "be fruitful and multiply."

Religion and Contraceptive Use

Organized religion can play a significant role in issues of reproductive health, and teachings and beliefs about contraception are often at the forefront of these discussions. But when it comes to actual usage of contraceptives—as opposed to official doctrine—does religion really matter? The quick answer is—maybe.

Studies of large national data sets have generally shown that religion is not a significant predictor of contraceptive use for adult women in the United States, although it may be significant for teenagers.[17] For example, while the Roman Catholic Church is well known for its forbidding stance on the use of artificial contraception, Catholic women in the United States use modern contraception at the same rates as the general population.[18] Among all women who have had sex, 99 percent have ever used a contraceptive method other than natural family planning; that figure is virtually the same—98 percent—among sexually experienced Catholic women.[19] There has also emerged a prominent organization, called Catholics for Choice, whose members are practicing Catholics who believe in reproductive freedom for Catholic women, including contraception and, in some cases, abortion.

There is, however, variation in what types of contraception are preferred and how effectively contraception is used among women of various religious backgrounds. Protestant women are more likely than Catholics to use highly effective contraceptive methods, with 73 percent of mainline Protestants and 74 percent of evangelicals using sterilization, hormonal methods, or IUDs. More than four in ten evangelicals rely on male or female sterilization, a figure higher than among the other religious groups.[20] Although the reasons for these differences are not fully understood, there are two basic sets of hypotheses: doctrine hypotheses, which suggest that differences stem from religious teachings and behaviors, and characteristics hypotheses, which suggest that the demographics of different religious groups drive the differences in contraceptive practices.[21] For example, education is known to decrease use of sterilization, and evangelicals are typically less educated than other Protestants in the United States.[22]

Data for non-Christian women in the United States are difficult to find, given the relatively small percentages of the population that they comprise. As a result, diverse religions such as Hinduism, Buddhism, and Judaism are often grouped into a meaningless "other" category. However, existing data on fertility patterns of religious minority groups, although limited, may offer some insight (Table 17.2). The low fertility rates for Jews, Hindus, and Buddhists suggest that they may use highly effective

TABLE 17.2 Total fertility rate in the United States by religion

RELIGION	RATE
Muslims	2.84
Hispanic Catholics	2.75
Black Protestants	2.35
Fundamentalist Protestants (excluding Black Protestants)	2.13
Non-Hispanic Catholics	2.11
Moderate Protestants (excluding Black Protestants)	2.01
Liberal Protestants (excluding Black Protestants)	1.84
Hindus/Buddhists	1.73
No Religion	1.66
Others	1.64
Jews	1.43
US Population Average	*2.08*

SOURCE: M. Blume, "Religions and Fertility in the US—GSS-Data," *Scilogs*, June 3, 2010, http://www.scilogs.eu/en/blog/biology-of-religion/2010-06-03/religions-and-fertility-in-the-us-gss-data.

contraceptive methods, whereas Muslims have higher fertility rates, suggesting less use of highly effective contraception or a cultural preference for larger families.

Prenatal Care

Prenatal care has been the cornerstone of health care for pregnant women in the United States since the early 1900s, when Mrs. William Lowell Putnam and Dr. Josephine Baker initiated the nation's first prenatal care programs in Boston and New York. Although the details of prenatal care have changed as medical science has advanced, the basic premise of regular check-ins with medical personnel throughout pregnancy has stayed the same. Prenatal care is widely accepted as beneficial—resulting in healthier mothers and babies[23] and reductions in neonatal and infant mortality and morbidity[24] (although the scientific literature on the impact of prenatal care in reducing low birth weight is somewhat equivocal)—and is the standard of care in the United States. There is little controversy—religious or otherwise—about its value.

But this doesn't mean that religion is irrelevant for issues of prenatal care. Actually, religions often speak to prenatal care. In Judaism, getting prenatal care is required as part of the stewardship of the body. Similarly, nearly all Christian groups in the United States, with the exception of Christian Scientists,[25] promote prenatal care. For Muslim women, prenatal care is widely used, but issues around modesty or hijab[26] are often of concern. Islam does not forbid medical providers of the opposite sex from examining a patient when necessary, but a Muslim woman will typically select a female midwife or obstetrician for her prenatal care and delivery. However, the inherently unplanned nature of childbirth means that a male provider may need to deliver her child or examine her in the hospital. Similarly, nurses or other medical personnel in a clinic or hospital may be male, compromising privacy and modesty. Other issues of hijab for Muslim women include dealing with skimpy medical gowns and the need to cover their heads. In a 2007 article on the topic of childbirth and modesty, one Muslim woman described having told the labor and delivery nurse that she wanted to accompany the baby when the child was taken out of the room and would need a few minutes to dress and cover her head. The nurse did not wait, and the woman ended up leaping out of bed despite her stitches, throwing on her coat over her medical gown, and quickly putting on her hijab (head cover). When she asked the nurse why she did not wait, the nurse responded that "the pictures are mandatory"—which, of course, did not answer the question.[27]

Abortion

Abortion may be the most heated, divisive issue in health care in the United States today. Religious mandates related to the morality of terminating a pregnancy dominate public policy discussions of reproductive health, creating an undercurrent of complexity and often animosity around topics ranging from the availability of contraceptives to prenatal genetic diagnosis. Although the Christian right in the United States has succeeded in equating religious piety with being "pro life"—that is, opposed to abortion—and no religion actually promotes abortion, a careful examination reveals a range of views on abortion among and even within various faiths (Table 17.3).

The intersection of religion and abortion has a long and complicated history, one that is not nearly as consistent as most people believe. Although many religions do stand staunchly against abortion, others have more nuanced views, as evidenced by the existence of the Religious Coalition for Reproductive Choice. Its forerunner, the Clergy Consultation Service on Abortion, was founded in 1967 with twenty-one ministers and rabbis and grew to include approximately 1,400 clergy members of

TABLE 17.3 Religious institutional policies regarding abortion

	DENOMINATION/SECT	STANCE ON ABORTION
Christianity	American Baptist Church	Permits abortion when not used as a primary means of contraception or without regard for its seriousness.
	Assemblies of God	Opposes abortion except when it is necessary to protect the life of the mother.
	Church of Jesus Christ of Latter-day Saints[a]	Permits abortion to protect the life of the mother, in cases of rape or incest, or in cases of severe fetal anomaly. Those seeking abortions outside of these reasons may be excommunicated.
	Southern Baptist Church	Opposes abortion except when it is necessary to protect the life of the mother.
	Episcopal Church	Permits abortion to protect the health of the mother, in cases of rape/incest, or cases of severe fetal anomaly.
	Evangelical Lutheran Church in America	Permits abortion to protect the life of the mother, in cases of rape or incest, or in cases of severe fetal anomaly. Opposes abortion after the point of fetal viability except when lethal abnormalities exist.
	Greek Orthodox Archdiocese of America	Opposes abortion except when it is necessary to protect the life of the mother.
	Presbyterian Church	No official opinion. Deems abortion a personal decision.
	Roman Catholic Church	Opposes all abortion.
	Seventh-day Adventist	Permits abortion to protect the life of the mother, when the mother's health is seriously jeopardized, in cases of rape or incest, or in cases of severe fetal anomaly.
	United Church of Christ	Permits abortion.
	United Methodist Church	Permits abortion unless used as a method of gender selection/birth control.
	Unitarian Universalist Association of Congregations	Permits abortion.
Judaism	Reform/Constructionist Judaism	Permits abortion.

continued

TABLE 17.3 *continued*

DENOMINATION/SECT	STANCE ON ABORTION
Conservative Judaism	Permits abortion when religious authorities determine it to be warranted under Jewish law (*Halakha*).
Orthodox/Hasidic Judaism	Varying positions. All permit abortion to save the life of the mother. Some consider threats to maternal health, such as mental health, to warrant abortion. Rabbinic authorization is required.
Islam	Varying positions. Most believe that abortion prior to 120 days gestation is acceptable to save the life of the mother. All Islamic legal schools prohibit abortion after 120 days gestation.
Hinduism	Opposes abortion except when it is necessary to protect the life of the mother.
Buddhism	Varying positions. Abortion is believed to incur the karmic burden of killing. Some believe that it may be justified for medical reasons or the well-being of the community.
Chinese Religions	Abortion is not encouraged but is sometimes viewed as a necessary evil.
Native Religions	Discretion is given to the women of the village; heavy reliance on the use of plants or herbs with abortifacient properties.

[a] There is debate whether the Church of Jesus Christ of Latter-day Saints should be considered a Christian denomination. Because Mormons self-describe as Christians, we include Mormonism under the Christian heading. SOURCES: Daniel C. Maguire, *Sacred Choices: The Right to Contraception and Abortion in Ten World Religions* (Minneapolis: Fortress Press, 2001) and *Sacred Rights: The Case for Contraception and Abortion in World Religions* (New York: Oxford University Press, 2003); P. Feldman, "Sexuality, Birth Control and Childbirth in Orthodox Jewish Tradition," *CMAJ* 146, no. 1 (1992): 29–33; Pew Forum on Religion and Public Life, "Religious Groups' Official Positions on Abortion," Pew Research Center, January 16, 2013, http://www.pewforum.org/Abortion/Religious-Groups-Official-Positions-on-Abortion. aspx; J. J. Hughes, "Buddhism and Abortion: A Western Approach," in *Buddhism and Abortion*, ed. D Keown (London: Macmillan, 1999), 183–198.

various denominations throughout the United States. Today, the Religious Coalition for Reproductive Choice continues to support the right of women of all religions to make their own determinations about all healthcare issues—including abortion.[28]

In stark contrast, we see examples of religious institutions and clergy opposing abortion for any reason and under any circumstances. This has been a particularly difficult stance for Roman Catholic hospitals, which have at times been forced to choose between adhering to the Church's teaching and saving a woman's life. The case of St. Joseph's Hospital and Medical Center in Phoenix, Arizona, is illustrative of the difficulties. In November 2009, a 27-year-old pregnant woman was admitted to the hospital for heart failure resulting from acute pulmonary hypertension brought on by her pregnancy. The fetus, at eleven weeks gestation, also appeared to be dying because the mother's condition was preventing enough oxygen from reaching the placenta. If she continued the pregnancy, the mother was told, she would almost certainly die. Sister Margaret Mary McBride, Vice President of Mission Integration and a member of the hospital's ethics committee, gave her approval for surgeons to remove the placenta from the mother, knowing this would end the life of the fetus—and save the life of the mother. Bishop Thomas J. Olmsted concluded that the hospital had performed an abortion. He excommunicated Sister McBride and revoked St. Joseph's status as a Catholic institution, ending a one-hundred-year relationship.[29]

Clearly, abortion is a contentious issue for many people and institutions of faith. Deeply held convictions about the value, origins, and meaning of life are often involved. Most religions provide their followers with beliefs about the origin of life, including the point in development when human life begins. In the Catholic, Hindu, and many Protestant faiths, life begins at the moment of conception. Many other faiths view the acquisition of human personhood as a process that develops over time. Islam is a good example; the Qur'an offers no single, clear answer on the subject of when exactly life begins, leaving the question open to different interpretations.[30] The Islamic perspective generally separates fetal development into pre- and post-ensoulment periods, with abortion being generally permissible prior to 120 days.[31] Similarly, Lutherans view conception as the first step in a four-month process of becoming human.[32]

As with many aspects of religion, a plurality of beliefs can be seen within some groups. For Jews, Talmudic law offers different answers on the subject, with abortions being allowed by some prior to forty days of gestation (*Yebamoth* 69b) and by others before eighty days (*Niddah* 30b).[33] Similarly, some groups within the Presbyterian Church believe life begins at conception, while others see this occurring when a fetus is viable outside of the uterine environment (at approximately twenty-four weeks of gestation).[34]

Most religions prescribe the conditions, if any, under which a woman can choose to end her pregnancy and remain in good standing with her faith community; even in faiths where abortion is typically banned, many allow an exception when the health or life of the mother is at risk. In Judaic law, the fetus is not viewed as a separate entity from the mother, and the moral imperative is to protect the life of the mother by ending a pregnancy that is putting her at risk.[35] This is in direct contrast to the Catholic perspective demonstrated by the story of St. Joseph's hospital. In what may be seen as a bit of an internal contradiction, a Catholic woman may receive medical treatment if a part of her own body is causing her to be ill, even if it indirectly ends a pregnancy; this allows a woman to have a tubal pregnancy removed or to undergo a hysterectomy for uterine cancer while pregnant.[36] The Lutheran perspective on abortion takes a pragmatic, two-pronged approach: while the act is considered morally wrong, most sects of the church—except the more conservative branch—recognize the necessity for government to regulate and define the provision of this service.[37]

Some faiths, such as the Christian Reformed Church in North America[38] and the more liberal branches of Judaism,[39] recognize threats to the mother's mental and emotional health as well as her physical health as acceptable motivation for abortion. This is particularly applicable when the pregnancy has resulted from rape or incest,[40] also recognized as a sufficient reasons for abortion under Islam.[41] In direct contrast, the Catholic Church argues that abortion itself causes mental or emotional damage to a woman and the circumstances surrounding conception do not matter.[42] Economic hardship is not considered sufficient reason to allow abortion by either Catholicism or mainstream Judaism,[43] although some liberal Judaic and Islamic rulings have permitted abortion for reasons of poverty.[44] In general, religious communities that place a higher emphasis on the parental obligation to provide more for their children than simply food and shelter are more likely to view abortion in this situation as necessary or at least the lesser evil.[45]

Prenatal Diagnosis and Screening

Religious perspectives on disability, which are inconsistent at best, are intertwined with the debate surrounding genetic diagnosis. Many faiths stress the importance of compassion, charity, and patience in dealing with disabled persons, and some even view disability as a gift and disabled people as worthy of special treatment.[46] In the Qu'ran, the Prophet Mohammed is admonished by Allah for being impatient toward a person who is blind.[47] For Christians, Jesus' compassion and healing of people suffering from various forms of disability and illness (Matthew 15:30–31) demonstrates this principle.[48]

Despite this, Christians in the Middle Ages viewed people with disabilities as possessed by the devil; some were even burned as witches.[49] Biblical verses such as Leviticus 21:17–24, which bans anyone "who has any defect" from entering certain holy places, lent credence to a pervasive belief in the "wrongness" of people with physical differences.[50] The Hindu concept of karma, described in the Laws of Manu, adds further complexity to this idea by implying that a disability is the result of past wrongdoing.[51] A belief in karma can also contribute to a sense of shame a family may feel after the birth of a child with a genetic condition.[52] Viewed in this light, a disability is something to be feared.

How these beliefs about disability translate into action depends on the balance between community and individual values. Religious faiths that emphasize the needs of the community and society often view prenatal diagnosis and abortion of a fetus with a malformation or genetic disease as the lesser of two evils, to be accepted in the context of the societal need for healthy children.[53] From a Judaic perspective, for example, the mandate to care for people with disabilities is viewed as compatible with the use of prenatal testing, as both can fulfill the obligation of responsibility toward the next generation.[54] However, in Orthodox Judaism, abortion of a fetus with a nonlife-threatening condition is not permitted, unless the impact on the mother is considered sufficiently harmful; cases are often considered individually based on their particular circumstances, and a rabbi may be involved in the decision-making process along with medical providers.[55] Buddhists may also view abortion after prenatal diagnosis as more compassionate than allowing the birth of a child who will experience a disproportionate amount of suffering.[56]

Religious proscriptions on prenatal diagnosis are also sometimes influenced by the intention of the mother. For example, amniocentesis is forbidden by the Catholic Church if the intention is to have an abortion in the event a malformation is detected.[57] However, if the intention is to diagnose a condition so that the family can intervene on behalf of the unborn child, the procedure is permissible.[58] With the growing field of fetal surgery, this option is becoming more relevant for Catholics and others holding this view.

Pre-implantation genetic diagnosis (PGD), an in vitro fertilization process in which embryos are transferred selectively, so that only those that have been tested and found not to have a particular genetic condition are implanted, is another topic of controversy. Many conservative religious groups, such as Catholics and evangelical Christians, oppose the use of PGD because the process results in the destruction of embryos with a particular genetic trait. The reasons for these objections are largely related to the churches' opposition to abortion.[59] For others, the fact that affected embryos are not transferred for implantation into the uterus renders the procedure allowable, because no abortion is needed. As an example, many rabbis would support a couple's choice to use PGD to achieve a healthy pregnancy, in part because any embryos that are destroyed during the process are at a very early stage not seen by Judaism as having achieved personhood.[60] PGD has largely been embraced by the Jewish community as an acceptable way for a couple with genetic risks to fulfill the mandate to have children while acting to protect the health and well-being of their future offspring.[61]

Preconception Genetic Carrier Screening

Over time, the frequency of a genetic disease often increases among religious or ethnic groups that tend to intermarry. For example, the Ashkenazi Jewish population is at increased risk for Tay-Sachs disease, a devastating genetic syndrome that causes progressive disability followed by death, usually by two years of age. Religious institutions can play an important role in population-based efforts to prevent these conditions through preconception genetic carrier screening. The story of a program called Dor Yeshorim illustrates this point.

Hasidic Rabbi Josef Ekstein had experienced more than his fair share of suffering. He and his wife had taken the command to "be fruitful and multiply" seriously, resulting in the births of four children with Tay-Sachs disease.[62] Tay-Sachs is an autosomal recessive condition, resulting from a child inheriting a broken gene from each parent. Both parents are healthy carriers who have one broken copy of the gene, but another working copy masks the presence of the nonworking one.[63] The only way for a person to learn if he or she is a carrier is to have a test done or to bear a child with the disease. Rabbi Ekstein was determined to find a way to increase the number of people who had carrier screening to prevent the kind of suffering he and his wife had endured.

He started Dor Yeshorim ("upright generation") in New York in 1983. To sidestep Orthodox Jewish prohibitions against contraception, prenatal diagnosis, and abortion, Dor Yeshorim offers voluntary, anonymous carrier screening. Rather than being given their screening results, participants are given a number. A couple considering marriage contacts the program with their screening numbers. Dor Yeshorim then informs the couple whether they are compatible or—in cases where both are carriers—not. Because most Hasidic Jews have arranged marriages, the majority of couples informed that they are incompatible choose not to marry. Dor Yeshorim has resulted in a more than 90 percent reduction in the number of children born with Tay-Sachs disease in this group.[64] Today, all people of Jewish descent are encouraged by religious leaders and medical providers to have carrier screening for a growing number of genetic diseases.[65]

This concept is echoed by the Orthodox Church in Cyprus, where the Church has taken on a major role in preventing thalassemia (a genetic form of severe anemia that leads to blood transfusion dependence, chronic illness, and often early death) by requiring couples seeking marriage to present certificates indicating both members have been tested and counseled about their results.[66] While the couple is aware of their carrier status, the priests are not because it is not listed on the certificate; as long as a couple has been screened, the marriage is allowed to proceed. Carrier couples in Cyprus, who have often developed a strong emotional bond prior to testing, tend to use prenatal diagnosis and abortion to prevent the births of affected children.

Both the Dor Yeshorim and thalassemia examples occur at the intersections of religion, health, and ethnicity, suggesting that the development of beliefs and practices also parallels real issues of genetic heritage as they have become understood for these communities. This entwined relationship of religion with other determinants yields an increasingly complex pathway for understanding the impact of religion in these cases.

Infertility

Fertility is often portrayed in monotheistic religious texts as a sign of God's favor or a blessing. Examples can be found in Jewish and Christian as well as Muslim texts (Genesis 17:16; Psalms 139, 1 Samuel 1:17–20; Luke 13–14; Qur'an 42.49–50). But what happens if a woman is unable to become pregnant? On average, 7 percent of married women in the United States struggle with infertility, defined as the inability to conceive for twelve months in the absence of contraceptives.[67] Infertility rates are increasing because many women now delay childbearing beyond the years of peak fertility.[68] Epidemiological data examining the influence of religion on infertility and its treatments are scarce, but responses to this issue do differ among religions.

Surrogacy may be one of the oldest methods for overcoming infertility: In Genesis, female slaves were enlisted as surrogates (Genesis 16:1–12, Genesis 30:1–13). A surrogate is "a woman who agrees to become pregnant using a man's sperm and her own egg. The child will be genetically related to the surrogate and the male partner. After birth, the surrogate will give up the baby for adoption by the parents."[69] Judaism,[70] Hinduism, and many Protestant faiths support surrogacy as a means of addressing infertility.[71] In Islam, however, surrogacy is considered adultery and is, therefore, forbidden,[72] while Catholic doctrine forbids surrogacy on the basis that the resulting child is not created in a natural manner.[73]

Sperm and egg donation are also treated differently by various religious groups. In Judaism, the prohibition against male masturbation, which is the standard way in which donor semen is obtained, prevents sperm donation from being a viable option for Orthodox couples when the male partner is infertile.[74] In Islam, both sperm and ovum donation are unacceptable means of achieving a pregnancy, because they involve using gametes from someone other than the husband and wife, thereby constituting adultery. Most other faiths, however, permit the use of gamete donation to achieve pregnancy.

Artificial reproductive technologies can also help overcome physical barriers to natural conception, adding further complexity to religious interpretations of its permissibility. As one example, intracytoplasmic sperm injection is a technique used when a man's sperm may have difficulty fertilizing an ovum, often related to problems with the quality or number of sperm. With intracytoplasmic sperm injection, a sperm is injected directly into an ovum with a micro-needle to increase the chances of successful fertilization. Orthodox Jewish and Catholic men may not feel this is an option, given the fact that sperm is often obtained via masturbation.[75] However, for some men, sperm are blocked from expulsion during ejaculation by a physical barrier in the vas deferens, requiring extraction of sperm via a needle. For those men who have religious objections to masturbation, this procedure may be an option if they are willing to undergo needle extraction. Similarly, if a physical barrier in a woman prevents sperm from reaching an ovum, Catholics can take advantage of a procedure called gamete intra-fallopian transfer, in which sperm can be collected from the uterus after sexual intercourse and transferred to the fallopian tubes, where fertilization can occur, sidestepping the prohibition on masturbation.[76]

Conclusion

We only begin to scratch the surface of the interactions between religion and reproductive health; there are many other examples—both positive and negative from the perspective of public health—that should be considered as this discussion continues, including female genital mutilation[77] and health risks associated with traditional circumcision rites,[78] two widely practiced religious traditions that remain controversial. Furthermore, religion is not a freestanding influence, but one intertwined with other determinants of health. So, if a woman's religion doesn't fully determine her reproductive choices, why should we consider religion as a social determinant for reproductive health? The answers fall into the grey areas.

While much has been made about the increasingly secular nature of America, religion is alive and well in the United States. The majority of Americans report that religion plays a "very important" role in their lives.[79] The majority of women of reproductive age (between the ages of 15 and 44) report that they have a religious affiliation, that they attend religious worship at least once a month, and that religion is important in their daily lives.[80] Our own research has shown that religion translates into all areas of life, including health decision-making.[81] While a Catholic woman may be as likely as a Jewish woman to use some method of family planning, her beliefs about building a family, priorities about motherhood and career, concerns about the acceptability of her and her partner's family-planning choices, access to education, and many other factors may differ, resulting in different priorities for preventing or encouraging a pregnancy. These priorities and beliefs are rooted in a woman's cultural, and often religious traditions and background.

Positive or negative—religion matters. Reproductive health is complicated. Decisions and behaviors are multifaceted and intertwined with education, income, culture, geography—and religion. It will take considerable work to continue to disentangle these determinants of health, but a full understanding of reproductive health in the United States requires consideration of all of these contributors.

Notes

1. Abu Dawood Hadith no. 2050; classed as saheeh by al-Albaani in Saheeh Abi Dawood, 1805.
2. Warren B. Miller, "Personality Traits and Developmental Experiences as Antecedents of Childbearing Motivation," *Demography* 29, no. 2 (1992): 265–285; William D. Mosher, Linda B. Williams, and David P. Johnson, "Religion and Fertility in the United States: New Patterns," *Demography* 29, no. 2 (1992): 199–214.
3. L. M. Gaydos, W. W. Thompson, and C. J. Rowland Hogue, "Does Faith Affect How Southern African-American Women Use Contraception?," paper presented at the American Public Health Association Annual Meeting, Philadelphia, November 2009; J. S. Hirsch, "Catholics Using Contraceptives: Religion, Family Planning, and Interpretive Agency in Rural Mexico," *Studies in Family Planning* 39, no. 2 (2008): 93–104; A. Lifflander, L. M. Gaydos, and C. J. Hogue, "Circumstances of Pregnancy: Low Income Women in Georgia Describe the Difference between Planned and Unplanned Pregnancies," *Maternal and Child Health Journal* 11, no. 1 (2007): 81–89; A. Srikanthan and R. L. Reid, "Religious and Cultural Influences on Contraception," *Journal of Obstetrics and Gynaecology Canada* 30, no. 2 (2008): 129–137.
4. Amy Adamczyk, "The Effects of Religious Contextual Norms, Structural Constraints, and Personal Religiosity on Abortion Decisions," *Social Science Research* 37, no. 2 (2008): 657–672; Marc Galanter, Peter Buckley, Alexander Deutsch, Richard Rabkin, and Judith Rabkin, "Large Group Influence for Decreased Drug Use: Findings from Two Contemporary Religious Sects," *American Journal of Drug and Alcohol Abuse* 7, nos. 3–4 (1980): 291–304; Gunter Runkel, "Sexual Morality of Christianity," *Journal of Sex & Marital Therapy* 24, no. 2 (1998): 103–122; M. Young, L. Ponder, and J. Reed, "Effects of an Anabolic Steroid on Sexual Performance in Male Albino Rats," *Psychological Reports* 45, no. 1 (1979): 281–282.
5. L. B. Finer and S. K. Henshaw, "Disparities in Rates of Unintended Pregnancy in the United States, 1994 and 2001," *Perspectives on Sexual and Reproductive Health* 38, no. 2 (2006): 90–96.
6. A. Conde-Agudelo and J. M. Belizan, "Maternal Morbidity and Mortality Associated with Interpregnancy Interval: Cross Sectional Study," *BMJ* 321, no. 7271 (2000): 1255–1259; V. Setty-Venugopal and U. D. Upadhyay, "Birth Spacing: Three to Five Saves Lives," *Population Reports Series L* 13(2002): 1–23.
7. A. Conde-Agudelo, A. Rosas-Bermudez, and A. C. Kafury-Goeta, "Birth Spacing and Risk of Adverse Perinatal Outcomes: A Meta–Analysis," *JAMA* 295, no. 15 (2006): 1809–1823.
8. Pope Paul VI, *Encyclical of Pope Paul VI, Humanae Vitae, on the Regulation of Birth, and Pope Paul VI's Credo of the People of God*, Study club ed. (Glen Rock, NJ: Paulist Press, 1968).
9. A. Barrick, "Most Evangelical Leaders Ok with Birth Control," *Christian Post*, June 9, 2010.
10. R. Shorto, "Contra–Contraception," *New York Times*, May 7, 2006.
11. C. Adams and M. Leverland, "The Effects of Religious Beliefs on the Health Care Practices of the Amish," *Nurse Practitioner* 3, no. 58 (1986): 63–67.

12. Dawn Stacey, "What Do Religions Say about Birth Control and Family Planning?: Buddhism," January 30, 2014, http://contraception.about.com/od/additionalresources/ss/religion_8.htm.

13. Dawn Stacey, "What Do Religions Say About Birth Control and Family Planning? Hinduism?: Hinduism," January 30, 2014, http://contraception.about.com/od/additionalresources/ss/religion_5.htm.

14. Avicenna, *The Canon of Medicine of Avicenna*, ed. O. Cameron Gruner (Birmingham, AL: Classics of Medicine Library, 1984).

15. Rachel Anne Codd, "A Critical Analysis of the Role of Ijtihad in Legal Reforms in the Muslim World," *Arab Law Quarterly* 14, no. 2 (1999): 112–131.

16. There is ongoing debate among Orthodox Jews concerning the use of condoms to prevent sexually transmitted infections. While it is clear that condoms are not allowed for prevention of pregnancy, many have argued that condoms are permissible to prevent harm to the body because preserving life is paramount.

17. Michael R. Kramer, Carol J. Hogue, and Laura M. Gaydos, "Noncontracepting Behavior in Women at Risk for Unintended Pregnancy: What's Religion Got to Do with It?," *Annals of Epidemiology* 17, no. 5 (2007): 327–334.

18. A. Chandra, G. M. Martinez, W. D. Mosher, J. C. Abma, and J. Jones, "Fertility, Family Planning, and Reproductive Health of U.S. Women: Data from the 2002 National Survey of Family Growth," *Vital Health Statistics* 23, no. 25 (2005): 1–160.

19. R. K. Jones and J. Dreweke, *Countering Conventional Wisdom: New Evidence on Religion and Contraceptive Use* (New York: Guttmacher Institute, 2011).

20. J. Dreweke, "Contraceptive Use Is the Norm among Religious Women," April 13, 2011, http://www.guttmacher.org/media/nr/2011/04/13/.

21. J. P. Marcum, "Explaining Fertility Differences among U.S. Protestants," *Social Forces* 60(1981): 532–543.

22. L. Bumpass, E. Thompson, and A. Godecker, "Women, Men and Contraceptive Sterilization," *Fertility and Sterility* 73, no. 5 (2000): 937–946; Pew Research Center, "Evangelicals and Education," *Daily Number*, April 18, 2008, http://www.pewresearch.org/daily-number/evangelicals-and-education/.

23. M. Terris and M. Glasser, "A Life Table Analysis of the Relation of Prenatal Care to Prematurity," *American Journal of Public Health* 64, no. 9 (1974): 869–875; H. Heins, N. Nance, B. McCarthy, and C. Efird, "A Randomized Trial of Nurse-Midwifery Prenatal Care to Reduce Low Birth Weight," *Obstetrics and Gynecology* 73, no. 3 (1990): 341–345.

24. M. A. Herbst, B. M. Mercer, D. Beazley, N. Meyer, and T. Carr, "Relationship of Prenatal Care and Perinatal Morbidity in Low-Birth-Weight Infants," *American Journal of Obstetrics and Gynecology* 189, no. 4 (2003): 930–933.

25. R. Anderson, "Religious Traditions and Prenatal Genetic Counseling," *American Journal of Medical Genetics Part C: Seminars in Medical Genetics* 15, no. 151c (2009): 52–61; A. M. Kaunitz, C. Spence, T. S. Danielson, R. W. Rochat, and D. A. Grimes, "Perinatal and Maternal Mortality in a Religious Group Avoiding Obstetric Care," *American Journal of Obstetrics and Gynecology* 150, no. 7 (1984): 826–831.

26. Hijab refers to both the Muslim concept of modesty in general and the head covering worn by Muslim women.

27. Amel S. Abdulla, "When a Muslim Woman Is Giving Birth, How Does She Tackle Issues Related to Modesty?," *InFocus News*, December 5, 2007.

28. Religious Coalition for Reproductive Choice, "Clergy Consultation Service on Abortion: A Brief History," 2007, http://rcrc.org/homepage/about/history/.

29. Jerry Filteau, "Catholic Status Revoked," *National Catholic Reporter* 47, no. 6 (2011): 1–14.

30. Daniel C. Maguire, *Sacred Choices: The Right to Contraception and Abortion in Ten World Religions* (Minneapolis: Fortress Press, 2001); M. Stephens, C. F. Jordens, I. H. Kerridge, and R. A. Ankeny, "Religious Perspectives on Abortion and a Secular Response," *Journal of Religion and Health* 49, no. 4 (2010): 513–535.

31. Stephens et al., "Religious Perspectives on Abortion."

32. Stephens et al., "Religious Perspectives on Abortion."

33. Stephens et al., "Religious Perspectives on Abortion."

34. Anderson, "Religious Traditions and Prenatal Genetic Counseling"; Stephens et al., "Religious Perspectives on Abortion."

35. Stephens et al., "Religious Perspectives on Abortion"; Anderson, "Religious Traditions and Prenatal Genetic Counseling."

36. Stephens et al., "Religious Perspectives on Abortion."

37. Stephens et al., "Religious Perspectives on Abortion."

38. Anderson, "Religious Traditions and Prenatal Genetic Counseling."

39. Stephens et al., "Religious Perspectives on Abortion."

40. Anderson, "Religious Traditions and Prenatal Genetic Counseling."

41. Stephens et al., "Religious Perspectives on Abortion."

42. Stephens et al., "Religious Perspectives on Abortion."

43. Stephens et al., "Religious Perspectives on Abortion."

44. Maguire, *Sacred Choices*; Stephens et al., "Religious Perspectives on Abortion."

45. Maguire, *Sacred Choices*.

46. Deborah Selway and Adrian F. Ashman, "Disability, Religion and Health: A Literature Review in Search of the Spiritual Dimensions of Disability," *Disability & Society* 13, no. 3 (1998): 429–439; M. Miles, "Some Historical Texts on Disability in the Classical Muslim World," *Journal of Religion, Disability & Health* 6, no. 2–3 (2002): 77.

47. M. Miles, "Disability in an Eastern Religious Context: Historical Perspectives," *Disability & Society* 10, no. 1 (1995): 49–69.

48. All biblical quotations in this chapter refer to the New International Version.

49. Selway and Ashman, "Disability, Religion and Health."

50. Avi Rose, "'Who Causes the Blind to See': Disability and Quality of Religious Life," *Disability & Society* 12, no. 3 (1997): 395–405.

51. Miles, "Disability in an Eastern Religious Context."

52. Vidya Bhushan Gupta, "How Hindus Cope with Disability," *Journal of Religion, Disability & Health* 15, no. 1 (2011): 72–78.

53. Maguire, *Sacred Choices*.

54. Aviad E. Raz, *Community Genetics and Genetic Alliances: Eugenics, Carrier Testing, and Networks of Risk* (New York: Routledge, 2009).

55. Stephens et al., "Religious Perspectives on Abortion."

56. Maguire, *Sacred Choices*.

57. Stephens et al., "Religious Perspectives on Abortion"; Anderson, "Religious Traditions and Prenatal Genetic Counseling."

58. Anderson, "Religious Traditions and Prenatal Genetic Counseling."

59. John H. Evans, "Religious Belief, Perceptions of Human Suffering, and Support for Reproductive Genetic Technology," *Journal of Health Politics, Policy & Law* 31, no. 6 (2006): 1047–1074.

60. J. G. Schenker, "Assisted Reproductive Practice: Religious Perspectives," *Reproductive Biomedicine Online* 10, no. 3 (2005): 310–319.

61. Schenker, "Assisted Reproductive Practice"; Mark Popovsky, "Jewish Perspectives on the Use of Preimplantation Genetic Diagnosis," *Journal of Law, Medicine & Ethics* 35, no. 4 (2007): 699–711.

62. J. Ekstein and H. Katzenstein, "The Dor Yeshorim Story: Community-Based Carrier Screening for Tay-Sachs Disease," *Advances in Genetics* 44(2001): 297–310.

63. M. M. Kaback and R. J. Desnick, "Hexosaminidase a Deficiency," in *GeneReviews*, ed. R. A. Pagon, M. P. Adam, T. D. Bird, C. R. Dolan, C. T. Fong, and K. Stephens (Seattle: University of Washington, 1993), http://www.ncbi.nlm.nih.gov/pubmed/20301397.

64. Ekstein and Katzenstein, "The Dor Yeshorim Story."

65. Willard Cates, "Family Planning: The Essential Link to Achieving All Eight Millennium Development Goals," *Contraception* 81, no. 6 (2010): 460.

66. R. S. Cowan, "Moving Up the Slippery Slope: Mandated Genetic Screening on Cyprus," *American Journal of Medical Genetics Part C: Seminars in Medical Genetics* 151C, no. 1 (2009): 95–103; B. Prainsack and G. Siegal, "The Rise of Genetic Couplehood? A Comparative View of Premarital Genetic Testing," *BioSocieties* 1, no. 1 (2006): 17–36.

67. Chandra et al., "Fertility, Family Planning, and Reproductive Health."

68. Chandra et al., "Fertility, Family Planning, and Reproductive Health."

69. Centers for Disease Control and Prevention, "Infertility FAQs: Surrogacy," February 12, 2013, http://www.cdc.gov/reproductivehealth/Infertility/.

70. Rabbi Elie Kaplan Spitz, "On the Use of Birth Surrogates," *EH* 1, no. 3 (1997): 1–22.

71. A. Mufti, *Islamic Principles on Family Planning* (Agra Area, India: Oswal, 1999).

72. Mufti, *Islamic Principles on Family Planning*.

73. Schenker, "Assisted Reproductive Practice."

74. Schenker, "Assisted Reproductive Practice."

75. Schenker, "Assisted Reproductive Practice."

76. Schenker, "Assisted Reproductive Practice."

77. See, for instance, World Health Organization Study Group on Female Genital Mutilation and Obstetric Outcomes, "Female Genital Mutilation and Obstetric Outcome: WHO Collaborative Prospective Study in Six African Countries" *Lancet* 367 (2006): 1835–1841; World Health Organization, *Eliminating Female Genital Mutilation: An Interagency Statement* (Geneva: World Health Organization, Department of Reproductive Health and Research, 2008).

78. See, for instance, Thomas Zambito, "Infant's Death at Maimonides Hospital Linked to Circumcision," *New York Daily News*, March 3, 2012, http://www.nydailynews.com/new-york/infant-death-maimonides-hospital-linked-circumcision-article-1.1032432.

79. Mufti, *Islamic Principles on Family Planning*.
80. Chandra et al., "Fertility, Family Planning, and Reproductive Health of U.S. Women."
81. Gaydos, Thompson, and Hogue, "Does Faith Affect How Southern African-American Women Use Contraception?"; Lifflander, Gaydos, and Hogue, "Circumstances of Pregnancy."

18 | Religion and Physical Health from Childhood to Old Age

ELLEN IDLER

I N 1974, IN HIS BOOK *Who Shall Live?*, a study of the links between health and economic status, Stanford University health economist Victor Fuchs compared the health of two geographically close populations, the residents of the western US states of Utah and Nevada. He called the section "A Tale of Two States"—the title cleverly captured the contrast of the best and the worst when it came to state-level health indicators.[1] Utah and Nevada are alike in many respects. They have a similar climate and geography and, at the time of Fuchs's writing, similar statistics for race, ethnicity, and socioeconomic status, including education, income, and the availability of medical care. Yet the mortality rates for these two states were quite different.

If there were differences in resources, they tended to fall in Nevada's favor, but the death rates were higher in Nevada for men and women, boys and girls, and even babies. For men aged 40–49, the death rate in Nevada was 54 percent higher than in Utah, and for women of the same age, it was 69 percent higher. Infant mortality was 42 percent higher for male babies and 35 percent higher for females. When Fuchs compared deaths specifically due to cirrhosis of the liver and respiratory cancer, the mortality rate in Nevada was 590 percent that of Utah for men aged 30–39 and 443 percent for women of the same age. What explained these dramatic differences?

Fuchs's primary theme in the book was that human behaviors have health consequences. He was making what was at the time a novel argument—that the way that people live their lives and the communities and social structures in which they live them have more impact on the health of populations than the quality or availability of their medical care, as important as that might be. Compared with the residents of Nevada, many more residents of Utah were born in the state, had lived in the same place for at least five years, and were married. Also, as was suggested by the extremely high rates for smoking- and alcohol-related causes of death in Nevada, the people of Utah generally had far healthier lifestyles.

As Fuchs observed, underlying these differences in the stability of communities and the behaviors of the people living in them was the predominance of the Church of Jesus Christ of Latter-day Saints (LDS), whose members made up a majority of Utah's population. The religious beliefs of LDS members proscribe them from smoking, or drinking alcohol; they have high marriage and fertility rates and fewer sexual partners and, in general, "lead quiet, stable lives."[2] Thus, although Fuchs's book was not in any way about the specific subject of religion as a determinant of population health, he identified the Mormon religion as a defining element in Utah's "extraordinary" lifestyle differences, which were reflected in the mortality rates for residents of all ages.

What does the picture look like today, forty years later? Are the health indicators for Utah and Nevada as different as they were in 1974? The answer is, largely, yes. Utah's population health is among the best in the nation; it is tied with the state of Washington for the lowest infant mortality rate in the country—4.9 deaths for every 1,000 live births—while Nevada is tied for fifteenth, with 6.2 deaths per 1,000.[3] Utah's overall age-adjusted mortality rate is among the lowest five (with Arizona, California, Hawaii, and Minnesota) while Nevada's rate ranks thirty-fifth.[4] Utah has by far the lowest smoking rate among the fifty states, with just 9.1 percent of adults current smokers—a full 3 percentage points lower than the second lowest state, California, at 12.1 percent; Nevada's smoking rate is more than twice that of Utah, at 21.3 percent.[5] As in 1974, the proportion of Utah's population that is married is significantly higher and its proportion of adults who have had a drink of alcohol in the past month significantly lower than Nevada's.[6] Also, the majority of Utah's population is still Mormon, a factor that seems to tie these other lifestyle factors together. Altogether, the picture that Victor Fuchs painted—of patterns of living that lead to better health indicators for Utah compared with Nevada—has remained in place.

Is religion a factor in population health? Does it belong among the group of social determinants of health, now primarily thought of as social structural, political, and socioeconomic? We saw in chapter 1 that, as conceptualized by the UN Commission on the Social Determinants of Health, the social determinants framework focuses on inequalities—in income, opportunities, status, wealth, and education—as determinants of health. But the commission defined social determinants broadly as "the circumstances in which people are born, grow up, live, work, and age,"[7] and religion is, for many, one of those circumstances. This chapter addresses the exclusion of religion from the social determinants framework by reviewing epidemiological research on religion as a factor in health, focusing specifically on studies that employ population-based data.

There are now thousands of articles in the research literature under the general topic of "religion and health." This literature was surveyed comprehensively in 2000 by Harold Koenig and colleagues,[8] who reviewed more than 1,200 studies published to that point. In 2012, in preparing a revision of their 2000 study, Koenig and colleagues identified more than 3,700 articles published through 2010.[9] Other systematic reviews of the literature include those of McCullough and colleagues,[10] Powell and colleagues,[11] Chida and colleagues,[12] and Idler.[13] Many or even most of the studies included in all of these reviews except the last, however, are studies of small and nonrandom samples, and their findings are not generalizable to larger populations. Studies based on samples of patients in healthcare settings, convenience samples from community or religious groups, or other nonrandomly selected samples, while interesting for clinical or other reasons, are less relevant to our question about religion's role as a large-scale determinant of population health because their samples are not representative of any group beyond the study subjects.

We consider studies of the link between religion and health outcomes to be strong evidence for the status of religion as a social determinant of health only if the data come from vital statistics (a complete enumeration of the population) or from probability samples that allow the data to be generalized to the population from which it is drawn. The population-based measure of health that has been most often studied for its association with religion is mortality from all causes or from specific causes (based on vital statistics and individual death records), but there are also studies of the prevalence of major chronic diseases, functional disability, and subjective ratings of overall health (from population-based surveys). Our purpose is to describe the relationship of religion to these measures of health, both as an independent social determinant and as one that may be related to and intertwined with the other important determinants of health.

The illustration provided by Fuchs in "The Tale of Two States" is just that—an illustration, albeit one that draws on population statistics; it is not a well-controlled study. There are potential confounding variables at work. The recent recession, the housing crisis, and unemployment have hit Nevada much harder than they have Utah. Also, while the racial and ethnic distributions of their populations were quite similar in 1970, when Fuchs wrote, today Utah remains a very homogeneous, largely white state, and Nevada has become much more diverse.

But the illustration is nevertheless a useful way to begin this chapter for several reasons. First, it prefigures a set of epidemiological studies published in the 1970s and 1980s that compared the mortality rates of several sectarian religious groups (including Mormons) with the mortality rates of the larger populations in their region. Studies like these (and the comparison of Utah and Nevada) compare one group's rate for a health indicator like mortality to another group's. Such studies are informative, but they are criticized because they tell us only about the rates for the groups and do not provide any information on relationships between factors at the individual level, as surveys do. We will review the literature for both the group-level studies of mortality and the more frequently cited individual-level studies, in which social and health indicators can be studied jointly.

Health across the Life Course

A second reason to begin this chapter with Fuchs's observation is that he includes comparisons of infant, child, and adolescent mortality in his account. Social determinants affect health throughout the life course, from birth to death—as "people are born, grow up, live, work, and age." This has been an essential aspect of the social determinants approach—to understand the way in which the (unequal) social and economic conditions of early life shape human health across the life course. The life course approach to understanding the social determinants of health began to take shape in the 1990s, with the availability of longitudinal studies such as the British Birth Cohort studies, which allowed researchers to link early life circumstances with later life outcomes.[14] These long-running studies, which began tracking children at birth, have allowed researchers to test ideas about the impact of good or poor childhood health on later economic outcomes and explore questions such as whether childhood poverty or inadequate schooling have an impact on health in adulthood.

Taking this life course approach, researchers have found that beginning life as a member of a certain social or economic group has a long-term effect in later life.[15] Each additional advantage in early life provides a cumulative protective effect on health as the individual ages; similarly every social *dis*advantage also remains part of the accumulating social influence. Lifetime exposures to advantages and disadvantages are structured by the social, economic, and political institutions within which individuals live their lives—their families, schools, neighborhoods, clubs, peer groups, and friendship networks. These are the social structures that provide individuals with both material resources and resources of social identity that tell them who they are—for good or ill. Mel Bartley, a leading researcher in the field of health inequalities, contends that such identities may either constrain or promote individual economic opportunities. Societies that provide individuals with opportunities for the "stable occupation of the 'central life roles' . . . , such as worker, partner or parent, and/or acceptance in a reasonably stable community" support strong identities and social ties, but at the same time they may restrict individual freedom, mobility, and creativity.[16] From this perspective, social institutions that individuals join early in life and to which they maintain attachments throughout their lives would be especially consequential in opening and supporting social and economic opportunities and in creating and maintaining an individual's identity.

The life course approach to understanding health inequalities points in particular to periods of transition as moments when the individual is especially vulnerable to his or her advantaged or disadvantaged circumstances. Thus, in addition to the framework of accumulating risk and protection over the life course, it is important to consider critical developmental periods, such as the first year of life or puberty, as moments when social circumstances have a heightened influence on health.[17] These may be moments not only of rapid biological growth but also of social development, with the adoption of new social roles, new social identities, and new social expectations and responsibilities. Thus, the life course perspective has become increasingly important to the understanding of health in adulthood as a product of an individual's life circumstances from the moment of birth or even before. Religious institutions have been a constant influence in the lives of most individuals, bringing regular repetitions of ritual observance and significant social identities that are often adopted during life course transitions. As we noted in chapter 1, however, the research literature on the social determinants of health and particularly the research undertaken with a life course framework rarely if ever mentions religion or religious institutions as either an advantage or disadvantage for health.

Religion across the Life Course

In Part I of this book, we offered a set of insiders' perspectives on their experience of religious rituals or practices, including, among others, fasting, meditating, and singing. Ritual practices are religious actions that are performed in the same way, time after time; they mark individuals as members of one specific religious group and not another, and thus they provide a strong underpinning for identity and membership in a community.[18] For most religions, ritual observances begin at birth and continue throughout the life course to death and after.[19] They are physical, material practices—they are things that people *do* with their bodies—with their voices, their hands, and their feet. When they experience these practices, they take that experience in through their senses—their hearing, sight, taste, smell, and touch. The body is inextricably involved.

There is more to religions than their rituals, of course. Religions have doctrines and beliefs, ethics and morals, holy texts and stories, and spiritual dimensions. These nonmaterial dimensions of religions have gotten considerable attention from religion and health researchers who have focused on measuring subjective or internal concepts such as intrinsic religiosity, religious coping, forgiveness, or the importance of religiousness and spirituality and their association with various measures of health.[20] The more subjective dimensions of religion cannot be separated from the material, observable religious practices that, after all, have as their purpose the bringing of the individual into the subjective experience of the sacred. By contrast with the field's heretofore predominant focus on the subjective, we want to draw attention to the public health consequences of the observable, physically enacted ritual practices in which millions of people engage throughout their lives.

The cyclical timing of religious practice gives it a natural relevance to the life course.[21] Some religious rituals are practiced every day (some more than once a day), every week, or every year; others occur just once in a life course, usually marking a transition. The cycles of religious rituals thus include the nearly continuous, the repetitive, the occasional, and the rarely experienced, and it is useful to think of these cycles as mapping themselves onto the life course. We might think of an individual's potential for participation in ritual religious practices over their lifetime on a graph, with the x axis tracking the human life course from birth to adolescence, to adulthood, to old age and death, and the y axis showing the occurrence of religious rituals, from those, like puberty rituals, that occur at most only once in a lifetime (for instance, the Roman Catholic confirmation), to those that happen every year (the Hindu Diwali), or every week (the Jewish Sabbath), every day, or even several times per day (Muslim ablutions and prayers).

A person born into a religiously observant family who begins practicing the rituals of his or her faith at an early age could conceivably fill this imaginary graph with symbols representing those ritual performances. The rare events would be at the bottom and the increasingly frequent observances at the top, continuing throughout the life course. On the other hand, an individual with a nonreligious upbringing and a completely secular life might have a blank graph. There could be many patterns. Annual or one-time religious observances conforming to family expectations but no daily or weekly practice would leave scattered symbols at the bottom of the graph, throughout the life course, but none at the top. One side of the graph could be blank, if a person with a secular family and no religious observance in early life became a devout, practicing convert in adulthood. Thus our imaginary graph shows the potential for religious ritual performance over the life course.

The other aspect of such a graph that connects religious practice to the life course and, ultimately, to health is the regularity of the repetition. Religious practices are a recurring part of life for many people. Some, like Easter for Christians, may be accompanied by a significant period of daily preparation and anticipation but do not recur again for a year. Others, like dietary practices or giving thanks before eating, recur at every meal, so that there is little time between them and failing to observe them would represent a distinct change in the daily patterns of the person's life.

Altogether, there is the potential for an individual to be exposed through a significant proportion of his or life to an immense variety of physical, embodied religious practices. Religious practices alter—sometimes slightly, sometimes profoundly—a person's state of consciousness through their action on the body: they take the participant to a different place both physically and spiritually, and in this experience the physical and the spiritual are united. To the extent that these practices involve the body, that they take place in a physical and social environment in contact with air and water and other people, and—most of all—that they happen in the same structured way for people around the world and have done so for centuries, such practices are an intrinsic part of the social environment and an important determinant of health that must be considered along with the other socially patterned determinants of health across the life course.

Religion is not independent of the other social determinants of health. In addition to providing the warm helping-hands-and-carrots type of social support and the maybe not-so-friendly-sticks type of social control, religious groups offer the social capital of membership in a group that can act as a mediating structure between the individual and the large, impersonal institutions of the wider society. Belonging to a religious group exposes one to these influences, for better or for worse. It is important to note that membership and participation are at least to some extent voluntary, even for highly sectarian groups like the Mormons. As Fuchs commented in 1974, individuals who did not wish to conform to the restrictive Mormon lifestyle could have and presumably already had selected themselves out of the LDS Church and maybe out of the state of Utah. At the same time, the growth of Mormonism suggests that many or even most who were born into the church remained there, and others have chosen to convert and move to Utah. This self-selected group, embracing a restrictive lifestyle enforced by church doctrine, creates a social context that, over generations, has produced one of the healthiest state-level populations in the United States.

In chapter 1 we argued that, in addition to the direct influences of social support, social control, and social capital, religion also has a complex relationship with the more well-studied economic and political determinants of health. We suggested that religion may reduce economic inequality by encouraging charitable and compassionate giving, by encouraging concern for others who are less fortunate, or by advocating for social justice. We also proposed that religion might act to reduce, not the inequality itself, but the perception of that inequality by substituting a different set of values, orienting individuals away from a perspective that privileges outward, material signs of status and achievement. Finally, we considered a third possibility, that religions could operate through status or caste systems to reinforce economic inequality, thereby producing a negative influence on population health. Until religion is included in the research on the social determinants, we cannot know how these relationships actually work out, but it is interesting to note that Utah has the second lowest level of income inequality in the United States (behind Alaska); in other words, it has among the smallest proportion of people at the top of the income ladder compared with those at the bottom (Gini coefficient for Utah = 0.414, Nevada = 0.433, United States = 0.469).[22] In Utah's case, it would seem that a high level of religious observance is found together with a relatively low level of economic inequality, producing a unified and long-term positive effect on population health.

The potential impact of religion as a determinant of health in infancy, childhood, adolescence, adulthood, and old age is likely to be registered in different ways. The relevant indicators of population health and the mechanisms by which religion might be operating to influence it will differ at each stage. While there is a great deal of research in the field now known as "religion and health," it is largely concentrated on studies of adults and the elderly. But religions are relevant to human health at every stage of the life course, and they operate through an evolving but persisting set of influences to produce health outcomes in middle and old age to be sure, but in earlier periods of the life course as well. In the following sections, I review the epidemiological evidence for the association of religion with population health indicators at each stage of the life course.

Religion and Health in Infancy and Childhood

All religions show concern for infants. Children are highly significant to the wider social circles they are born into—their immediate and extended families, villages, neighborhoods, and religious groups—because social groups have a natural interest in perpetuating themselves. The care of orphans has been a particular concern of religious groups historically, and especially since the HIV/AIDS epidemic has left so many children without parents.[23] The founding of orphanages and innovative programs for caring for these children (some examples are given in chapter 22) demonstrate the mission of faith communities to care for the vulnerable and at the same time for their own future.

Religious rituals that take place at the time of birth are many and varied.[24] They include baptism for some Christian children, the cutting of the Hindu child's hair, the circumcising of Jewish male infants, and the saying of the call to prayer (*adhan*) into the right ear of the newborn Muslim boy before his head is shaved.[25] Naming rituals exist in most religions. The ceremonial speaking of the name, in the social context of family and religious group, extends the community's recognition that the infant is a member of the group and bears its identity as part of his or her own.

Reviewing the Research

This careful ritual attention to infants, together with the extensive role of religion's influence on reproductive health and health care (discussed in chapter 17), might lead one to expect that there would be a substantial number of studies of religion's role in the health of infants and children. But in fact there are surprisingly few such studies, especially population-based studies. We have mentioned Fuchs's observation of the considerably lower infant mortality rates for Utahans compared with Nevadans in 1974, a difference that persists. A more precise study comparing the birth outcomes of Norwegian members of the Seventh-day Adventist Church (SDA) with matched controls in the population found significantly greater birth weight and length in SDA infants at the same gestational age.[26] Another example is a recent study of child survival in India that addresses the puzzle of the Muslim advantage over Hindus, despite their socioeconomic disadvantage and the higher fertility of Muslim women; by the age of 5, Muslim children are 2.3 percent more likely to have survived than their socioeconomically advantaged Hindu counterparts, a difference that has existed for decades. The authors of this study argue that religion may "encapsulate unobservable behaviours or endowments that influence health," such as stronger social networks or personal hygiene related to religious ritual practice.[27] But for the most part, extremely few intergroup studies make age-specific comparisons for infants and children.

The other major type of research design in the study of religion and population health is survey based. In this research design, rather than comparing vital statistics for a religious group with another group, data are collected from a probability sample of individuals selected from a larger population on factors potentially related to health, sometimes including measures of religious involvement. This form of research has yielded a large number of studies of the health of adults, elderly persons, and even adolescents. But children and infants cannot complete survey forms, so again there are few studies to review.

Some recent analyses of data from large US samples of pregnant women, however, do focus on religion. In the US National Survey of Family Growth, researchers found that pregnant and postpartum women who attended religious services more frequently were significantly less likely to smoke cigarettes, drink alcohol, or smoke marijuana than women who attended services less often.[28] Using data from the US Fragile Families and Child Wellbeing study, other researchers have shown that mothers' religious attendance is significantly associated with lower odds of cigarette smoking and poor nutrition during pregnancy and also lower odds of low birth weight in infants; these authors argue that the benefits of religious involvement for the health of the mother extends to the next generation.[29] Another analysis of the same data showed that mothers who attended religious services more often were more likely to initiate breastfeeding than nonattenders and those with no religion; the same was true for mothers who were Muslim or who belonged to some other non-Christian or conservative Christian groups.[30] But with research in this area barely begun, the influence of parental religious involvement on infant and child health must be said to remain unknown.

On the negative side, there is an important public health concern regarding religious objections to immunizations, a clear example of parental religious influence on the health of children. Nearly all states in the United States allow exemptions from vaccinations for infants and children on religious grounds.[31] The failure to immunize children from the infectious diseases of childhood jeopardizes not only those children for whom the decision is made but also younger children who may not be fully immunized in their own and other families to whom they may be exposed. In communities where vaccination rates are very high, a small number of nonvaccinating families may not change the incidence of disease. But if the numbers of unvaccinated children grow—as one might expect if the motivation is socially (religiously) influenced rather than idiosyncratic—there could be a real resurgence of serious childhood diseases.

Overall, it would seem that, given the prominence of the life course perspective in understanding the social determinants of health, it would be prudent for researchers to be comprehensive in approaching the entire range of early-life influences. At this point, with few exceptions, we know little about the impact of family religious involvement on the health of infants and children, despite the influence of many religions on daily life activities that would profoundly affect growing children, such as a religious prohibition on smoking that reduces the child's exposure to secondhand smoke or a religious admonition to adhere to a vegetarian diet. Taking this reality in combination with the particular focus of ritual attention on infants, it would seem important not to exclude religion from the set of social determinants of health at the earliest stages of the life course.

Religion and Health in Adolescence

If many or even most religions mark the birth of a child with ritual practices and ceremonies, the transition from childhood to adolescence may be seen as even more significant. The young person reaching puberty and beginning to reach his or her adult size and capabilities has clearly survived the vulnerability of infancy and childhood and is ready to become a productive member of society. There is a lot for a society to celebrate in the successful nurturing of an infant through childhood to the brink of adulthood. What has until this point been mostly a one-way street of care and support is about to become a two-way street, as the adolescent begins to take on adult responsibilities. So coming-of-age rituals mark a moment of great significance both for the young person and for the society in which he or she is about to become a full member.

Classic anthropological accounts of rituals in the world's religions place heavy emphasis on rites of passage for adolescents. The term rites of passage was given by van Gennep to ceremonies accompanying life crises; he identified the three major ritual phases of separation, transition, and incorporation.[32] Some rituals that take place at the time of puberty involve the young person literally leaving his or her family or village to live elsewhere, as for some Buddhists who send their sons to live as novices in monasteries; puberty rituals may also involve periods of intense training and initiation into religious doctrine, as in the Jewish bar mitzvah (for boys) and bat mitzvah (for girls). The young person undergoes a period of testing—of knowledge or physical endurance or courage—and then is welcomed back into the family and religious group as an adult member, with new privileges, such as being able to share the bread and wine in the Christian sacrament of the Eucharist or, in traditional societies, to wear the clothing of adults or become sexually active.

Reviewing the Research

As for children and infants, there is little population-based research on religion's influence on the health status or mortality of young people. A review of work on religion, spirituality, and adolescent health outcomes from 1999 to 2009 identified just four studies of physical health outcomes,[33] and Koenig and colleagues found only three.[34] Both reviews did identify large numbers of studies of religion and adolescent *mental health* outcomes, the subject of the next chapter in this volume.

Serious illness or death from disease are rare among adolescents in many societies, which is why external, behaviorally caused deaths from violence, automobile accidents, and suicide—for which rates are higher among adolescents—are of such concern. The higher rates of adolescent mortality that Fuchs observed in Nevada were most likely a combination of these causes. But even within the Utah LDS church, rates of suicide for young men have been shown to differ by their level of religious commitment; non-LDS adolescents and those with lower levels of religious commitment had suicide risks more than three times those of the most highly committed.[35] The US National Longitudinal Study of Adolescent Health (Add Health) found that private religiosity was associated with a lower likelihood of having had suicidal thoughts or attempted suicide;[36] a similar study in Canada also found that adolescent respondents' reports of how important religion was to them were related to fewer instances of suicidal ideation but for females only.[37]

In other contexts, however, religion can increase the risk of suicide, as Emile Durkheim noted in his nineteenth-century studies.[38] A twenty-first-century review of suicide rates in developing countries (where rates for adolescents and young adults are higher than those for other age groups, just as they are in developed countries) found that religions that sanction suicide may increase suicide rates in areas where they are predominant.[39] Another matched control study of adolescent and young adult suicides in China in 2008 found religiosity to be somewhat higher for the suicides than for the controls, not lower.[40] A study in the United Kingdom found that students in schools where their own religious affiliation was in the minority were two to four times more likely to attempt suicide or self-harm.[41] In short, the relationship of religion to suicide and suicidal behavior in adolescents is complex and context dependent but unquestionably significant.

By contrast with the small number of studies measuring adolescent health *status*, there is a very large body of research assessing the association of religion and spirituality with health *practices*, of both the risky and protective types. Adolescence is a critical period for the formation of daily life habits concerning dietary practices, alcohol consumption, smoking, and sexual activities. Decisions made by young people at this period of rapid development and self-discovery may have both short- and long-term impacts on health. Social conditions, including parental and sibling relationships, peer group influences, and neighborhood and community contexts, affect these choices—and have lasting consequences.

Smoking is of particular importance because of its long-term risks for the most serious chronic illnesses, but also because it is most likely to be initiated in adolescence if it is initiated at all. Unlike the rates for adults in the United States, which have been in a long decline, the rates for adolescents have stopped decreasing, according to a 2012 US Surgeon General's report.[42] A review of studies of religion and adolescent tobacco use found that religion was significantly related to lower lifetime, occasional, and regular use of tobacco, but the authors concluded that the primary negative effect of religion was on preventing the initiation of smoking in the first place.[43] Koenig and colleagues cite twenty population-based studies of religion and smoking among adolescents, nearly all of which show that smoking rates are lower among more religiously observant adolescents.[44] Religion may also have an influence on the use of smokeless tobacco, which presents its own health risks; a 2009 US study showed that among men aged 17–29, frequent attenders at religious services were only half as likely as infrequent attenders to use smokeless tobacco products.[45] A 2011 analysis of the National Survey on Drug Use and Health linked the inverse association of religious affiliation with tobacco use to the healthy norms among reference groups of peers and family in the adolescent's social network.[46] Smoking initiation is more likely to take place in adolescence than at any other time in the life course; if religion prevents adolescents from smoking at this vulnerable point in their lives, it alters lifetime risk in a profound way.

There is similarly extensive research on the subject of religiosity and adolescent substance use, including alcohol, marijuana, and other drugs. Substance use may be considered an even more serious risk than smoking because it exposes young persons not only to the risk of the substance itself, but also to criminal penalties that could be dramatically life changing. As in the research literature for cigarette smoking, the research on adolescent substance use overwhelmingly shows that the individual adolescent's level of religiousness and the religiousness of his or her social environment line up very strongly with lower rates of nicotine addiction, binge drinking, and illegal drug use. A recent meta-analysis of twenty-two studies published between 1995 and 2007 showed significantly lower use of cigarettes, alcohol, marijuana, and other illicit drugs among religiously observant adolescents.[47] These associations are similar for white, African American, Hispanic, and American Indian youth in the United States, although the relationships seem to be strongest for highly religious whites.[48] Similar findings linking religiosity to lower adolescent substance use have been found internationally, in studies from Mexico City,[49] Bulgaria,[50] Trinidad,[51] and Jerusalem.[52] These findings have been tied to the dampening effect of religiosity on thrill seeking,[53] the ability of religiosity to buffer the effects of stress on substance use,[54] higher levels of self-control and more negative attitudes toward deviance observed among religious adolescents,[55] and the role of close friends with similar religious values.[56]

Understanding the Patterns

An important advance in understanding the strong relationship between religion and positive health decisions was made in a multilevel analysis of data from an ongoing US national survey of high school students, the Monitoring the Future Study. It found that an adolescent's individual level of religiosity was linked to lower substance use but that the religious context of the school he or she attended was also important, over and above the individual level, underscoring the fact that religion is an important feature of communities and not simply a characteristic of individuals.[57]

We note, however, that most of the surveys cited here are cross-sectional assessments of patterns of adolescent religiosity and substance use. In other words, the research is measuring both things at the same time, and a correlation between the two could be the result of different directions of influence. One scenario, the one that is implicit in most of the interpretations of the data offered in the publications, is that the religious participation of adolescents dampens their enthusiasm for cigarettes, alcohol, or other drugs, and that the lower rates are the result of the adolescent's religious involvement. Given that adolescents are still minor children and subject to the religious influence of their parents, it is not unreasonable to think of the religious influence being present prior to the desire or opportunity to smoke, drink, or use drugs.

But adolescents are on the verge of adulthood. They are forming identities in the crucible of homes and schools and communities where pressures to conform to behavioral norms may be conflicting, even diametrically opposed. What parents expect of a "good kid" may line up nicely with the norms of the priest or youth group at church, but the "cool kids" at school may have a very different set of norms and offer a very desirable kind of social approval. Thus, there is a different possible interpretation of the cross-sectional correlation of religious participation and lower rates of substance use, and that is that adolescents who begin to smoke or use drugs and who experience the disapprobation of parents or religious group members as a result may in response reduce their religious involvement. They thus select themselves out of groups to whose expectations they no longer conform. In more severe circumstances, they may even be shut out of, shunned by, or excommunicated from a strict religious group that will not tolerate their behavior. This would be an extreme example of social control. But whether it is voluntary or involuntary, the separation of the adolescent from the religious group that he or she may have been a part of from birth would result in just the same data pattern of "insiders" with lower rates of substance use and "outsiders" with higher rates. With studies taken at a single point in time, it is impossible to know which of the two directions of influence is operating or which is predominant.

Regardless of whether religious social influence, social selection, or both are playing a role in substance use, religious involvement is clearly associated with lower risk. The setting of that pattern in adolescence may have profound consequences for health over the entire life course.

However, the role of religion for another adolescent health risk—sexual behavior—is more complex and potentially more negative. Religion's impact on many indicators of sexual behavior, including age at first intercourse, oral versus vaginal sex, the viewing of Internet pornography, the number of sexual partners, the prevalence of sexually transmitted diseases, and the use of contraception, have all been studied in samples of adolescents. In a recent review of the literature, Mark Regnerus notes that in the United States, both denominational differences (such as Catholic vs. Protestant) and religiosity per se (that is, participation in services) are influential in the timing of first sexual intercourse.[58] He also notes that the association between religiousness and delay in the initiation of sexual activity is stronger for whites than for African Americans. In his analysis of the Add Health study data, he finds that whites, African Americans, and Hispanics who attended church most often and who said that religion was very important to them were the least likely to have experienced first sexual intercourse during the course of the study.[59]

These data are longitudinal, not cross-sectional, and thus less subject to a selection interpretation, since the adolescent's report of the importance of religion was made prior to the initiation of sexual activity. In an analysis of a different set of data from the first wave of National Study of Youth and Religion, this one cross-sectional, Regnerus finds similar associations of religious attendance and importance of religion with having had sexual intercourse, having had oral sex, and the frequency of using Internet porn, and also that evangelical Protestants and black Protestants are more likely than Catholics and mainstream Protestants to have had sex.[60] Thus, there is some evidence that adolescent religious involvement plays a positive, protective role by significantly delaying the young person's entry into sexual activity.

But the effects of religion may not be protective once sexual activity has (inevitably for most adolescents) begun. In an analysis of data from the National Survey of Family Growth, Kramer and colleagues found denominational differences in the rate of contraceptive use among adolescent girls (but not adult women): rates of not using any contraception were fifteen times higher among Catholics, five times higher among fundamentalist Protestants, and nine times higher among those with no religious affiliation, compared with mainstream Protestants.[61] Bearman and Brückner studied the practice of virginity pledges sponsored by the Southern Baptist Church and found that, while such pledges had a significant delaying effect in initiating intercourse, when they eventually did have intercourse, pledgers were less likely to use contraception than nonpledgers.[62] In a further analysis of data from Add Health, they found that pledgers, although they started being sexually active later, rapidly caught up with nonpledgers in their rates of acquiring human papilloma virus, chlamydia, gonorrhea, and trichomoniasis, and they were less likely to have ever seen a doctor for these conditions.[63] These findings are all from US data where the risk is for serious but treatable non-life-threatening conditions. But similar findings of the importance of religious group membership for abstinence (but not condom use) are reported from the Zimbabwe Demographic and Health Survey,[64] where the risk for HIV is much greater. As with other issues, the role of religion in the sexual behavior of adolescents is complex and multifaceted but clearly intertwined with other factors, and it is incumbent upon researchers to include religion in their research if they are to have a full view of the social context of adolescent sexual behavior and decision making.

Thus far, this section has summarized research on religion's association with specific health *risk* behaviors common among adolescents. Good health behaviors, however, include not only risk avoidance but also the promotion of positive practices like eating regular nutritious meals, getting exercise, and getting enough sleep. Wallace and Forman published a wide-ranging analysis of religion's role in both avoiding risk and promoting health; their findings from the Monitoring the Future study of US high school seniors showed that higher levels of religious importance and religious attendance were significantly associated with lower risk of carrying a weapon, getting into fights, driving while drinking, smoking cigarettes, binge drinking, and smoking marijuana.[65] At the same time, religious attendance and reporting that religion is important were also associated with the positive, health-promoting behaviors of eating breakfast, having green vegetables and fruit in their diets, exercising frequently, using seatbelts, and getting at least seven hours of sleep.[66] A more recent systematic review of studies of religion and both positive and risk-reducing health behaviors among adolescents found that, after adjustments for other variables, more than 75 percent of the studies showed a significant beneficial association of religion with more positive and fewer risky behaviors.[67] Such studies give us a bigger picture of the range of health behaviors and their individual associations with adolescent religiosity, but more research is needed to show how and if such behaviors cluster in groups to form the basis of healthy or unhealthy lifestyles that are carried from adolescence into adulthood.

The period of adolescence is of tremendous importance in understanding the determinants of health over the life course. Adolescents are developing rapidly—physically, socially, emotionally, cognitively—and they are extremely vulnerable to the environment in which that development takes place. Adolescent brain development, particularly in the prefrontal cortex, according to Candace Alcorta, "creates a unique developmental window" for the "experiential sculpting of our social and moral brains."[68]Alcorta goes on to argue that religions create emotionally evocative experiences through the use of music and ritual; these experiences trigger neuronal processes in those rapidly developing areas, linking emotional value and reward with the religious frameworks that "reduce indecision and anxiety and promote in-group cooperation."[69]

Kuh and colleagues speak of adolescent development as the period of the development of "personal capital,"[70] when consequential decisions—not only about healthy lifestyles but also about education, work, friendships, and social group membership—are made. Those decisions are made in socially advantaged or disadvantaged contexts of families, schools, and communities that may be widely different in societies like the United States that have high levels of income inequality. The association of religion with (mostly) protective health behaviors in the studies reviewed here is over and above the influence of other social factors and would be especially salient for adolescents with weaker supports from other social institutions. This is the groundwork for understanding the cumulative effect of factors influencing health in adulthood and old age.

Religion and Health in Adulthood

The conditions of childhood and adolescence—physical and socioeconomic—have a profound effect on health in adulthood. This is the underpinning of the social determinants perspective, which argues that the effects of the environment work themselves out over years and decades and that the conditions of early life have a special and far-reaching impact. So the groundwork for health in adulthood has already been laid in early life—and the payoff, so to speak, really comes when individuals reach adulthood and especially middle age. We have been arguing that religion is an influence on the lives of most individuals from childhood and often continues through adolescence and young adulthood. For many, the direct experience of religious practice and involvement begins in early childhood and is repeated at regular intervals in expanding cycles, and, for some people, it occupies significant amounts of time in adulthood.

The most important life course ritual in adulthood for most people is certainly marriage. Not all people get married, and not all marriage ceremonies are religious, but in many societies both of these proportions are quite high, and marriage remains a time when even otherwise secular people are often exposed to religious practices. Because all religions have an interest in perpetuating themselves, the event of a new, potentially procreative union is an occasion of significance to a religious group. "Blessing" the marriage implies the support of the witnessing community for the couple (and their future offspring). In religiously homogeneous societies, most marriages would necessarily take place between individuals of the same religion; even in religiously heterogeneous societies like the United States, the majority of first marriages are between individuals of the same or closely related religions.[71]

A far less frequent but nevertheless important religious ritual of adulthood would be an individual's induction into a religious order or ordination to the priesthood. In some cases, this has been an alternative to marriage, for instance in the case of religions in which clergy or members of religious orders are celibate, such as Roman Catholicism or Buddhism. These rituals of adulthood are rare but repeatable events. Certainly people can be married more than once. A Catholic priest could leave the priesthood, or a monk could leave his order to get married and then become an ordained Episcopalian priest. Some individuals could live secular lives and never marry and therefore not experience any of these life course adulthood rituals directly. The embarking of the young adult into a marriage or a dedicated religious life implies a major commitment of time and self into old age.

Reviewing the Research

Research on religion and measurable population health indicators among adults has proliferated since the 1980s, and there are also many reviews of this literature. In this section, we undertake a new review of studies of religion and mortality specifically focused on the population-based literature, drawing on and updating all of the previous reviews and using a graphical approach. We review both group-level studies comparing specific religious groups and individual-level studies based on surveys. Studies included in this survey met several criteria:

- All were published in English in peer-reviewed sources.
- The work reported was based on vital statistics, complete population census, or probability-based representative national or regional samples.

- The studies took mortality from all causes as the outcome.
- Findings were reported in the form of standardized mortality ratios, hazard ratios, risk ratios, or odds ratios.

Sometimes multiple publications drawing on the same sample met the criteria; to save space, we included only the publication with the longest follow-up period and/or the full sample. In the individual-level studies, we report the findings from the fully adjusted models, after sociodemographic and health status covariates are included and potential explanatory mechanisms have been tested. The findings reported here are thus the most conservative estimates of the effects of religion on mortality.

We identified thirteen group-level studies of the Amish, Seventh-day Adventists, Mormons, and various clergy groups reported in eleven publications.[72] This list, which draws primarily from Idler with some more recent studies added,[73] includes published reports that began appearing in the late 1970s and 1980s, when the National Institutes of Health had a program of research on "low-risk populations." The graph shows the standardized mortality ratio (SMR) for mortality from all causes and statistical significance as reported in each study, usually for males and females separately (Figure 18.1). The values show the ratio of the age-adjusted death rate of

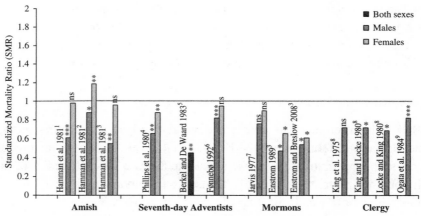

Note: SMR = 1.0 *if the mortality rate of the religious group is not different from the reference population. SMRs less than 1.0 mean the religious group has a lower mortality rate than the comparison population.* *p<.05, **p<.01, ***p<.001

Reference populations:

1. *Non-Amish in county, ages 40–69*   4. *American Cancer Society study*   7. *Population of Alberta, Canada*
2. *Non-Amish in county, ages 70+*   5. *Dutch population*   8. *US white males*
3. *US whites*   6. *European population*   9. *Japanese males*

Source: *Idler 2011 and updated reviews of PubMed and Medline.*

FIGURE 18.1 Standardized mortality ratios (SMRs) for specific religious groups compared to standard populations.

members of the religious group to the rate for the population of the county, state, or nation. (The comparison group used in the study is indicated in the chart notes.) If the SMR value in the study is less than 1.0, then the SMR for the religious group is less than the larger population's rate; if it is higher than 1.0, the religious group has a higher mortality rate. Almost all of the bars fall below the center line, showing a consistent pattern of lower mortality for those who are members of these three religious groups or the clergy compared with the standard populations. For example, the study by Berkel and de Waard[74] showed that Dutch Seventh-day Adventists had an SMR of just 45, or less than half that of the Dutch population in general.

Overall, most of the studies show mortality rates for the Amish, Seventh-day Adventists, and Mormons in the United States, Canada, and Europe that are 20 to 40 percent lower than the rate for comparison populations. In addition, there is a mortality advantage for males compared with females in every case where gender-specific findings are reported. The overall pattern is striking and even more so in that the comparison is being made with populations in wealthy, industrialized societies with high life expectancies, and in the United States at least, the comparison is made to a general population that is itself religiously observant. Note the exception for Amish women, whose rate was scarcely different from that of women in the surrounding communities.[75]

Fuchs's observation of Mormon mortality rates back in the 1970s noted that the differences between Utahans and Nevadans were present at every age, but the differences increased from infancy to childhood to adolescence, peaked in middle age, and then declined again. Systematic age-specific studies of both Mormons[76] and Seventh-day Adventists[77] show a similar pattern, with the biggest contrasts between the religious groups and comparison populations occurring in adulthood. Many of these studies also reported cause-specific mortality findings that are not shown here to save space; those additional findings are summarized in Idler.[78] The predominant causes of death are from cardiovascular disease and cancer, and many of the studies report cause-specific rates for the religious groups far lower than those for the comparison populations. To return to Fuchs's original point, the primary causes of death in modern societies are related to lifestyles and behaviors that have health consequences; because it takes decades for those health effects to accumulate, the point of impact is in middle age.

Age is important in another way as well. Researchers with access to SDA church records have examined the impact of a person's age at the time of entry into the church; several studies have found that, even within these strict churches with overall lower mortality rates, those who were born into the religion and remained in it had lower mortality rates than those who joined later in life.[79] In the Fønnebø study in Norway, men and women who joined the SDA church before they were 19 years old had overall mortality rates that were just 69 and 59 percent, respectively, that of the Norwegian population; those who joined after the age of 35 had SMRs of 89 percent and 103 percent, a much smaller advantage for later-joining men compared with earlier-joining men and a rate for women that was actually slightly higher than that for other Norwegian women.[80] This is a paradigmatic illustration of a life course epidemiological impact. Because religion is a lifelong influence for many in these religious groups and because they have such strict low-health-risk lifestyles, the mortality differences with the general population are dramatic. Moreover, even within these groups, there are internal differences that privilege those with the longest involvement.

We next examine findings for the other type of study, those that analyze individual-level mortality data for adults who participated in random-sample surveys that asked about religious participation. Using the list in Idler and a more recent review of Medline and PubMed, we identified twenty-three studies reported in twenty-two publications.[81] In these studies (summarized in Figures 18.2–18.4), large numbers of randomly chosen adults reported on their religious involvement—usually defined by attendance at religious services—at the beginning of the study; the participants were then followed over time. This type of study focuses on the association of the individual's level of religiousness (no matter which religious tradition, if any) with his or her survival over time; this study design can thus link reports of religious observance made by the individual with health outcomes that take place years later. Another advantage is that such studies can adjust for individual health status at the start of the study, thereby reducing to some extent the likelihood that the findings are due to self-selection or dropping out rather than to the influence of religion itself. Individual-level studies are also different from group-level studies in that there is little attention to the particular religion or faith tradition to which an individual belongs. Religious affiliation is often not even known; the only indicator of religious involvement in many studies is the level of religious participation through attendance at services, as reported by the respondent. Thus the dimension of religiousness that is being considered in these studies is the extent of participation or involvement in religion (if any), while the specific content of that involvement—the beliefs or practices engaged in—is unknown.

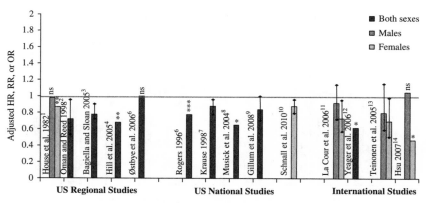

Note: *Hazard, relative risk, or odds ratio = 1.0 if the mortality risk of those with frequent religious attendance is not different from that of the reference group (those with no/low religious attendance). Values below 1.0 signify a lower hazard of mortality for frequent attenders; values higher than 1.0 indicate a higher hazard. Statistical significance was reported in studies by 95% Confidence Intervals or *p<.05, **p<.01, ***p<.001, ns = not significant*

Study samples representing:

1. *Tecumseh County, MI, ages 35–69*
2. *Marin County, CA, ages 55+*
3. *NC, CT, MA, IA, ages 65+*
4. *TX, CA, NM, AZ, CO, ages 65+*
5. *UT, ages 65+*

6. *US, ages 55+*
7. *US Medicare, ages 65+*
8. *US, ages 25+*
9. *US, ages 40+*
10. *US women, ages 50–79*

11. *Glostrup, Denmark, age 70*
12. *Taiwan, ages 70+*
13. *Finland, ages 65+*
14. *Taiwan, ages 65+*

Source: *Idler 2011 and updated reviews of PubMed and Medline.*

FIGURE 18.2 Adjusted hazard, relative risk, or odds ratios for all causes of mortality for those with highest rates of religious attendance.

The studies in Figure 18.2 calculated risk of mortality for people who report a high level of religious participation compared with those who reported attending services infrequently or not at all; the center grid line at 1.0 represents the risk of mortality for respondents who reported little or no religious participation. The bars show the risk of mortality and its statistical significance for respondents who attended services the most frequently, taking into account their age, health status, and other important social factors at the start of the study. Most of the studies show a reduced risk for those who report high levels of religious engagement. For example, Schnall and colleagues found that US women in the Women's Health Initiative study who attended religious services frequently had a statistically significant 12 percent lower risk of all-cause mortality over the following seven years than those who did not.[82] While not many of these studies differentiated their findings by gender (by contrast with the group-level studies summarized earlier), it appears that women show lower mortality risks than men at the same level of religious attendance, thereby appearing to benefit more from religious participation.

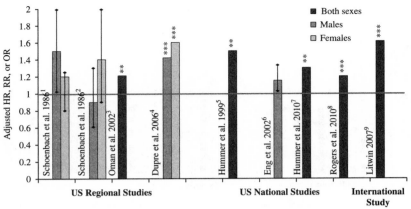

Note: *Hazard, relative risk, or odds ratio = 1.0 if the mortality risk of those with no/low religious attendance is not different from that of the reference group (those with frequent religious attendance). Values above 1.0 indicate a higher hazard of mortality for no/low attenders; values lower than 1.0 indicate a lower hazard.*
Statistical significance was reported in studies by 95% Confidence Intervals or *p<.05, **p<.01, ***p<.001, ns = not significant

Study samples representing:
1. *GA, whites ages 15+*
2. *GA, blacks ages 15+*
3. *Alameda County., CA, ages 21+*
4. *NC, ages 65+*

5. *US, ages 18–89*
6. *US health professionals, ages 40–75*
7. *US, ages 51–61*
8. *US, ages 18+*

9. *Israel, ages 70+*

Source: *Idler 2011 and updated reviews of PubMed and Medline.*

FIGURE 18.3 Adjusted hazard, relative risk, or odds ratios for all causes of mortality for those with lowest rates of religious attendance.

Another group of studies made those who attended services most frequently the reference group (Figure 18.3). In this group of studies, the bars show the mortality risk for individuals who attended religious services *least* often, with values above the center line representing higher risks of mortality. As in Figure 18.2, most of the studies show a higher risk for those with less frequent attendance after taking into account individual health status and social and demographic factors at the start of the study. For example, with data from US respondents aged 51–61 in the Health and Retirement Survey from 1992 to 2000, after all other factors were taken into account, Hummer and colleagues found that those who never attended services had a 34 percent higher hazard of mortality during that eight-year period than those who attended religious services once a week or more.[83] Gender-specific results are more mixed in this group, but women who never attended services show a consistently higher risk of mortality than women who did.

Attendance at services is not the only possible indicator of religiousness; other measures of religiousness include the degree to which a person looks to a religious perspective as a way to cope with stress (religious coping); the personal sense of the importance of religion; the frequency of attention to religious media, such as TV or radio programs; the strength of religious belief; the frequency of prayer, or engagement in other private religious practices. Together, these constitute a set of indicators of more private, personal, internal experiences of religion by comparison with the social participation of public observances. Some of the studies reported in earlier figures collected data about one or more of these indicators in addition to attendance at religious services and calculated mortality risks for those who reported the most private religious experiences compared to those who reported few or none (Figure 18.4). The center line in this graph represents the risk for those with no or low levels of private religiousness. In this chart there is no consistent pattern; some of the bars are below the line, indicating a lower risk for those with greater private religiousness, but some are above, indicating a higher risk, and almost none show a statistically significant effect. For example, in the study of the Women's Health Initiative data, Schnall and colleagues found that those who reported

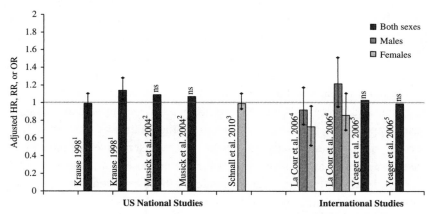

Note: Hazard, relative risk, or odds ratio = 1.0 if the mortality risk of those with a high level of private religiousness is not different from that of the reference group (those with low private religiousness). Values above 1.0 indicate a higher hazard of mortality for those with high levels of private religiousness; values lower than 1.0 indicate a lower hazard. Bars represent different studies or different measures of private religiousness (nonorganizational religiosity, religious coping, importance of religion, watching religious TV or listening to radio, religious beliefs, private religious practices) in the same study.
Statistical significance was reported in studies by 95% Confidence Intervals or *p<.05, **p<.01, ***p<.001, ns = not significant

Study samples representing:
1. US Medicare, ages 65+   4. Glostrup, Denmark, age 70
2. US, ages 25+   5. Taiwan, ages 65+
3. US women, ages 50–79

Source: Idler 2011 and updated reviews of PubMedand Medline.

FIGURE 18.4 Adjusted hazard, relative risk, or odds ratios for all causes of mortality for those with high levels of private religiousness.

receiving a great deal of strength and comfort from religion had only a 1 percent lower hazard of mortality than those who reported none.[84] Similarly, Musick and colleagues found that there was no distinguishable difference in mortality between those who (i) reported a high level of subjective spirituality or (ii) reported engaging in more private devotional activities and those who were less spiritual or did not report a high level of private devotional activity.[85] Here again, where gender-specific findings are reported, women have somewhat lower hazards than men.

To this point, we have focused on studies of mortality. There are also many studies in the scientific literature of other health outcomes, including the incidence and prevalence of chronic disease (especially cardiovascular disease and cancer), infectious disease, and disability. Some of these disease (also called morbidity) studies come from strict religious groups. As long ago as 1959, Wynder and colleagues identified significantly lower rates of both cancer and coronary artery disease among Seventh-day Adventists by reviewing hospital records in California, Illinois, Washington, DC, and Massachusetts.[86] A recent study of new cases (incidence) of cancer among the Ohio Amish found that the age-adjusted rate for all new cancers among the Amish was just 60 percent of the rate for all adults in Ohio, meaning it was 40 percent lower; for tobacco-related cancers, the incidence was an extremely low 37 percent, or 63 percent lower than that of all adults in the state.[87]

However, most of the studies of religion and disease rates come from individual-level survey-based studies. The systematic reviews by Powell, Shahabi, and Thoresen[88] and Koenig, King, and Carson[89] take a disease-based approach in their organization, grouping studies by diagnosis. Both reviews also include many studies of nonrepresentative (often patient-based) samples that are less relevant for our purposes, but the sampling is clearly identified, and we refer the reader to these excellent sources, along with Koenig, McCullough, and Larson's original *Handbook*.[90]

Powell, Shahabi, and Thoresen concluded in their systematic review with a levels-of-evidence approach, that the research finding that religious attendance is protective against overall mortality was "persuasive."[91] There was no similarly strong judgment for any other disease or disability outcome or any other (non-attendance-based) measure of religiousness. For example, for cardiovascular disease, they found, on the basis of four representative studies, "some" evidence that religion or spirituality was protective. Koenig, King, and Carson's more recent review lists thirty-eight representative, population-based studies that analyze the association of some measure of religiousness with cardiovascular disease, hypertension, inflammatory indicators, and cerebrovascular disease.[92] Of the thirty-eight, nineteen studies find a protective effect for religiousness, eleven show no significant association, seven show a significant association of religiousness with poorer outcomes, and one study had mixed findings.

For diabetes and endocrine function, Koenig, King, and Carson list fourteen population-based studies.[93] Four of these showed that some measure of religiousness (usually attendance at services) was associated with lower incidence or prevalence; seven showed no association; and two showed a negative association, while one simply compared rates for Indian Hindus and Muslims (Hindus had higher rates). For cancer incidence and prevalence, there were just two population-based studies; one showed no association between religious attendance and cancer, and the other showed lower cancer rates for those who attended more often. Among ten studies of religiousness and pain, two found religion associated with less pain, four found religion associated with more pain, two studies had mixed findings, and in two there was no association. Overall, this cursory summary of Koenig, King, and Carson's[94] recent findings shows them to be similar to the earlier conclusions of the Powell, Shahabi, and Thoresen[95] review—that the evidence for an association of religiousness with any specific disease diagnosis is mixed. More studies have been done, and there are more significant outcomes for cardiovascular and related diseases than for other disease groups, but overall the findings are inconsistent.

In many ways it is easier to study mortality than it is to study new cases or current cases of disease, and it is especially easier in the United States, where death records are centralized but health records are not. Death records are also official, having been completed and signed by appropriate professionals, while surveys that ask respondents to report on their own conditions may vary in accuracy. Moreover, some important causes of death, such as suicide or homicide or other external causes, are not related to disease. Thus, for many reasons, mortality records present a more complete and valid health outcome for study. Studies of religious attendance and mortality are also necessarily longitudinal studies, with clear time ordering and the opportunity to control for health and other important demographic characteristics at the start of the study, while many disease-outcome studies are cross-sectional with all factors measured at the same time.

Koenig, King, and Carson rated all of the studies in the *Handbook* for quality;[96] the twelve best-rated studies examining mortality as an outcome all had a measure of religious attendance (as opposed to a more subjective aspect of religion) at the start of the study. Among those twelve studies, 92 percent found that religious attendance was associated with a lower risk of mortality. The persuasive evidence from all of these studies, like those reviewed in this chapter, is that more frequent participation in public religious observances is associated with lower risk of mortality over periods of years or even decades. All of these studies adjusted for age and other demographic characteristics—gender, race/ethnicity, marital status, education, income, and, most important, health status—at the start of the study, so that the statistical association of religious attendance with mortality was independent of such potential confounders. Together, they show a pattern of longer life expectancy for those who actively participate in religious services. This is not particular to adherents to one religion or another but true for members of all of the religious traditions present in the societies where these population-representative studies took place. It is true that most of the studies have been performed in the United States, but the United States is a highly religiously diverse nation. Studies are beginning to appear from other countries, even very secular ones. There is now a solid body of evidence that, by the time of midlife, when adults have settled into patterns of religious observance or nonobservance, those exposures matter for life expectancy.

Understanding the Patterns

The advantage that the individual-level studies (Figures 18.2–18.4) have over the group-level studies (Figure 18.1) is that the survey interviews from which these data come ask for information not only about religious involvement but also about some of the practices or social conditions to which religion might be linked. That could help explain the association over time. All of these studies controlled for such factors, taking many of the possible mechanisms or intervening pathways by which religion might impart an advantage into account. So what are these mechanisms or pathways?

Building on Durkheim's work exploring the benefits of social engagement—including religious engagement—for health, we can describe the possible explanations as being based on social support, social control, and social capital. The first is probably the most obvious. Social support comes from a connection to a caring community that anchors an individual in relationships that provide tangible, instrumental support, expressive comfort, and intimacy. Face-to-face meetings and participation in religious activities expose an individual to a whole set of people whom he or she might not otherwise meet. Thus, individuals who belong to religious congregations have an additional potential to build friendships and social ties above and beyond those that they have through other venues. Moreover, ties to a religious congregation are positively correlated with having more of other types of ties—to family and other community organizations.[97]

There is evidence that the warm, friendly, helping-hand functions of religious groups—the "carrots" of social interaction—provide a distinct health benefit. In a study of the population of Alameda County, California, Strawbridge and colleagues found that individuals who attended religious services once a week or more at the start of the study were more likely to (i) increase the number of close friends and relatives whom they saw during the course of the study, (ii) increase their nonreligious community group memberships, and (iii) stay married to the same person throughout the course of the study.[98] Those who attended religious services once per week or more had a 36 percent lower hazard of mortality over the following twenty-eight years compared with those who attended services infrequently or not at all; when ties to friends, relatives, community groups, and spouses were included, this difference was reduced to 31 percent—still a significant difference, but it shows that some of the benefit of religious group membership over time came through its association with other forms of social connection that have their own independent protective effect.

The "sticks" of social regulation or social control that religious groups appear to wield over members' behavior is a second possible explanation for the association of religious observance with better health. In some religious groups, there may be explicit teachings about avoiding certain health risks such as smoking; in others, there may simply be normative patterns of less risk-prone behavior. Regardless, the research literature shows a strong tendency of adolescents who are religiously observant not to smoke, use drugs, or engage in other risky health behaviors. Perhaps to some extent because of the patterns established in adolescence, religiously observant adults show similarly lower levels of smoking both in the United States and internationally.[99] Moreover, in a large US sample, religious attendance was the only type of social contact significantly associated with a lower likelihood of smoking.[100] Similar patterns are evident with regard to substance use in adulthood; adults who had never used cannabis were less likely to start using it if they attended religious services regularly than if they did not.[101] Alcohol use is also strongly inversely associated with religion; a recent analysis of the US Health and Retirement Survey showed that 79.6 percent of alcohol abstainers but just 36.4 percent of those who drink more than three drinks per day said that religion was very important to them.[102] However, in this study and many others, the lowest mortality risk is found for those in the middle, who drink a moderate amount of alcohol, making complete abstinence due to religion an added, not a reduced risk.

The practices associated with religious observance do help to explain the association of religion with better health. Strawbridge and colleagues showed that, even though religious attenders were less likely to be smokers in the first place, those who did smoke and who also attended religious services at the start of the study were more likely to quit smoking during the course of the follow-up than smokers who were not attending services, and this reduction in risk partially explained the overall lower mortality hazard of the frequent attenders.[103] Schnall and colleagues, in the Women's Health Initiative Study, found an initial adjusted hazard for mortality that was 20 percent lower for those who attended religious services more than once per week, compared with those who had not attended in the last month, but when they took smoking and alcohol use into account, the difference was reduced to 11 percent.[104] Again, as with social support, the lower rate of smoking and alcohol consumption among frequent religious attenders partially (although not completely) explains their higher rate of survival.

The third major reason for an association of religious observance with better health is social capital. Health inequality that is tied to income inequality has a complicated relationship to religion. Religion may be seen as increasing income inequality, decreasing it, or changing how people perceive it. Religious origins and influences may have an indirect effect on health inequality through the profound influence of income inequality. Economically advantaged adults have more of the things that promote good health: a safe neighborhood to live in, good food to eat, clean air to breathe, and pure water to drink. In the United States (although to a lesser extent elsewhere), access to health insurance and affordable, quality medical care is a function of economic advantage. Koenig, King, and Carson[105] report on forty-four studies examining the relationship between religion and spirituality and disease screening and twenty-seven studies on the association between religion and adherence to treatment. In both groups, a majority of studies showed a positive association between higher religiousness and greater use of medical care. For example, Benjamins and Buck, reporting on a study in Mexico, found that survey participants who attended services frequently were 42 percent more likely to have had blood pressure screening and 40 percent more likely to have had diabetes screening than those who did not attend services.[106]

In another study, the influence of religion on screening behavior appeared to be direct and not a function of access to health insurance;

research on 320 Muslim Iranian women showed that women who agreed that trying to keep one's health is a Muslim responsibility were significantly more likely to have had mammography.[107] Knowledge of, access to, and appropriate use of the healthcare system represents a type of social capital, and it has an obvious and direct impact on health, even in the short term. Over a lifetime, preventive services and monitoring of health and lifestyle patterns can have profound effects on health—and middle age is the period when accumulated risks result in premature mortality.

Religious social capital is intertwined with secular social and economic capital in complex ways that unfold over the life course and have their greatest effects on health in middle age, where all mortality is premature. Kuh and Ben-Shlomo develop the concept of "health capital" to convey the "accumulation of biological resources, inherited and acquired during earlier stages of life, which determine current health and future health potential, including resilience to future environmental insults."[108] The health capital that one holds in adulthood began accumulating or failing to do so in infancy and childhood, according to individual circumstances of advantage or disadvantage. Then, as with savings accounts or pensions—some of which may even have been begun before birth with family trust funds—decades of deposits, small or large, result in dramatically different amounts of capital by middle age. This is not just a metaphor; there is strong evidence that the same social determinants that benefit individuals with more financial capital will produce more health capital as well. The linkage between health capital and "real" capital, in other words, is not metaphorical at all.

Our point is that religion is important as a social determinant of health because, while it mostly aligns with better health, it does not necessarily align with greater economic and social advantage. Religious social capital may play its most important role precisely for those individuals and in those communities where there is little secular capital. The research reviewed thus far shows religion to be an independent influence in health, one that may promote, undercut, or mitigate the effects of other social determinants. The picture of the social determinants of health is simply not complete without it.

Religion and Health in Old Age and at the End of Life

Old age is the outcome of a life lived with sufficient health and resources to be sustained for seven decades or more. Unlike the life stages that have gone before, however, most of the world's religious traditions have no rituals to mark the onset of old age and signify the transition to a new stage of life, despite the fact that this stage has distinctly new challenges and patterns. One exception to this is the Hindu recognition of sannyasi, a state that some older persons may achieve by giving up their possessions and living a life of asceticism. But a religious marking of the entry into a specific old-age role is an exception, even within Hinduism. The religious practices and rituals that we tend to think of in the context of old age are those that take place at the end of life—marking not entry into this final stage of life but exit from it. However, the rites associated with death, to be found in some form in all religions, are not age specific. Thus, unlike the beginnings of the life course stages of childhood, adolescence, and adulthood, there are no widely practiced rituals that open or even distinctively close the period of late life.

Even in the absence of rituals specifically to mark old age, many older adults do continue engaging in annual, weekly, and daily religious practices until the very end of life. Religious involvement in old age is likely to be a continuation of patterns of religious participation in midlife. There are many studies of the forms and frequency of religious participation in old age in the United States (although few in other societies); they tend to show that adults aged 65 and older attend religious services more often than younger persons, in addition to professing deeper religious beliefs and engaging in the private practice of religion more often.[109] The weekly practice of attending religious services (common to all of the major religions in the United States) is particularly important; older persons attend services at a higher rate than any younger age group.[110] In a longitudinal study of the religious practices and beliefs of older persons in New Haven, Connecticut, researchers found that the average level of weekly religious attendance fell hardly at all among surviving members of the sample from 1982 to 1994.[111] In the last six months of life, attendance did decline somewhat, but respondents still attended services an average of twice per month.[112]

Regular attendance at religious services provides the older person with a repeated opportunity to experience the ritual of religious worship in all its many facets. The weekly cycle of attendance breaks the routine of other days of the week, which for many older people may be marked by social isolation and lack of structure. Religious congregations often provide transportation and accommodations for the disabled or elderly that are unmatched by other social institutions; reaching out to those in need is a part of the mission of the institution. One of the most notable benefits of including older and socially isolated persons in religious services is that it brings them into an intergenerational social setting. This mixing of people at all stages of the life course is in stark contrast to the narrowly age-segregated settings in which many, even most, elderly persons in industrial societies live.

A religious institution, in fact, is the only social institution—perhaps besides the family—where infants and the extremely aged and everyone in between congregate on a regular basis for the same purpose, with common values, traditions, and practices. Long-time members of religious groups have watched each others' families be born, grow up, and then have families of their own. They have participated in and observed each others' life events, both happy and sad, providing a sense of continuity and meaning and a larger context for daily joys and sorrows. The practice of religious ritual in extreme old age draws a thread through years and decades of life, linking the individual to those who have gone before and those who follow, undergirding a sense of identity and integrity despite the inevitable losses of this phase of the life course.

Many religious groups also provide care to their members through institutions established specifically for the care of the widowed, the ill, the infirm, and the dying. Most if not all nineteenth-century homes for the aged in the United States were started by Christian and Jewish groups, and even in the mid-twentieth century, most remained under religious auspices.[113] Perhaps most notable among these religiously motivated institutions is the hospice movement, which provides care for the dying. This innovative institution was conceived by its founder, Dame Cicely Saunders, as a quasi-religious, quasi-medical institution; the spiritual care of the dying was at the center of its mission, along with a scientific approach to pain and symptom management.[114]

The life cycle for everyone ends in death, and in industrialized societies this occurs most often in old age, increasingly in middle to late old age. Bereavement is a crisis of existence that breaks into the normal routines of everyday life. Death is a threat to individuals and but it is also a threat to their social groups. Rituals that take place at the time of death bring comfort to the bereaved through the response of the community.

Religious rituals provide comfort in one sense because they offer a guide for what to do and what to say in a strange and threatening situation, telling us exactly how to rise to the occasion with a dignity befitting its seriousness. They also offer a strategy to cope with the profound unknown represented by death. In rituals around death, families and religious communities come together both to remember the one who is gone and to assert the existence and vitality of the social group despite its loss. As Alain de Botton writes, religious rituals "give us lines to recite and songs to sing while they carry us across the treacherous regions of our psyches."[115] The religious community acts together, using words and songs that were given by generations long ago, and representing its collective existence for the future.

Religions also attend to the more practical side of death. They have long performed a function of utmost importance to the health of the community by providing direction for the disposal of the corpse. In the earliest human civilizations, there is evidence of religion's relevance to death through burial practices and goods deposited with the deceased to accompany them on their journey to the other world.[116] Dead bodies must be disposed of in a way that is respectful of the deceased and will not spread infection among the living. Cremation is practiced by Hindus (see chapter 13), Sikhs, and increasingly Christians, while burial is most common in other religions, but all religious traditions connect death rituals with their fundamental beliefs about life and what happens afterward. As in birth and marriage rituals, the religious community asserts its agency, manifesting itself in the lives of even the most secular individuals in even the most secular societies.

The Jewish ritual of mourning provides an example of an extensive ritual. It begins with the funeral, which must be held within twenty-four hours of the death and is followed by the family's seven days of sitting *shiva*, during which they mourn their loss and receive the respects of the community. That ritual is followed by thirty days of reduced responsibilities for family members; the grieving period culminates in the unveiling of the deceased's headstone, one year after the death. This extended ritual evokes the support of the community and provides a set of stages for the bereaved to move through and a guide to the meanings that they are to absorb, with a clear destination—the eventual resumption of everyday life.

Reviewing the Research

The research on religion and mortality in old age is an extension of the research on religion in adulthood. If we go back to Fuchs's observation of age-specific death rates in Utah and Nevada, the biggest contrasts were among the middle-aged, but there were still significant survival advantages among Utahans aged 65 and older. One might reason that the losses due to mortality among the less religious could have played themselves out by the time people reach old age, and therefore the differences would be reduced. On the other hand, one might expect a continuing influence as the causes of death shift even more toward chronic disease and the life course influences on health mount.

Some of the studies described thus far reported results on middle-aged adults only;[117] many reported results for all adults, including the elderly and middle-aged and even adults as young as 15,[118] while the rest reported on elderly respondents specifically.[119] The large number of studies of religious involvement and mortality that are limited to elderly persons reflects the recognition of both the importance of social factors in general as determinants of the health of elderly persons and the important role of religious group membership in particular among those social connections.

Only one group-level study that we surveyed reports results specifically for the aged population (Figure 18.1). Hamman and colleagues' study of Amish men and women over age 70 showed a smaller difference between Amish men and the standard population than any other study in this group, and the SMR for Amish women was actually higher than it was for non-Amish elderly women.[120] In this single group-level study, the mortality advantage for the Amish does not seem to extend into old age. For the individual-level studies, however, the results are different. Both the largest and smallest reductions in mortality in the individual-level studies that we survey come from studies of elderly-only populations (Figure 18.2), making the results for old-age populations not very different from those for middle-aged populations, where those who attended religious services more frequently almost always showed a lower risk of mortality than those who never attended. In studies exploring risk for those with low levels of religious participation (Figure 18.3), the two studies that examined only the elderly—one focused on persons older than 65[121] and another on those older than 70[122]—were the two studies with the biggest differences; in both, respondents with low religious attendance had significantly greater risks of mortality than those who attended more frequently. When the dimension of religion examined was private activity or subjective feelings rather than public attendance (Figure 18.4), a majority of the studies had old-age samples; however, these studies found few or no significant differences in mortality over time between those who scored high on private religiousness and those who scored low. As in middle age, the aspect of religious participation that appears to be associated with lower mortality rates among older people is regular attendance at religious services; other dimensions, such as watching religious programs on television, feeling that religion is important, or using religion to cope with life problems, do not appear to have much effect. From visual inspection, then, it appears that the influence of religious involvement on mortality is not contingent on age and that the reduced risk of mortality for those with higher levels of attendance at religious services continues into old age.

Although we have not emphasized specific causes of death in this account, special mention should be made of suicide, a voluntary and tragic cause of death that occurs at higher rates in elderly males in the United States than in any other age/gender group. Since Durkheim's study of suicide,[123] religion has been shown to be a protective factor for people of all ages in studies from around the world. Two recent studies confirm the particular importance of religion as a factor in reducing suicides among the elderly. Nisbet and colleagues[124] studied all US deaths in 1993 using data from the National Mortality Followback Study and found that the odds of suicide compared with other causes of death were 4.34 times greater for men and women aged 50 and over who never attended religious services, compared with persons in the same age group who attended religious services frequently. A study in Switzerland of men aged 65–94 years found the rates of suicide were 40 percent lower for Catholics and 96 percent higher for the nonaffiliated, compared with Protestants; there were significant differences for older women as well, with Catholic women's rates 33 percent lower and the rates of the nonaffiliated 163 percent higher than those of older Protestant women.[125] Although these studies were not included in the earlier examination because they examined only a single cause of death, their findings are similar to those that we did examine: membership in a religious group provides protection against all types of mortality in old age, particularly from suicide.

In the section on adulthood, we discussed studies of disease or morbidity rates and religious involvement, in which we saw mixed findings and significant limitations, including cross-sectional designs, nonrepresentative samples, and self-reported diagnoses. We do not need to repeat the summary here since many of the study samples included older persons. There is, however, one disease-related outcome that is very important in studies of health and aging populations, and that is the measure of disability, often referred to as limitations in activities of daily living. Such measures are widely used in longitudinal studies of aging because they capture and calibrate the impact of serious chronic illnesses on the health of older persons and the impairment in an older person's ability to care for him- or herself. These measures are especially important because many older persons suffer from more than one chronic condition, and the co-occurrence or interplay of those conditions or comorbidity, can create additional vulnerabilities.

There are a number of studies of religious involvement and disability in older persons. In the Koenig, King, and Carson review,[126] there are ten studies of representative samples of elderly persons in which some form of religious involvement was studied for its association with disability. In three of these studies, there was no association between religiousness and disability, in one the findings were mixed; in two religiousness was associated with greater disability, and in four religiousness was associated with lower levels of disability. In Idler and Kasl's study of elderly persons in New Haven, attendance at religious services was associated with less disability over six years of follow-up after researchers adjusted for disability at the start of the study.[127] Interestingly, new instances of disability caused only a small, short-term effect on attendance at religious services during the next year, while the effect of religious attendance on subsequent disability was much stronger and more sustained. Some have argued that poor health in old age is itself the reason for lower religious attendance; when older persons have trouble with mobility, for example, they may not be able to continue with social activities. But our longitudinal study showed the reverse—that new disability hardly affected later attendance levels, and those who maintained their attendance levels also kept their functional ability levels high. This is an important area for further investigation because levels of disability relate so obviously to the quality of life of older persons and their ability to remain in their homes and communities.

Another important type of morbidity in old age that is increasingly becoming a cause of death is Alzheimer's disease and related dementias. Research on religious involvement as a factor in the incidence and prevalence of dementia is just beginning. In their review, Koenig, King, and Carson list just four studies with representative samples; in all four, however, participation in religious services was associated with lower rates of dementia.[128] The diagnosis of dementia in an older person has profound consequences for his or her family, who must become the primary caregivers. A recent small study of sixty-four patients with Alzheimer's disease and their caregivers in Italy found that after a twelve-month follow-up period, patients with high religiosity had significantly less decline in their cognitive scores, and their caregivers reported significantly less stress.[129] We discuss religion and the epidemic of Alzheimer's disease and dementia in chapters 7 and 26 of this book; we mention it here because, in the consistency of its performance over time, religious practice offers dementia patients a tie to the past. By involving the body and the senses, rituals provide multiple routes to meaning for those whose usual cognitive avenues are blocked. Thus, this connection with religion in very late life, in the midst of physical and mental impairment, underscores for us the crucial life course dimension of the influence of religious participation on health and well-being.

Finally, we turn to an interesting set of studies on the timing of death around religious holidays and holy days that seem to indicate that some individuals have some level of control over the exact day of death. These studies began with the work of David Phillips, who found significantly fewer deaths of Jewish residents of California in the week before Passover compared with the week after, while no such patterns were found among Asians, blacks, and Jewish infants, for whom the period would not have been meaningful.[130] Phillips and Smith[131] also found significantly fewer deaths among Chinese Americans in the week before the Harvest Moon Festival compared with the week after. Anson and Anson[132] showed a similar pattern among adult and elderly Jewish Israelis around the weekly Sabbath, but not around annual religious holidays. In the data from Idler and Kasl's religiously diverse sample in New Haven, researchers saw significantly fewer deaths in the thirty days before Christian holidays of Christmas and Easter among Christians but not among Jews and significantly fewer deaths among Jewish males and the more religiously observant (but not among Jewish females, the less observant, or Christians) in the thirty days before the Jewish holidays of Passover, Yom Kippur, and Rosh Hashanah.[133]

All of these studies suggest an ability of persons near the end of their lives to extend life by a short time to celebrate one final ceremonial occasion. This observation of the capacity of older persons to time their deaths in a meaningful way has often been noted by individual families, but these studies and a small number of others consistently find a statistically significant pattern. Persons whose death was impending were able to delay that death until after a significant religious observance had been completed, making that participation one of the final acts of their lives.

The cumulative impact of religious participation in old age is something only the very old can experience. The significance of religious ritual is that it brings people together and brings dignity and significance to pivotal moments of the life course. That significance may be seen more clearly by elderly persons than by their children and grandchildren, because they have seen more occasions of it. Rituals in general but especially the annual rituals of holiday celebrations, with all of their music and special foods and family gatherings, draw a thread through the life course, connecting the present with the long-ago past in a singular way. Elderly family members celebrate the holidays with one, two, or, even in some families, three generations. But also present in their memories as they eat familiar foods and hear familiar music are generations past—parents with whom they may share memories with their children, or the grandparents or even great-grandparents only they remember.

There is an additional reason for emphasizing the importance of religious practice as a marker of the life course. There is no other social institution that is more age-inclusive. Other than the family, no regular gathering of people in modern societies so consistently includes people of all ages. Our places of business, schools, stores, clubs, associations, and even many of our neighborhoods all have direct or indirect age criteria for entrance and membership. Many, like schools or active adult communities, quite narrowly define who can enter and even who must leave because of age. At a religious service, however, you can find a regular social gathering that includes newborns and centenarians and everyone in between, on a regular basis. And all who are present are valued members of equal worth.

Conclusion

In this chapter, we have reviewed studies that capture religious practice in early life, midlife, and old age and find religious participation to be positively associated with survival over years or even decades, into later adulthood and old age. Much more research remains to be done. We may have some understanding of the sticks of behavior control and the carrots of social support, but much is unexplained. The complex sorting of individuals into and out of religious groups is surely responsible for some of the patterns. Religious practice in adulthood is a function of religious practice in earlier periods of the life course: the religious or secular environment into which one is born, grows up, and grows old. This form of capital is just as lifelong an influence as economic and social capital and therefore needs to be considered with them in any complete enumeration of the social determinants of health.

Notes

1. Victor Fuchs, *Who Shall Live? Health, Economics, and Social Choice* (New York: Basic Books, 1974), 52–54.
2. Fuchs, *Who Shall Live?*, 53.
3. National Center for Health Statistics, *Health, United States, 2011: With Special Feature on Socioeconomic Status and Health* (Hyattsville, MD: US Department of Health and Human Services, 2011), 101, http://www.cdc.gov/nchs/data/hus/hus11.pdf, Table 18.
4. National Center for Health Statistics, *Health, United States, 2011*, 110, Table 23.

5. Centers for Disease Control and Prevention, "Tobacco Use, 2011: Adults Who Are Current Smokers," *Prevalence and Trends Data,* http://apps.nccd.cdc.gov/brfss/list.asp?cat=TU&yr=2011&qkey=8161&state=All.

6. Centers for Disease Control and Prevention, "Alcohol Consumption—2011: Adults Who Have Had at Least One Drink of Alcohol in the Past 30 Days," *Prevalence and Trends Data,* http://apps.nccd.cdc.gov/brfss/list.asp?cat=AC&yr=2011&qkey=8361&state=All.

7. Commission on the Social Determinants of Health, *Closing the Gap: Health Equity through Action on the Social Determinants of Health: Commission on Social Determinants of Health Final Report* (Geneva: World Health Organization, 2008).

8. Harold Koenig, Michael McCullough, and David Larson, *Handbook of Religion and Health* (New York: Oxford University Press, 2000).

9. Harold Koenig, Dana King, and Verna Carson, *Handbook of Religion and Health,* 2d ed. (New York: Oxford University Press, 2012).

10. Michael E. McCullough, William T. Hoyt, David B. Larson, Harold G. Koenig, and Carl Thoresen, "Religious Involvement and Mortality: A Meta-Analytic Review," *Health Psychology* 19, no. 3 (2000): 211–222.

11. Lynda H. Powell, Leila Shahabi, and Carl E. Thoresen, "Religion and Spirituality: Linkages to Physical Health," *American Psychologist* 58, no. 1 (2003): 36–52.

12. Yoichi Chida, Andewq Steptoe, and Lynda H. Powell, "Religiosity/Spirituality and Mortality: A Systematic Quantitative Review," *Journal of Psychotherapy and Psychosomatics* 78, no. 2 (2009): 81–90.

13. Ellen Idler, "Religion and Adult Mortality: Group- and Individual-Level Perspectives," in *The International Handbook of Adult Mortality,* ed. Richard Rogers and Eileen Crimmins (New York: Springer, 2011), 345–377.

14. Mel Bartley, *Health Inequality: An Introduction to Theories, Concepts and Methods* (Cambridge, UK: Polity Press, 2004).

15. Diana Kuh and Yoav Ben-Shlomo, *A Life Course Approach to Chronic Disease Epidemiology,* 2d ed. (Oxford: Oxford University Press, 2004).

16. Bartley, *Health Inequality,* 18. See also Johannes Siegrist, "Place, Social Exchange and Health: Proposed Sociological Framework," *Social Science & Medicine* 51, no. 9 (2000): 1283–1293.

17. Kuh and Ben-Shlomo, *A Life Course Approach to Chronic Disease Epidemiology.*

18. Roy Rappaport, *Ritual and the Making of Humanity* (Cambridge: Cambridge University Press, 1999).

19. Frank A. Salamone, *The Routledge Encyclopedia of Religious Rites, Rituals, and Festivals* (New York: Routledge, 2010).

20. Ellen L. Idler, Marc A. Musick, Christopher G. Ellison, Linda K. George, Neal Krause, Marcia G. Ory et al., "Measuring Multiple Dimensions of Religion and Spirituality for Health Research: Conceptual Background and Findings from the 1998 General Social Survey," *Research on Aging* 25, no. 4 (2003): 327–335.

21. Ellen L. Idler, "Ritual and Practice" in *Handbook of Psychology, Religion, and Spirituality,* Vol. 1, ed. Kenneth Pargament and James Jones (Washington, DC: American Psychological Association, 2013), 329–348.

22. Amanda Noss, "Household Income for States: 2008 and 2009," *American Community Survey Briefs,* September 2010, http://www.census.gov/prod/2010pubs/acsbr09-2.pdf.

23. Michael Barnett and Janice Gross Stein, *Sacred Aid: Faith and Humanitarianism* (New York: Oxford University Press, 2012).

24. Vernon Reynolds and Ralph Tanner, *The Social Ecology of Religion* (Oxford: Oxford University Press, 1995).

25. Salamone, *The Routledge Encyclopedia of Religious Rites, Rituals, and Festivals.*

26. Vinjar Fønnebø, "The Healthy Seventh-day Adventist Lifestyle: What Is the Norwegian Experience?," *American Journal of Clinical Nutrition* 59, no. 5 Suppl (1994): 1124S–1129S.

27. Sonia Bhalotra, Christine Valente, and Arthur van Soest, "The Puzzle of Muslim Advantage in Child Survival in India," *Journal of Health Economics* 29, no. 2 (2010): 191.

28. Robin L. Page, Christopher G. Ellison, and Jinwoo Lee, "Does Religiosity Affect Health Risk Behaviors in Pregnant and Postpartum Women?," *Maternal and Child Health Journal* 13, no. 5 (2009): 621–632.

29. Amy M. Burdette, Janet Weeks, Terrence D. Hill, and Isaac W Eberstein, "Maternal Religious Attendance and Low Birth Weight," *Social Science & Medicine* 74, no. 12 (2012): 1961–1967.

30. Amy M. Burdette and Natasha V. Pilkauskas, "Maternal Religious Involvement and Breastfeeding Initiation and Duration," *American Journal of Public Health* 102, no. 10 (2012): 1865–1868.

31. Koenig, King, and Carson, *Handbook of Religion and Health*, 2d ed.

32. Arnold Van Gennep, *Rites of Passage* (Chicago: University of Chicago Press, 1960).

33. Sian Cotton, Meghan E. McGrady, and Susan L. Rosenthal, "Measurement of Religiosity/Spirituality in Adolescent Health Outcomes Research: Trends and Recommendations," *Journal of Religion and Health* 49, no. 4 (2010): 414–444.

34. Koenig, King, and Carson, *Handbook of Religion and Health*, 2d ed.

35. Sterling C. Hilton, Gilbert W. Fellingham, and Joseph L. Lyon, "Suicide Rates and Religious Commitment in Young Adult Males in Utah," *American Journal of Epidemiology* 155, no. 5 (2002): 413–419.

36. James M. Nonnemaker, Clea A. McNeely, and Robert W. Blum, "Public and Private Domains of Religiosity and Adolescent Health Risk Behaviors: Evidence from the National Longitudinal Study of Adolescent Health," *Social Science & Medicine* 57, no. 11 (2003): 2049–2054.

37. Daniel Rasic, Steve Kisely, and Donald B. Langille, "Protective Associations of Importance of Religion and Frequency of Service Attendance with Depression Risk, Suicidal Behaviours and Substance Use in Adolescents in Nova Scotia, Canada," *Journal of Affective Disorders* 132, no. 3 (2011): 389–395.

38. Emile Durkheim, *Suicide: A Study in Sociology*, trans. Joseph Swain (1897; repr. New York: Free Press, 1951).

39. Lakshmi Vijayakumar, Sujit John, Jane Pirkis, and Harvey Whiteford, "Suicide in Developing Countries (2): Risk Factors," *Journal of Crisis Intervention and Suicide Prevention* 26, no. 3 (2005): 112–119.

40. Jie Zhang, William F. Wieczorek, Yeates Conwell, and Xin Ming Tu, "Psychological Strains and Youth Suicide in Rural China," *Social Science & Medicine* 72, no. 12 (2011): 2003–2010.

41. Robert Young, Helen Sweeting, and Anne Ellaway, "Do Schools Differ in Suicide Risk? The Influence of School and Neighbourhood on Attempted Suicide, Suicidal Ideation and Self-Harm among Secondary School Pupils," *BMC Public Health* 11, no. 1 (2011), 874, http://www.biomedcentral.com/1471-2458/11/874.

42. Teddi D. Johnson, "Youth Tobacco Use an Epidemic, Surgeon General Report Warns," *Nation's Health* 42, no. 4 (2012): 1–20.

43. Andrew J. Weaver, Kevin J. Flannelly, and Adrienne L. Strock, "A Review of Research on the Effects of Religion on Adolescent Tobacco Use Published between 1990 and 2003," *Adolescence* 40, no. 160 (2005): 761–776.

44. Koenig, King, and Carson, *Handbook of Religion and Health*, 2d ed.

45. Frank Gillum, Thomas O. Obisesan, and Nicole C. Jarrett, "Smokeless Tobacco Use and Religiousness," *International Journal of Environmental Research and Public Health* 6, no. 1 (2009): 225–231.

46. Jan Gryczynski and Brian W. Ward, "Social Norms and the Relationship between Cigarette Use and Religiosity among Adolescents in the United States," *Health Education & Behavior* 38, no. 1 (2011): 39–48.

47. Jerf W. Yeung, Yuk-Chung Chan, and Boris L. Lee, "Youth Religiosity and Substance Use: A Meta-Analysis from 1995 to 2007," *Psychological Reports* 105, no. 1 (2009): 255–266.

48. John M. Wallace Jr., Jorge Delva, Patrick M. O'Malley, Jerald G. Bachman, John E. Schulenberg, Lloyd D. Johnston, and Christopher Stewart, "Race/Ethnicity, Religiosity and Adolescent Alcohol, Cigarette and Marijuana Use," *Social Work in Public Health* 23, nos. 2–3 (2007): 193–213; ManSoo Yu and Arlene Rubin Stiffman, "Culture and Environment as Predictors of Alcohol Abuse/Dependence Symptoms in American Indian Youths," *Addictive Behaviors* 32, no. 10 (2007): 2253–2259.

49. Corina Benjet, Guilherme Borges, Marina E. Medina-Mora, Jeronimo Blanco, Joaquin Zambrano, Ricardo Orozco et al., "Drug Use Opportunities and the Transition to Drug Use among Adolescents from the Mexico City Metropolitan Area," *Drug and Alcohol Dependence* 90, no. 2–3 (2007): 128–134.

50. Iliana V. Kohler and Samuel H. Preston, "Ethnic and Religious Differentials in Bulgarian Mortality, 1993–1998," *Population Studies* 65 (2011): 91–113.

51. Steve C. T. Rollocks, Natasha Dass, Randy Seepersad, and Linda Mohammed, "The Role of Religiosity in Influencing Adolescent and Adult Alcohol Use in Trinidad," *Journal of Drug Education* 38, no. 4 (2008): 367–376.

52. Miriam Schiff, "Living in the Shadow of Terrorism: Psychological Distress and Alcohol Use among Religious and Non-Religious Adolescents in Jerusalem," *Social Science & Medicine* 62, no. 9 (2006): 2301–2312.

53. W. Alex Mason and Richard L. Spoth, "Thrill Seeking and Religiosity in Relation to Adolescent Substance Use: Tests of Joint, Interactive, and Indirect Influences," *Psychology of Addictive Behaviors* 25, no. 4 (2011): 683–696.

54. Thomas A. Wills, Allison M. Yaeger, and James M. Sandy, "Buffering Effect of Religiosity for Adolescent Substance Use," *Psychology of Addictive Behaviors* 17, no. 1 (2003): 24–31.

55. Carmella Walker, Michael G. Ainette, Thomas A Wills., and Don Mendoza, "Religiosity and Substance Use: Test of an Indirect-Effect Model in Early and Middle Adolescence," *Psychology of Addictive Behaviors* 21 (2007): 84–96.

56. Neharika Chawla Chawla, Clayton Neighbors, Melissa A. Lewis, Christine M. Lee, and Mary E. Larimer, "Attitudes and Perceived Approval of Drinking as Mediators of the Relationship between the Importance of Religion and Alcohol Use," *Journal of Studies on Alcohol and Drugs* 68, no. 3 (2007): 410–418.

57. John M. Wallace, Ryoko Yamaguchi, Jerald G. Bachman, Patrick M. O'Malley, John Schulenberg, and Lloyd D. Johnston, "Religiosity and Adolescent Substance Use: The Role of Individual and Contextual Influences," *Social Problems* 54, no. 2 (2007): 308–327.

58. Mark D. Regnerus, "Religion and Adolescent Sexual Behavior," in *Religion, Families, and Health: Population-Based Research in the United States*, ed. Christopher G. Ellison and Robert A. Hummer (New Brunswick, NJ: Rutgers University Press, 2010), 61–85.

59. Regnerus, "Religion and Adolescent Sexual Behavior."

60. Regnerus, "Religion and Adolescent Sexual Behavior."

61. Michael R. Kramer, Carol J. Hogue, and Laura M. Gaydos, "Noncontracepting Behavior in Women at Risk for Unintended Pregnancy: What's Religion Got to Do with It?," *Annals of Epidemiology* 17, no. 5 (2007): 327–334.

62. Peter S. Bearman and Hannah Brückner, "Promising the Future: Virginity Pledges and First Intercourse," *American Journal of Sociology* 106, no. 4 (2001): 859–912.

63. Hannah Brückner and Peter Bearman, "After the Promise: The STD Consequences of Adolescent Virginity Pledges," *Journal of Adolescent Health* 36, no. 4 (2005): 271–278.

64. William Sambisa, Sian L. Curtis, and C. Shannon Stokes, "Ethnic Differences in Sexual Behaviour among Unmarried Adolescents and Young Adults in Zimbabwe," *Journal of Biosocial Science* 42, no. 1 (2010): 1–25.

65. John M. Wallace and Tyrone A. Forman, "Religion's Role in Promoting Health and Reducing Risk among American Youth," *Health Education & Behavior* 25, no. 6 (1998): 721–741.

66. Wallace and Forman, "Religion's Role in Promoting Health and Reducing Risk."

67. Lynn Rew and Y. Joel Wong, "A Systematic Review of Associations among Religiosity/Spirituality and Adolescent Health Attitudes and Behaviors," *Journal of Adolescent Health* 38, no. 4 (2006): 433–442.

68. Candace S. Alcorta, "Religious Behavior and the Adolescent Brain," in *The Biology of Religious Behavior: The Evolutionary Origins of Faith and Religion*, ed. Jay R. Feierman (Santa Barbara, CA: Praeger, 2009), 112–113.

69. Alcorta, "Religious Behavior and the Adolescent Brain," 119.

70. Kuh and Ben-Shlomo, *A Life Course Approach to Chronic Disease Epidemiology*, 380.

71. Linda J. Waite and Alisa C. Lewin, "Religious Intermarriage and Conversion in the United States," in Ellison and Hummer, *Religion, Families, and Health*, 148–163.

72. On the Amish, R. F. Hamman, J. I. Barancik, and A. M. Lilienfeld, "Patterns of Mortality in the Old Order Amish," *American Journal of Epidemiology* 114 (1981): 845–861. On Seventh-day Adventists, J. Berkel and F. de Waard, "Mortality Pattern and Life Expectancy of Seventh-day Adventists in the Netherlands," *International Journal of Epidemiology* 12 (1983): 455–459; Fønnebø, "The Healthy Seventh-day Adventist Lifestyle"; and R. L. Phillips, J. W. Kuzma, W. L. Beeson, and T. Lotz,

"Influence of Selection versus Lifestyle on Risk of Fatal Cancer and Cardiovascular Disease among Seventh-day Adventists," *American Journal of Epidemiology* 112 (1980): 296–314. On Mormons, James E. Enstrom, "Health Practices and Cancer Mortality among Active California Mormons," *Journal of the National Cancer Institute* 81 (1989): 1807–1814; James E. Enstrom and Lester Breslow, "Lifestyle and Reduced Mortality among Active California Mormons, 1980–2004," *Preventive Medicine* 46 (2008): 133–136; and G. K. Jarvis, "Mormon Mortality Rates in Canada," *Social Biology* 24 (1977): 294–302. On clergy members, H. King and F. B. Locke, "American White Protestant Clergy as a Low-Risk Population for Mortality Research," *Journal of the National Cancer Institute* 65 (1980): 1115–1124; H. King, G. Zafros, and R. Hass, "Further Inquiry into Protestant Clerical Mortality Patterns," *Journal of Biosocial Science* 7 (1975): 243–254; F. B. Locke and H. King, "Mortality among Baptist Clergymen." *Journal of Chronic Disease* 33 (1980): 581–590; and M. Ogata, M. Ikeda, and M. Kuratsune, "Mortality among Japanese Zen Priests," *Journal of Epidemiology and Community Health* 38 (1984): 161–166.

73. Idler, "Religion and Adult Mortality"; H. C. Hsu, "Does Social Participation by the Elderly Reduce Mortality and Cognitive Impairment?," *Aging & Mental Health* 11 (2007): 699–707; Robert A. Hummer, Maureen R. Benjamins, Christopher G. Ellison, and Richard G. Rogers, "Religious Involvement and Mortality Risk among Pre-retirement Aged US Adults," in Ellison and Hummer, *Religion, Families, and Health*, 273–291; Howard Litwin, "What Really Matters in the Social Network–Mortality Association? A Multivariate Examination among Older Jewish-Israelis" *European Journal of Ageing* 4 (2007): 71–82; Richard G. Rogers, Patrick M. Krueger, and Robert A. Hummer, "Religious Attendance and Cause-Specific Mortality in the United States," in Ellison and Hummer, *Religion, Families, and Health*, 292–320; Eliezer Schnall, Sylvia Wassertheil-Smoller, Charles Swencionis, Vance Zemon, Lesley Tinker, Mary Jo O'Sullivan, Linda Van Horn, and Mimi Goodwin, "The Relationship between Religion and Cardiovascular Outcomes and All-Cause Mortality in the Women's Health Initiative Observational Study," *Psychology and Health* 25 (2010): 249–263; Timo Teinonen, Tero Vahlberg, Raimo Isoaho, and Sirkka-Liisa Kivela, "Religious Attendance and 12-Year Survival in Older Persons," *Age & Ageing* 34, no. 4 (2005): 406–409.

74. Berkel and de Waard, "Mortality Pattern and Life Expectancy of Seventh-day Adventists in the Netherlands."

75. Hamman, Baranick, and Lilienfeld, "Patterns of Mortality in the Old Order Amish."

76. James E. Enstrom, "Cancer Mortality among Mormons in California During 1968–1975," *Journal of the National Cancer Institute* 65, no. 5 (1980): 1073–1082.

77. Wieslaw Jedrychowski, Beata Tobiasz-Adamczyk, Antoni Olma, and Piotr Gradzikiewicz, "Survival Rates among Seventh Day Adventists Compared with the General Population in Poland," *Scandinavian Journal of Public Health* 13, no. 2 (1985): 49–52.

78. Idler, "Religion and Adult Mortality."

79. Ivar Heuch, Bjarne K. Jacobsen, and Gary E. Fraser, "A Cohort Study Found That Earlier and Longer Seventh–day Adventist Church Membership Was Associated with Reduced Male Mortality," *Journal of Clinical Epidemiology* 58, no. 1 (2005): 83–91; Fønnebø, "The Healthy Seventh–day Adventist Lifestyle."

80. Fønnebø,"The Healthy Seventh–day Adventist Lifestyle."

81. E. Bagiella, V. Hong, and R. Sloan, "Religious Attendance as a Predictor of Survival in the EPESE Cohorts," *International Journal of Epidemiology* 34 (2005): 443–451; M. E. Dupre, A. T. Franzese, and E. A. Parrado, "Religious Attendance and Mortality: Implications for the Black–White Mortality Crossover," *Demography* 43 (2006): 141–164; P. M. Eng, E. B. Rimm, G. Fitzmaurice, and Ichiro Kawachi, "Social Ties and Change in Social Ties in Relation to Subsequent Total and Cause-Specific Mortality and Coronary Heart Disease Incidence in Men," *American Journal of Epidemiology* 155 (2002): 700–709; R. Frank Gillum, D. E. King, T. O. Obisesan, and Harold G. Koenig, "Frequency of Attendance at Religious Services and Mortality in a US National Cohort," *Annals of Epidemiology* 18 (2008): 124–129; Terrence D. Hill, Jacqueline L. Angel, Christopher G. Ellison, and Ronald J. Angel, "Religious Attendance and Mortality: An 8-Year Follow-Up of Older Mexican Americans," *Journal of Gerontology: Social Sciences* 60, no. 2 (2005): S102–109; James S. House, Carolyn Robbins, and Howard L. Metzner, "The Association of Social Relationships and Activities with Mortality: Prospective Evidence from the Tecumseh Community Health Study," *American Journal of Epidemiology* 116 (1982): 123–140; H. C. Hsu, "Does Social Participation by the Elderly Reduce Mortality and Cognitive Impairment?"; Hummer et al., "Religious Involvement and Mortality Risk among Pre-Retirement Aged US Adults"; R. A. Hummer, R. G. Rogers, C. B. Nam, and C. G. Ellison, "Religious Involvement and US Adult Mortality," *Demography* 36 (1999): 273–285; Neal Krause, "Stressors in Highly Valued Roles, Religious Coping, and Mortality," *Psychology and Aging* 13 (1998): 242–255; P. La Cour, K. Avlund, and K. Schultz-Larsen, "Religion and Survival in a Secular Region: A Twenty Year Follow-Up of 734 Danish Adults Born in 1914," *Social Science and Medicine* 62 (2006): 157–164; Howard Litwin, "What Really Matters in the Social Network–Mortality Association?"; Marc A. Musick, James S. House, and David R. Williams, "Attendance at Religious Services and Mortality in a National Sample," *Journal of Health and Social Behavior* 45 (2004): 198–213; D. Oman, J. H. Kurata, W. J. Strawbridge, and R. D. Cohen, "Religious Attendance and Cause of Death over 31 Years," *International Journal of Psychiatry in Medicine* 32 (2002): 69–89; D. Oman and D. Reed, "Religion and Mortality among the Community-Dwelling Elderly," *American Journal of Public Health* 88 (1998): 1496–1475; T. Østbye, K. M. Krause, M. C. Norton, J. Tschanz, L. Sanders, K. Hayden et al., "Ten Dimensions of Health and Their Relationships with Overall Self–Reported Health and Survival in a Predominately Religiously Active Elderly Population: The Cache County Memory Study," *Journal of the American Geriatrics Society* 54 (2006): 199–209; Richard G. Rogers, "The Effects of Family Composition, Health, and Social Support Linkages on Mortality," *Journal of Health and Social Behavior* 37 (1996): 326–338; Rogers, Krueger, and Hummer, "Religious Attendance and Cause-Specific Mortality in the United States"; Schnall et al., "The Relationship between Religion and Cardiovascular Outcomes and All-Cause Mortality"; V. J. Schoenbach, B. Kaplan, L. Fredman, and D. Kleinbaum, "Social Ties and Mortality in Evans County, Georgia," *American Journal of Epidemiology* 123 (1986): 577–591; Teinonen et al., "Religious Attendance and 12-Year Survival in Older Persons"; and D. M. Yeager, D. A. Glei, M. Au, H.-S. Lin, R. P. Sloan, and M. Weinstein, "Religious Involvement and Health Outcomes among Older Persons in Taiwan," *Social Science and Medicine* 63 (2006): 2228–2241.

82. Schnall et al., "The Relationship between Religion and Cardiovascular Outcomes and All-Cause Mortality."

83. Hummer et al., "Religious Involvement and Mortality Risk among Pre-Retirement Aged US Adults."

84. Schnall et al., "The Relationship between Religion and Cardiovascular Outcomes and All–Cause Mortality."

85. Musick, House, and Williams, "Attendance at Religious Services and Mortality in a National Sample."

86. Ernest L. Wynder, Frank R. Lemon, and Irwin J. Bross, "Cancer and Coronary Artery Disease among Seventh-day Adventists," *Cancer* 12 (1959): 1016–1028.

87. Judith A. Westman, Amy K. Ferketich, Ross M. Kauffman, Steven N. MacEachern, J. R. Wilkins III, Patricia P. Wilcox et al., "Low Cancer Incidence Rates in Ohio Amish," *Cancer Causes Control* 21, no. 1 (2010): 69–75.

88. Powell, Shahabi, and Thoresen, "Religion and Spirituality."

89. Koenig, King, and Carson, *Handbook of Religion and Health*, 2d ed.

90. Koenig, McCullough, and Larson, *Handbook of Religion and Health*.

91. Powell, Shahabi, and Thoresen, "Religion and Spirituality."

92. Koenig, King, and Carson, *Handbook of Religion and Health*, 2d ed.

93. Koenig, King, and Carson, *Handbook of Religion and Health*, 2d ed.

94. Koenig, King, and Carson, *Handbook of Religion and Health*, 2d ed.

95. Powell, Shahabi, and Thoresen, "Religion and Spirituality."

96. Koenig, King, and Carson, *Handbook of Religion and Health*, 2d ed.

97. Robert Putnam, *Bowling Alone: The Collapse and Revival of American Community* (New York: Simon and Schuster, 2000).

98. William J. Strawbridge, Richard D. Cohen, Sarah J. Shema, and George A. Kaplan, "Frequent Attendance at Religious Services and Mortality over 28 Years," *American Journal of Public Health* 87, no. 6 (1997): 957–961. This study is not included in our survey because Oman et al., "Religious Attendance and Cause of Death Over 31 Years," analyze the same data with a longer follow-up.

99. Gillum et al., "Frequency of Attendance at Religious Services and Mortality in a US National Cohort"; Melani Prinsloo, Lynne Tudhope, Leyland Pitt, and Colin Campbell, "Using Demographics to Predict Smoking Behavior: Large Sample Evidence from an Emerging Market," *Health Marketing Quarterly* 25, no. 3 (2008): 289–301; Hua-Hie Yong, Stephen L. Hamann, Ron Borland, Geoffrey T. Fong, and Maizurah Omar, "Adult Smokers' Perception of the Role of Religion and Religious Leadership on Smoking and Association with Quitting: A Comparison between Thai Buddhists and Malaysian Muslims," *Social Science & Medicine* 69, no. 7 (2009): 1025–1031.

100. Jim P. Stimpson, "Smoking by Frequency and Type of Social Contact," *American Journal of Health Behavior* 34, no. 3 (2010): 322–327.

101. Arpana Agrawal and Michael T. Lynskey, "Correlates of Later-Onset Cannabis Use in the National Epidemiological Survey on Alcohol and Related Conditions (NESARC)," *Drug and Alcohol Dependence* 105, nos. 1–2 (2009): 71–75.

102. Sei J. Lee, Rebecca L. Sudore, Brie A. Williams, Karla Lindquist, Helen L. Chen, and Kenneth E. Covinsky, "Functional Limitations, Socioeconomic Status, and All-Cause Mortality in Moderate Alcohol Drinkers," *Journal of the American Geriatrics Society* 57, no. 6 (2009): 955–962.

103. Strawbridge et al., "Frequent Attendance at Religious Services and Mortality over 28 Years."
104. Schnall et al., "The Relationship between Religion and Cardiovascular Outcomes and All-Cause Mortality."
105. Koenig, King, and Carson, *Handbook of Religion and Health*, 2d ed.
106. Maureen R. Benjamins and Anna C. Buck, "Religion: A Sociocultural Predictor of Health Behaviors in Mexico," *Journal of Aging & Health* 20, no. 3 (2008): 290–305.
107. Effat Hatefnia, Shamsaddin Niknami, Mohsen Bazargan, Mahmood Mahmoodi, Minoor Lamyianm, and Nasrien Alavi, "Correlates of Mammography Utilization among Working Muslim Iranian Women," *Health Care for Women International* 31, no. 6 (2010): 499–514.
108. Kuh and Ben-Shlomo, *A Life Course Approach to Chronic Disease Epidemiology*, 374.
109. Ellen Idler, "Religion and Aging," in *Handbook of Aging and the Social Sciences*, 6th ed., ed. Robert H. Binstock and Linda K. George (San Diego, CA: Elsevier, 2006), 277–300.
110. Idler et al., "Measuring Multiple Dimensions of Religion and Spirituality."
111. Ellen L. Idler and Stanislav V. Kasl, "Religion among Disabled and Nondisabled Persons I: Cross-Sectional Patterns in Health Practices, Social Activities, and Well-Being," *Journal of Gerontology: Series B* 52, no. 6 (1997): S294–S305.
112. Ellen L. Idler, Stanislav V. Kasl, and Judith C. Hays, "Patterns of Religious Practice and Belief in the Last Year of Life," *Journal of Gerontology: Series B* 56, no. 6 (2001): S326–S334.
113. Paul Maves, "Aging, Religion, and the Church," in *Handbook of Social Gerontology: Societal Aspects of Aging*, ed. Clark Tibbitts (Chicago: University of Chicago Press, 1960), 698–749.
114. Shirley du Boulay, *Cicely Saunders: Founder of the Modern Hospice Movement* (London: Hodder and Johnson, 1984).
115. Alain de Botton, *Religion for Atheists* (New York: Pantheon Books, 2013), 63.
116. Allan Kellehear, *A Social History of Dying* (Cambridge: Cambridge University Press, 2007).
117. Hamman, Barancik, and Lilienfeld, "Patterns of Mortality in the Old Order Amish"; House, Robbins, and Metzner, "The Association of Social Relationships and Activities with Mortality"; Hummer et al., "Religious Involvement and Mortality Risk among Pre-Retirement Aged US Adults."
118. Musick, House, and Williams, "Attendance at Religious Services and Mortality in a National Sample"; Gillum et al., "Frequency of Attendance at Religious Services and Mortality in a US National Cohort"; Schnall et al., "The Relationship between Religion and Cardiovascular Outcomes and All-Cause Mortality"; Schoenbach et al., "Social Ties and Mortality in Evans County, Georgia"; Oman et al., "Religious Attendance and Cause of Death over 31 Years"; Hummer et al., "Religious Involvement and U.S. Adult Mortality"; Eng et al., "Social Ties and Change in Social Ties"; Rogers, Krueger, and Hummer, "Religious Attendance and Cause-Specific Mortality in the United States."
119. Hamman, Barancik, and Lilienfeld, "Patterns of Mortality in the Old Order Amish"; Oman and Reed, "Religion and Mortality among the Community-Dwelling El-

derly"; Bagiella, Hong, and Sloan, "Religious Attendance as a Predictor of Survival in the Epese Cohorts"; Hill et al., "Religious Attendance and Mortality"; Østbye et al., "Ten Dimensions of Health"; Rogers, "The Effects of Family Composition, Health, and Social Support Linkages on Mortality"; La Cour, Avlund, and Schultz-Larsen, "Religion and Survival in a Secular Region"; Krause, "Stressors in Highly Valued Roles, Religious Coping, and Mortality"; Yeager et al., "Religious Involvement and Health Outcomes among Older Persons in Taiwan"; Hsu, "Does Social Participation by the Elderly Reduce Mortality and Cognitive Impairment?"; Teinonen et al., "Religious Attendance and 12-Year Survival in Older Persons"; Dupre, Franzese, and Parrado, "Religious Attendance and Mortality"; Litwin, "What Really Matters in the Social Network–Mortality Association?"

120. Hamman, Barancik, and Lilienfeld, "Patterns of Mortality in the Old Order Amish."
121. Dupre, Franzese, and Parrado, "Religious Attendance and Mortality."
122. Litwin, "What Really Matters in the Social Network–Mortality Association?"
123. Durkheim, *Suicide*.
124. Paul A. Nisbet, Paul R. Duberstein, Yeates Conwell, and Larry Seidlitz, "The Effect of Participation in Religious Activities on Suicide versus Natural Death in Adults 50 and Older," *Journal of Nervous & Mental Disease* 188, no. 8 (2000): 543–546.
125. Adrian Spoerri, Marcel Zwahlen, Matthias Bopp, Felix Gutzwiller, and Matthias Egger, "Religion and Assisted and Non-Assisted Suicide in Switzerland: National Cohort Study," *International Journal of Epidemiology* 39, no. 6 (2010): 1486–1494.
126. Koenig, King, and Carson, *Handbook of Religion and Health*, 2d ed.
127. Idler and Kasl, "Religion among Disabled and Nondisabled Persons I."
128. Koenig, King, and Carson, *Handbook of Religion and Health*, 2d ed.
129. A. Coin, E. Perissinotto, M. Najjar, A. Girardi, E. M. Inelmen, G. Enz et al. "Does Religiosity Protect against Cognitive and Behavioral Decline in Alzheimer's Dementia?," *Current Alzheimer Research* 7, no. 5 (2010): 445–452.
130. David P. Phillips and Elliot W. King, "Death Takes a Holiday: Mortality Surrounding Major Social Occasions," *The Lancet* 332, no. 8613 (1988): 728–732.
131. David P. Phillips and Daniel G. Smith, "Postponement of Death until Symbolically Meaningful Occasions," *JAMA* 263, no. 14 (1990): 1947–1951.
132. Jon Anson and Ofra Anson, "Death Rests a While: Holy Day and Sabbath Effects on Jewish Mortality in Israel," *Social Science & Medicine* 52, no. 1 (2001): 83–97.
133. Ellen L. Idler and Stanislav V. Kasl, "Religion, Disability, Depression, and the Timing of Death," *American Journal of Sociology* 97, no. 4 (1992): 1052–1079.

19 | Religion, Spirituality, and Mental Health: Toward a Preventive Model Based on the Cultivation of Basic Human Values

BRENDAN OZAWA-DE SILVA

THESE ARE EXCITING TIMES FOR our understanding of mental health. Our knowledge is expanding, and long-held views and assumptions are giving way as recent discoveries highlight the ability of mental practices (including religious and spiritual practices) to affect brain, body, and behavior in ways that would have appeared impossible—perhaps even magical—just a few decades ago. Our conception of mental health is widening to include flourishing and positive well-being, and we are beginning to recognize the interrelation between the promotion of flourishing and the prevention of mental illness and dysfunction.

These changes have numerous implications—implications that go beyond what most of us can foresee. In this chapter, I examine a few of the implications for study of the relationship between religion and mental health. My focus will be on research that suggests that a significant factor in the relationship between mental health and religious belief, practice, and communal belonging has to do with the cultivation of moral emotions and ethical values. The implications of this research extend beyond religious people, because moral emotions and values can be cultivated by anyone and are relevant to the flourishing of everyone. The relationship between religion and mental health, therefore, has wide relevance to the promotion of flourishing and in the provision of preventive mental health care on both an individual and public health level.

"Mental Health" and Cartesian Dualism

Following the legacy of Descartes, modern thought in the West has until recently drawn a rigid line between the mental and physical realms. While the body has been seen as part of the physical, material, and mechanistic order of the universe, following natural laws and therefore available to study through observation, the mind has been seen as the seat of the soul and of free will, something immaterial, mysterious, and not constrained by the causal, deterministic nature of external reality. The legacy of this thinking still affects our thought and our disciplines. It continues to inform our understanding of physical and mental health; it is the reason that we have the mind/body problem and the "explanatory gap" in the cognitive and neurosciences, and it lies behind our division of the *Geisteswisssenschaften* (the humanities, social sciences, and religious studies) from the *Naturwissenschaften* (the "hard" sciences).

But Descartes's division of the world into two "substances" of mind and body, one extended and one not, has been thrown into question in recent years.[1] It is now widely accepted that mind and body are deeply interconnected and that this interconnectedness has deep implications for our understanding of mental and physical health.[2] Furthermore, rather than a distinct "substance" set apart from matter, consciousness can be understood as the subjective pole for the objective world of physical matter, meaning that subjectivity and objectivity mutually entail each other, like two sides of a sheet of paper. From a health perspective, thoughts, feelings, emotions, memories, hopes, and even the processes of meaning-making can no longer be considered exclusively mental phenomena; rather, they have a direct impact on our bodies and should therefore be incorporated into a holistic approach to health. We are similarly realizing that the conditions of our bodies affect our cognition, emotions, and decision-making processes in ways so powerful that they are calling into question our very notion of selfhood.[3]

The relationship between mind and body is relevant for understanding the relationship between religion and health for several reasons. For one thing, religion is typically placed within the realm of the Geisteswissenschaften. It is something that we associate with culture, with societies, with beliefs and the mind, not typically with physical objects and physical laws—although there is, of course, a very material and embodied dimension to religion and religious practice, a reality to which many of the chapters in Part I of this book give testimony. But religion is also of interest in this context because most religions understand health not merely in a negative sense—as the absence of disease and dysfunction—but also in a positive and holistic sense—as a state of well-being and flourishing. Indeed, the ultimate goal of many religious traditions is the attainment of what we could conceptualize as a complete state of physical and mental health—be it referred to as a state of complete harmony, enlightenment, liberation, salvation, sanctification, or resurrection.

This is important because, especially in fields related to mental health, there is a growing sense that a purely negative definition of health—that is, one that defines mental health as merely the absence of mental illnesses and disorders—is too narrow.[4] An absence of illness, we are discovering, is only part of the picture. The other part is the cultivation of constructive mental states and traits—such as compassion, gratitude, forgiveness, and generosity—and the presence of positive social relations, which not only give life greater meaning and value but also appear to serve as preventive factors for both mental and physical disease. The remarkable reception that the subdiscipline of positive psychology has received from the public and the increasing number of studies on compassion, empathy, gratitude, and other constructive emotions appearing each year serve as a testament to this growing awareness. This move away from the diagnosis and treatment of disorders—important as that will remain—toward the promotion of flourishing and positive mental health moves us into the realm of what could be or what should be for us as individuals and as societies. This begins to verge on territory that has long been considered the domain of religion and spirituality.

Religion and Spirituality

While numerous disciplines seek to envision a positive definition of health, a similar movement can be detected in medical anthropology and the medical humanities in the concern being shown for the increased medicalization of suffering, whereby existential problems such as loneliness, fear of death, dysphoria, and so on are seen as illnesses to be treated, rather than aspects of life to be confronted in a productive manner.[5] How, then, are we to recognize the relevance to our health of our minds and all that they entail—meaning, emotions, attitudes, ways of perceiving—without being limited to a negative definition of health?

Religions may offer resources to fulfill the basic emotional and social needs that are fundamental to our health and well-being as human beings and social animals. In examining these resources, it can be helpful to look not just at religion as an overarching concept but also at the specific dimensions of religion that may contribute to or impede health.[6] When we do so, we may find that some of the benefits and disadvantages of religious membership and practice may be factors that are not unique to religion. The putative benefits of church attendance for mental health, for example, may be due to a number of factors, including the benefits conferred by membership in a community and a sense of belonging, the social support offered by the religious group, the group's nonreligious practices or beliefs, or religious practices or beliefs held by the community. All of these might be beneficial to the mental health of individuals who belong to the community but only the last two would actually pertain directly to religion.

Many recent studies, such as Sharp's recent study on prayer,[7] have attempted to tease out the elements of religious membership and practice in just this way. In a longitudinal study of 114 Catholics and Protestants, Miller and colleagues found that those who reported that religion or spirituality was highly important to them had about one-fourth the risk of experiencing major depression ten years later compared with other participants; neither religious attendance nor denomination significantly predicted this outcome.[8] Remarkably, among those identified as being at high risk for developing depression (in this case due to having had a depressed parent), those who rated religion or spirituality as highly important had one-tenth the risk of experiencing major depression ten years later. If attendance at services and the type of religion practiced were not significant factors in this effect, then what aspect of religiosity or spirituality was protective?

As I have argued elsewhere,[9] it is quite possible that many of the protective and beneficial aspects of religious membership, practice, and belief for mental health may stem from what are essentially nonreligious factors that are effective because they tap into aspects of our embodied cognition—or "embodied cognitive logics"—that actually precede their adoption by the specific religion. Practices such as bowing and prayer, for example, are found across religious traditions; this is likely because they tap into aspects of embodied and grounded cognition that are cross-cultural and not irreducibly religious.[10] In other words, bowing (lowering oneself with regard to an object or person to whom one wishes to pay respect) is conducive to developing humility, respect, and devotion—values that most religions seek to inculcate in their members. It makes sense that religions would co-opt such practices or that particular practices would exapt—be drawn upon to fill a new purpose—in a religious setting; if so, they could also be once again removed from their religious contexts while still retaining some of their effects.

Some of these practices might have nothing to do with spirituality or religion, but others might be spiritual in a broad sense while not necessarily being religious—for example, the basic attitudes, values, and emotions that contribute to the mental health and flourishing of an individual may not necessarily be tied to a specific religion. In support of this view, McCullough and Willoughby argue that many of the health benefits of religiosity may be attributed to self-control and self-regulation, values that are taught by all major world religions but that are not, in themselves, necessarily religious values.[11]

This does not mean that religions have nothing to offer when it comes to our understanding of positive mental health. On the contrary, if religions have developed methods that foster the factors that promote flourishing, then there is all the more reason to study them. Moreover, although the study of these beneficial factors has increased in recent years, for example, in the rise of positive psychology, there remain interesting disparities between the ways that religions (and secularized practices drawn from religion) bolster these factors and the way that they are promoted through positive psychology interventions. The mental states and emotions considered constructive and beneficial in religious traditions are not necessarily the same as the "positive emotions" identified by psychology—at least if we understand those emotions in terms of positive affect. Indeed, religious traditions are often suspicious of the pursuit of *hedonia* (understood as good feelings, pleasure, and positive affect) and instead promote the pursuit of a vision of *eudaimonia* (a state of positive functioning, of being in right relationships with others and oneself). Moreover, negative affect, such as feelings of shame and sadness, are often intentionally induced in religious practices; while these feelings and practices produce a short-term reduction of hedonia, they ultimately—in the eyes of their adherents—lead to an increase of eudaimonia. The Japanese practice of *Naikan*, in which practitioners reflect on what they have received from others, what they have given to others, and what trouble they have caused others—a process that creates strong feelings of guilt and regret and yet leads to physical and emotional healing—is but one example.[12] These practices appear to spring from an understanding that some constructive emotions, such as compassion, depend on the ability to experience negative affect (sadness at seeing the suffering of another). Therefore, the paradigm of constructive versus destructive emotions in religious traditions does not correspond to the paradigm of positive versus negative emotions in contemporary psychology, and future research should attend to this difference.

More recently, the Dalai Lama has argued that certain constructive emotions and traits, such as self-control, compassion, gratitude, and forgiveness, comprise universal basic human values that can be drawn upon in constructing a "secular spirituality" or "secular ethics" for our pluralistic world.[13] These values, which are also skills that can be embodied and cultivated through training, are basic for human survival and contribute to both individual and social flourishing; moreover, they can be cultivated by individuals regardless of their religious tradition or lack thereof. For this reason, the Dalai Lama would likely be sympathetic to McCullough and Willoughby's argument. He has also urged scientists and researchers to examine the nature of these constructive values and emotions and their impact on health, focusing in particular on compassion.

It is important to note that the term "secular" here refers to a nonpartial attitude toward all religious and spiritual traditions and not to the rejection of religion. Secular in this sense is not the opposite of religious and does not mean not religious; rather, it is the opposite of the promotion of one religion over and above other viewpoints. We may distinguish between what could be called a full or pluralistic secularism model, in which members of diverse religious and cultural traditions are encouraged to show and express their distinctiveness in the public arena and diversity is acknowledged and celebrated, and a minimal secularism model, in which religious and cultural expressions and identities are kept out of public spaces. Both versions of secularism have their challenges: the challenge of a full secularism is to accommodate all religious and cultural views in a respectful way that does not privilege some over others; the challenge of a minimal secularism is that it may end up merely masking the values and beliefs that shape this supposedly religion-free space. Which route a society decides to take likely depends on how its history has been marked by religion.

Compassion, Social Cognition, and Mental Health

To evaluate whether the basic human values promoted in religions can contribute to flourishing, we need to engage in research that asks whether such values and moral emotions can be cultivated and whether their cultivation results in measurable physiological, psychological, and behavioral changes. Such research contributes not only to positive psychology and our understanding of physical and mental health but to the study of religion, since these values are of central importance to all of the world religions.

In 2005, Emory University launched a research program designed to address this question by examining the benefits of actively cultivating one such value, compassion, through a meditation protocol created by Geshe Lobsang Tenzin Negi. Drawn from a specific religion, Tibetan Buddhism, the practice was secularized by excluding any aspects that would be considered specifically Buddhist, such as belief in past and future lives, rebirth, enlightenment, divine or enlightened beings, spiritual teachers, the idea of karma, and so on. The protocol, called Cognitively Based Compassion Training (CBCT), can be seen as normative in that it promotes the cultivation of compassion for oneself and others and sets this cultivation as the goal of the practice.

Two studies by Pace and colleagues, one published in 2009 and the other in 2010, suggest that the practice of the CBCT protocol among undergraduates reduced neuroendocrine, inflammatory, and behavioral responses to psychosocial stress that are linked to the development of a large number of mental and physical illnesses.[14] Since this initial study, additional studies with adults, foster children aged 13–16, and elementary school children aged 5–9 suggest that compassion can be cultivated as a trainable skill and doing so may lead to a number of positive benefits, including increasing empathic accuracy and feelings of hopefulness, improving immune function, and reducing symptoms of depression.[15]

The idea of secular compassion training is of broad interest, because it reflects an attempt to draw from a religious tradition a specific practice that can contribute to mental and physical well-being and that can be employed by most, regardless of religious affiliation. The values of compassion, a sense of connection with others, forgiveness, gratitude, and responsibility toward others and the skills involved in intentionally cultivating these values can indeed be seen as religious in the sense that they lie at the heart of most, if not all, major religious traditions. At the same time, because they are not the exclusive domain of any one religion and because they can be cultivated by anyone, including nonreligious individuals, they can also be seen as entirely secular or as related to spirituality but not (necessarily) religion, if spirituality is understood as being comprised of the basic human values that are shared by diverse humanistic and religious traditions. This is not the most common definition of spirituality, but it is a useful one. Nancy Ammerman notes that spirituality is commonly understood in one of four ways: through a "theistic" package, an "extra-theistic package" of transcendence, an "ethical spirituality" focusing on everyday compassion, or a "belief and belonging" package tied to cultural notions of religiosity.[16] Secular programs like CBCT can be seen as cultivating "ethical spirituality." This aligns with the Dalai Lama's claim that the cultivation of compassion can serve as the basic for a "secular ethics" or "secular spirituality."[17]

The advantage of drawing upon contemplative practices in the teaching of ethical spirituality or basic human values is that it allows an approach that builds emotional and social skills that people can use for themselves, rather than simply telling them which values they should or should not have. In other words, it is about enhancing skills for moral decision-making, rather than simply telling people to be compassionate, generous, or kind. For example, in the CBCT programs for elementary school children, participants are taught basic mindfulness meditation so that they can notice thoughts, emotions, and feelings as they arise. The program then goes beyond basic mindfulness approaches by teaching children to recognize these mental events as being potentially destructive or constructive. Children are asked if they know what causes a forest fire and whether a forest fire can be easily put out before it causes destruction. Just as a spark can be easily put out if noticed early enough, they are taught, so can a destructive emotion be dealt with if one catches it early, before it results in harm to oneself and others. By learning to notice their inner mental states with greater clarity and to attend to what is helpful or harmful (which they are encouraged to choose for themselves), children learn skills that can contribute to their well-being and gain confidence in their ability to regulate their emotions and behaviors. This is how self-compassion is understood in the CBCT protocol. The participants learn to be forest rangers of their own minds, identifying and watching out for harmful sparks that could cause problems.

After one such class, a 5- or 6-year-old boy spontaneously commented, "I have a lot of forest fires in my life." One 13-year-old boy participating in another class explained the difference between noticing and putting out a forest fire (something harmful) and seeing a campfire that one wouldn't need to put out (something that wasn't necessarily harmful). In a similar way, games, plays, and stories are used to discuss other CBCT topics like impartiality, empathy and interdependence, which are then further reflected upon and internalized through meditation. The ability of young children to grasp topics like this, which have been the subject of religious practices for centuries, is most encouraging, and ongoing research is exploring the effects of these programs.[18]

Religious belief and belonging may play an important role in the establishment and cultivation of these values but may not be the only dimensions of religion that we wish to consider when examining the relationship between religion and mental health. After all, religious belief has been linked over the years with both mental health and mental illness, and religious belonging in groups with extremist or cult tendencies can be very harmful. Graham and Haidt[19] rightfully point out that a great deal of the attention paid to religion across various disciplines—not including religious studies itself but evident particularly in subdisciplines such as the cognitive science of religion[20]—has concentrated on the role of belief. Religions are understood as belief systems, and to be religious is to be someone who holds certain beliefs about the world. They note, however, that this comprises only one dimension of religion and that it misses the communal aspect of religion (being religious also typically means *belonging* to a community) and the element of religious practice (it also means *doing* certain things). Interestingly, Graham and Haidt stress the moral dimension of community membership: religion involves not being part of just any type of community, like participating in a book club or supporting a particular sports team but rather being part of a *moral* community, one that espouses certain values and aspires to embody them. In examining the health impact of such belonging, we should pay attention therefore not merely to the fact of belonging to a moral community but to the particular values held up by that community.

Cultural psychologists who have examined morality across cultures argue for five fundamental moral dimensions: harm/care, fairness/reciprocity, in-group/loyalty, authority/respect, and purity/sanctity.[21] Of these, the central and most universal would appear to be the dimension of harm/care, because this is the most basic moral dimension of human existence, one that we can easily translate not only across cultures but also across species. As Frans de Waal has argued, the evolutionary roots of morality cannot be seen as uniquely human but extend outward to include at least all bird and mammal species, because these species all rely on maternal care for their survival.[22] It is therefore no wonder that we see what may be the basis for higher-level morality and moral emotions such as compassion in the behaviors nonhuman primates. As a result, care and protection from harm do not represent a moral dimension separate from the most basic issue of survival, but rather one that is absolutely central to it—regardless of religious belief or lack thereof. Without compassion and an emotional bond, we would simply not be able to exist. Mothers would have no reason to bear their unborn children for nine months or to care for them after they were born. It is no wonder that our need for social connection runs so deep in our bodies and minds and that without it we languish and suffer, both mentally and physically.

While de Waal's approach is based on our evolutionary history and comparative psychology, Philippe Rochat arrives at conclusions very much aligned with de Waal's from a developmental psychological perspective.[23] Humans do not come into the world as fully formed adults with cognition that later takes into account other individuals and develops into social cognition; rather, our developmental trajectory begins in the womb and continues in infancy, where all cognition is inherently social. Ideas of selfhood and individual cognition emerge out of this fundamentally social matrix (of fetus in the womb and later infant dependent on caregiver), and not the other way around. Based on his research, Rochat argues that we have a basic affiliative need from birth that continues developmentally and that is central to our very conception of self. This need is so fundamental that our greatest fear is that of social rejection and social isolation, since these represent threats to our very survival.

In fact, a growing body of research is underlining the dangers of social isolation and social rejection for our mental and physical health, including a recent study of group suicides in Japan.[24] The fact that individuals would choose to commit suicide due to (or out of fear of) social rejection lends support to the argument that for many of us our greatest drive, even greater than the drive for physical survival, is for social connection and our greatest fear, even greater than the fear of death, is social rejection. In other words, the fact that for many social death is worse than physical death means that social bonds of love, compassion, acceptance, and care transcend concerns of mere physical survival. This is supported by evidence showing that populations who face parental and social rejection and discrimination have suicide rates much higher than the national average; in the case of gay, lesbian, and bisexual individuals, for instance, the rates can be two to eight times higher, and in the case of transgender and transsexual individuals, two hundred to three hundred times higher.[25]

The medical anthropologist Arthur Kleinman's recent work addresses concerns about the medicalization of human suffering, and his strong concern for social suffering leads him to address questions of morality and subjectivity, which for him, in line with Rochat's work, are inherently intersubjective. For Kleinman, experience itself is both inherently interpersonal and moral. It is interpersonal because, he writes, "It is a medium in which collective and subjective processes interfuse. We are born into the flow of palpable experience. Within its symbolic meanings and social interactions our senses form into a patterned sensibility, our movements meet resistance and find directions, and our subjectivity emerges, takes shape, and reflexively shapes our local world."[26] It is furthermore moral, he writes, "because it is the medium of engagement in everyday life in which things are at stake and in which ordinary people are deeply engaged stakeholders who have important things to lose, to gain, and to preserve."[27]

This perspective brings a richer context to the results of the studies on compassion reported previously: cultivating a greater sense of connection with others appears to affect us on a deep biological level because it touches upon something at the foundation of our survival as individuals and as a species. For too long we have seen compassion and positive social interaction as fringe elements of what it means to be an individual human being instead of realizing that it is the other way around: healthy individuals arise out of compassionate and caring social interactions, beginning—but not ending—with maternal care. Mental health therefore has to examine that basic need for connection, love, empathy, and compassion much more strongly. As research creates a more solid understanding of our need for such social connection and the emotions that support it, we will increasingly need resources that help repair social connection where it is missing and strengthen it where it exists. This is where religions can help and not only for those who are religious.

Although all major religious traditions emphasize the care/harm dimension of morality in injunctions to love one another, care for the poor, and live nonviolently, we must also remember that the inclusion by religions of a variety of other moral concerns and dimensions can mask this central core of morality or even subvert it. As Harris points out, "Religion allows people to imagine that their concerns are moral when they are not—that is, when they have nothing to do with suffering or its alleviation."[28] In other words, religious belief, membership, and practice can reinforce basic moral emotions like compassion, but they can also subvert those moral emotions if the religion's specific code of morality overrides the basic morality of care/harm. It is precisely when this happens that outsiders to a religious group look on its members with horror: because the group condones violence against people in the name of religion (for example, suicide bombers, stoning of women for infidelity) while violating the basic morality of harm/care, a morality so basic that it is not even unique to humans.

Ethics and Values

Exploring the connection between religion, ethical spirituality, and positive mental health is valuable from multiple perspectives. Research on how religious practices, beliefs, and communities contribute to the mental health of individuals in a "this-worldly" or secular sense improves our understanding of mental health itself. Furthermore, whereas psychology and psychiatry have typically focused on how to treat disorders and diseases, thereby bringing people from what we might call a subnormally functional state to a normally functional state, religions have typically attempted to lead believers and practitioners to states of well-being that go beyond the ordinary—to salvation, sainthood, enlightenment, liberation, for example—and to states of community that go so far beyond the ordinary that they may even appear utopian from a nonreligious perspective. This means that religions can be valuable resources for exploring the upper limits of human flourishing on both individual and collective levels.

At the same time, religions see a clear connection between the moral life and the fully healthy, flourishing life, a connection that has not been explored nearly enough in either the health sciences or emerging subfields like positive psychology. If we conceive of morality only through a religious lens, this connection becomes obscured, because religious morality is complex, multifaceted, and different across traditions. But if we see the issue of morality as being fundamentally about suffering and its alleviation—the harm/care dimension—the connection becomes clearer.

Current measures of flourishing look at emotional, social, and psychological well-being, but these measures could be improved by reflecting the importance of the harm/care dimension to individual and social flourishing—in other words, by including the dimension of ethical spirituality. Otherwise, such measures could fail to differentiate between genuine flourishing and facsimiles of flourishing. Take, for example, the instance of a young individual who feels alone and alienated but then joins a religious cult, an extremist group, or a violent gang. Many, if not most, of the current measures in positive psychology would rate such a person as showing a marked increase in flourishing, life satisfaction, and happiness after joining the group. His mood would be elevated, and he would feel more social support, a stronger sense of meaning and direction in life, greater self-esteem, and so on. On almost all measures of emotional, social, and psychological well-being, he would show a strong improvement. Most of us would agree, however, that a diagnosis of this individual as flourishing or as exhibiting positive mental health would be incorrect. We certainly do not consider members of cults and extremist groups to be flourishing, because we naturally rebel against the idea that someone who is engaging in activities that are harming or will harm others (and that will ultimately, therefore, harm themselves) and who is therefore leading a life that violates the most important dimension of morality—the care/harm dimension—could be truly flourishing. In this way, we implicitly include ethical spirituality in our practical assessments of others' well-being. Therefore it would be helpful to include this dimension and all that goes with it in formal assessments and research.

Developing a Culture of Compassion that Promotes Flourishing

Arguments over the costs and benefits of religion in the abstract for health and mental health are unlikely to be terribly fruitful. A top–down approach that sees religions as monolithic systems and mental health as a catalog of mental illnesses may not allow much rapprochement between religion and mental health, because religions at this level are not typically concerned with the treatment of mental illness or the this-worldly promotion of mental or physical health. I have attempted to outline a bottom–up approach that sees religions as complex systems that include nonreligious elements (some of which may draw upon embodied cognitive logics) and that sees the role that the cultivation of basic human values can play in promoting positive mental health, which in turn may protect against mental illness, suicide, and other problems. On this level, we see a close connection between the resources that religions have to offer and the pressing mental health needs that face us.

The vast majority of people in the world are religious, and—despite what many proponents of the secularization thesis thought a few decades ago—that seems unlikely to change in the near future. A way forward, therefore, is to identify the underlying features of religions that are beneficial for health and those that are not, especially those features that in themselves do not require religious belief or membership. The value of such an approach is that what we learn from it has practical implications: if certain practices in a religion contribute to the cultivation of basic human values such as compassion, gratitude, self-discipline, and a sense of connection with others, then those practices can be celebrated when they occur in religious contexts and can be adapted to nonreligious contexts where they can contribute to health beyond the confines of the religion.

This trend has already begun, of course. Yoga is now a popular practice engaged in by millions of people in the West, almost none of whom were born into a religious tradition associated with yoga or see it as a religious practice. That it began as a part of religious practice in specific religious contexts is commonly accepted. It has become, however, a secular practice. Moreover, the fact that it is a secular practice does not mean that its benefits are limited to physical health alone. Yoga practitioners—even those who are not religious—often see it as beneficial for achieving mental health and well-being and for cultivating positive values such as a sense of peace, stability, acceptance, forgiveness, and so on. Similarly, the practice of meditation techniques such as mindfulness meditation or CBCT adapted from Buddhism are becoming popular primarily among non-Buddhists. Although the earlier forms of meditation that became popular in the West were not explicitly normative, practices like CBCT explicitly aim to help practitioners cultivate moral emotions like compassion, and they do so while remaining secular in orientation.

Hopefully, this means that Western societies are beginning to realize that the category of religion need not be cordoned off from the rest of society. Rather, religions can contribute to our practice and understanding of well-being, even if what we take from them ends up in a secular form once it enters the public sphere. It also hopefully points to a recognition that issues of morality, ethics, and spirituality (understood as a basis of universal human values) need not be religious per se. The former are all likely to be essential components of a completely flourishing life and a flourishing society—something we cannot say (at least without giving up impartiality) of any one religion.

Because positive mental health appears, on the basis of a growing body of research, to play a strongly preventive role in future mental illness,[29] the most practical step of all would be to introduce the cultivation of basic human values in education. This would help children to develop resilience and aid them in leading truly meaningful and flourishing lives. At Emory, researchers have already begun adapting practices like CBCT for use in settings such as elementary schools, foster care facilities, hospitals, and prisons. The preliminary findings from such programs and interventions are promising.[30]

The use of such practices in public settings raises important questions that we must address collectively as a society. Are we comfortable with the teaching and training of moral emotions and values like compassion and empathy in secular settings, when such education is inherently normative? Are we able to separate out ethical spirituality from the practice of religion? Can we use science, reason, and collective experience and dialogue to come to a consensus on these issues, overcoming religious differences and ideologies for the purpose of promoting flourishing in a diverse, pluralistic society? Although these are very difficult questions, the alternative would appear to be worse: ignoring research that shows how important basic human values and moral emotions are for our physical and mental health and for our relationships and pretending that we can leave the question of ethics completely out of the public sphere—something that many, including myself, think is impossible. We already have a sense of secular ethics enshrined in our society in the form of the laws and norms by which we collectively abide; in future, these should also reflect our fullest scientific understanding of mental health and well-being.

Notes

1. Works in this area that have been highly influential for the arguments presented in this chapter include Antonio Damasio, *Descartes' Error: Emotion, Reason and the Human Brain* (New York: Penguin Books, 2005) and *The Feeling of What Happens: Body and Emotion in the Making of Consciousness* (Boston: Houghton Mifflin-Mariner Books, 2000); Francisco J. Varela, Evan T. Thompson, and Eleanor Rosch, *The Embodied Mind: Cognitive Science and the Human Experience* (Cambridge, MA: MIT Press, 1992).
2. Chikako Ozawa-de Silva and Brendan Ozawa-de Silva, "Secularizing Religious Practices: A Study of Subjectivity and Existential Transformation in Naikan Therapy," *Journal for the Scientific Study of Religion* 49, no. 1 (2010): 147–161.
3. Damasio, *The Feeling of What Happens.*
4. Corey L. M. Keyes, "Mental Illness and/or Mental Health? Investigating Axioms of the Complete State Model of Health," *Journal of Consulting and Clinical Psychology* 73, no. 3 (2005): 539–548, and "Promoting and Protecting Mental Health as Flourishing," *American Psychologist* 62, no. 2 (2007): 95–108.
5. Arthur Kleinman, *What Really Matters: Living a Moral Life amidst Uncertainty and Danger* (New York: Oxford University Press, 2006).
6. One problem that we face in drawing a connection between religion and mental health is that there is no such thing as "religion" in the singular independent of our historical and cultural conception of that term, which is not shared universally. The failure of numerous religious studies scholars to come up with an acceptable definition of religion led Jonathan Z. Smith to conclude, "While there is a staggering amount of data, phenomena, of human experiences and expressions that might be characterized in one culture or another, by one criterion or another, as religion—there is no data for religion. Religion is solely the creation of the scholar's study. It is created for the scholar's analytic purposes by his imaginative acts of comparison and generalization. Religion has no existence apart from the academy." Jonathan Z. Smith, *Imagining Religion: From Babylon to Jonestown* (Chicago: University of Chicago Press, 1988), 9. We can say a lot about the relationship between actual religious communities and mental health—say, for example, the relationship between church attendance and mental health—but "religion" is an analytical concept not shared by many other cultures, including, incidentally, many subcultures that we consider "religions" (see, for instance, Chikako Ozawa-de Silva's discussion of Shintoism in chapter 8 of this volume).

7. Shane Sharp, "When Prayers Go Unanswered," *Journal for the Scientific Study of Religion* 52, no. 1 (2013): 1–16.

8. L. Miller, P. Wickramaratne, M. J. Gameroff, M. Sage, C. E. Tenke, and M. M. Weissman, "Religiosity and Major Depression in Adults at High Risk: A Ten-Year Prospective Study," *American Journal of Psychiatry* 169, no. 1 (2012): 89–94.

9. Brendan Ozawa-de Silva and Brooke Dodson-Lavelle, "An Education of Heart and Mind: Practical and Theoretical Issues in Teaching Cognitive-Based Compassion Training to Children," *Practical Matters*, no. 4 (2011): 1–28.

10. For a general review of embodied and grounded cognition, see Lawrence Barsalou, "Grounded Cognition," *Annual Review of Psychology* 59(2008): 617–645.

11. Michael E. McCullough and Brian L. B. Willoughby, "Religion, Self-Regulation, and Self-Control: Associations, Explanations, and Implications," *Psychological Bulletin* 135, no. 1 (2009): 69–93.

12. Chikako Ozawa-de Silva, *Religion and Psychotherapy in Japan: The Japanese Introspection Practice of Naikan* (New York: Routledge, 2009).

13. Dalai Lama, *Ethics for the New Millennium* (New York: Riverhead, 1999), and *Beyond Religion: Ethics for a Whole World* (New York: Houghton Mifflin Harcourt, 2011).

14. Thaddeus W. W. Pace, Lobsang Tenzin Negi, Daniel D. Adame, Steven P. Cole, Teresa I. Sivili, Timothy D. Brown, Michael J. Issa, and Charles L. Raiso, "Effect of Compassion Meditation on Neuroendocrine, Innate Immune and Behavioral Responses to Psychosocial Stress," *Psychoneuroendocrinology* 34, no. 1 (2009): 87–98; Thaddeus W. W. Pace, Lobsang Tenzin Negi, Teresa I. Sivili, Michael J. Issa, Steven P. Cole, Daniel D. Adame, and Charles L. Raison, "Innate Immune Neuroendocrine and Behavioral Responses to Psychosocial Stress Do Not Predict Subsequent Compassion Meditation Practice Time," *Psychoneuroendocrinology* 35, no. 2 (2010): 310–315.

15. Gaëlle Desbordes, Lobsang T. Negi, Thaddeus W. W. Pace, B. Alan Wallace, Charles L. Raison, and Eric L. Schwartz, "Effects of Mindful-Attention and Compassion Meditation Training on Amygdala Response to Emotional Stimuli in an Ordinary, Non-Meditative State," *Frontiers in Human Neuroscience* 6 (2012): art. no. 292, http://journal.frontiersin.org/Journal/10.3389/fnhum.2012.00292/full; Jennifer S. Mascaro, James K. Rilling, Lobsang Tenzin Negi, and Charles L. Raison, "Compassion Meditation Enhances Empathic Accuracy and Related Neural Activity," *Social Cognitive and Affective Neuroscience* 8, no. 1 (2013): 48–55; Thaddeus W. W. Pace, Lobsang T. Negi, Brooke Dodson-Lavelle, Brendan Ozawa-de Silva, Sheethal Reddy, Steven Cole, Linda Craighaid, and Charles Raison, "Cognitively-Based Compassion Training Reduces Peripheral Inflammation in Adolescents in Foster Care with High Rates of Early Life Adversity," *BMC Complementary and Alternative Medicine* 12(2012): 175; Sheethal D. Reddy, Lobsang Tenzin Negi, Brooke Dodson-Lavelle, Brendan Ozawa-de Silva, Thaddeus W. W. Pace, Steve P. Cole, Charles L. Raison, and Linda W. Craighead, "Cognitive-Based Compassion Training: A Promising Prevention Strategy for At-Risk Adolescents," *Journal of Child and Family Studies* 22, no. 2 (2013): 219–230.

16. Nancy Ammerman, "Spiritual But Not Religious? Beyond Binary Choices in the Study of Religion," *Journal for the Scientific Study of Religion* 52, no. 2 (2013): 258–278.

17. Dalai Lama, *Beyond Religion.*
18. Brendan Ozawa-de Silva and Brooke Dodson-Lavelle, "An Education of Heart and Mind."
19. Jesse Graham and Jonathan Haidt, "Beyond Beliefs: Religions Bind Individuals into Moral Communities," *Personality and Social Psychology Review* 14, no. 1 (2010): 140–150.
20. Pascal Boyer, Religion Explained: The Evolutionary Origins of Religious *Thought* (New York: Perseus-Basic Books, 2001).
21. Jonathan Haidt and Jesse Graham, "When Morality Opposes Justice: Conservatives Have Moral Intuitions That Liberals May Not Recognize," *Social Justice Research* 20, no. 1 (2007): 98–116.
22. Frans de Waal, *The Age of Empathy: Nature's Lessons for a Kinder Society* (New York: Random House, 2010). De Waal's work also aligns in my view with contemporary work in moral psychology that argues for a nativist, rather than a purely empiricist, approach to morality. For more on this, see Samuel Fullhart, "Distinguishing Morality from Convention: Evidence for Nativism," *Journal of Cognition and Neuroethics* 1, no. 1 (2013): 1–37.
23. Philippe Rochat, *Others in Mind: Social Origins of Self-Consciousness* (New York: Cambridge University Press, 2009).
24. John T. Cacioppo and Louise C Hawkley, "Perceived Social Isolation and Cognition," *Trends in Cognitive Sciences* 13, no. 10 (2009): 447–454; Chikako Ozawa-De Silva, "Shared Death: Self, Sociality and Internet Group Suicide in Japan," *Transcultural Psychiatry* 47, no. 3 (2010): 392–418.
25. A. P. Haas, M. Eliason, V. M. Mays, R. M. Mathy, S. D. Cochran, A. R. D'Augelli, M. M. Silverman et al., "Suicide and Suicide Risk in Lesbian, Gay, Bisexual, and Transgender Populations: Review and Recommendations," *Special Issue: Suicide, Mental Health, and Youth Development*, edited by John P. Elia. *Journal of Homosexuality* 58, no. 1 (2010): 10–51.
26. Arthur Kleinman, "Experience and Its Moral Modes: Cultural, Human Conditions and Disorder," *The Tanner Lectures on Human Values* 20 (1999): 358–359, http://tannerlectures.utah.edu/_documents/a-to-z/k/Kleinman99.pdf.
27. Kleinman, "Experience and Its Moral Modes," 362. I do not know whether Kleinman would subscribe to the possibility of the "secular ethics" or "ethical spirituality" suggested by the Dalai Lama, but I am sure that if he were to, he would insist that it be grounded in an attention to ethnographic realities and a recognition of the diverse moralities of local worlds—that is, to shared "human conditions," as he puts it, rather than to a singular human nature. Without such attention, any secular ethics that we prescribe as universal may simply reflect our own unexamined assumptions and biases; the negative public health and clinical consequences of this error would likely be significant. If we simply use the term "human nature" to refer to those shared human conditions that can be investigated empirically (scientifically and ethnographically), rather than from some a priori notion of what a universal human nature must be, then I see no problem in the usage of this term. We should, however, recognize that it is often not used in this way.
28. Sam Harris, *Letter to a Christian Nation* (New York: Vintage, 2008), 25.

29. Corey L. M. Keyes, Satvinder S. Dhingra, and Eduardo J. Simoes, "Change in Level of Positive Mental Health as a Predictor of Future Risk of Mental Illness," *American Journal of Public Health* 100, no. 12 (2010): 2366–2371.

30. Current information on the latest research publications on CBCT is available at http://www.tibet.emory.edu/cbct/.

Religion and Public Health across the Globe

I N PART IV, WE enlarge our view to the role of religion in public health across the globe. For centuries, religious institutions have had an impact on the health of their own and sometimes other populations by establishing institutions to care for the sick and schools to train those who provide care. Today, the globalization of economies, the international spread of epidemic infectious disease, and major flows of philanthropic funding have made global health a fast-growing area of research and teaching in schools of public health around the world. The themes of social justice and humanitarian outreach that underlie these actors' commitment to improving health around the world might seem closely related to religious motivations and perspectives, but religion has been largely absent from emerging paradigms in global health.

Peter Brown opens the discussion with a history of global health as a field for research, teaching, and philanthropy. Evolving from nineteenth-century tropical medicine and twentieth-century international health, twenty-first-century global health has ridden a wave of funding from public and private sectors in developed countries, spurred by the AIDS epidemic and the Millennium Development Goals. From nineteenth-century missionary hospitals in colonial capitals, to faith-based aid organizations, to medical mission tourism, religious groups have been a critical part of the complex global health picture all along. In the next three chapters, we get a closer look at some of the topics that Brown raises.

In chapter 21, Matthew Bersagel Braley outlines the history of the Christian Medical Commission (CMC), the healthcare arm of the World Council of Churches, and its relationship with the World Health Organization (WHO), the healthcare arm of the UN. Braley traces theological developments that took place in the 1960s as this ecumenical body of churches considered the future direction of its medical missions. What emerged was a radical shift away from the traditional focus on hospital-based disease care to a theologically based emphasis on strengthening primary care in local, especially rural, communities. This new direction influenced thinking at the WHO that eventually led to its 1978 Alma-Ata Declaration on Primary Health Care.

Chapter 22 focuses on the creation of ingenious new public health institutions arising from religious origins. Ellen Idler tells the stories of several internationally recognized organizations, including the La Leche League International and Bangladesh's Dhaka Ahsania Mission, that arose in response to the public health problems of their time and place, addressing those problems with entirely new social structures that had religious ideas at their core. Some of these organizations, like the La Leche League International, do not now identify themselves as religiously motivated. For others, like the L'Arche Communities, the spiritual core has been a continuous key to their mission and identity.

Finally, in chapter 23, James Cochrane, Gary Gunderson, and Deborah McFarland write about the origins of the African Religious Health Assets Programme (ARHAP). An ingenious institution itself, with a decentralized network structure, ARHAP (now the International Religious Health Assets Programme) was founded in 2002 by Cochrane, Gunderson, and McFarland. With a focus on local strengths and resources, ARHAP has used community-based participatory research methods and geographical information systems to map and understand the role of religious assets in health.

Together, these chapters lift our focus from the health of individuals—as addressed in Part III—to the health of whole communities, manifested in their social institutions. The theological voices in this part bring a strong Christian perspective to these chapters—unavoidably, since caring for the sick was an essential aspect of nineteenth- and twentieth-century Christian missions around the world, and those missions introduced Western medicine wherever they went. Especially in the former colonial regions of Africa and Asia, this has left a complicated legacy and a lingering presence. As Karen Scheib and John Blevins in Part II and all of our Part IV chapters show, Christian theological views were centrally expressed through institution building in societies around the world. Many of those local, national, and international institutions—churches, religious orders, abbeys, clergy and laity associations, interfaith councils—were purely religious in their functions. But many also had a focus on healing the sick, one of the core messages of the Gospels. Care of the sick, of course, is important to other religions besides Christianity, and examples of ingenious religion and health institutions in Islam, Judaism, and Jainism can also be found in chapter 22.

There is a thick vein of critique of Western medicine running through these chapters as well. Just as John Wesley criticized the physicians of his day for their expensive and dangerous medicines, in the 1960s the CMC criticized the inaccessibility and unsustainable expense of the main form of healthcare delivery at that point: acute care hospitals in former colonial capitals. The mothers of the La Leche League bucked the tide of pediatricians' accepted practice in the 1950s by rejecting the then-standard recommendation to use manufactured infant formula fed with bottles. And Jean Vanier's impetus for creating the first L'Arche community was to rescue men from the asylum, the standard "treatment" for the mentally ill in the 1970s.

In each of these cases, the response to the critique was to (re)discover, promote, and support local knowledge and institutions. John Wesley distributed copies of *Primitive Physic*, a manual of remedies for common illnesses, to Methodist laypeople everywhere he traveled, including in the American colonies. The CMC set out to find examples of primary care delivery that depended more on traditional healing and local knowledge than on high-tech diagnostic equipment and complex pharmaceuticals. The La Leche League mothers organized meetings to teach other new mothers in their communities the art of breastfeeding. L'Arche homes were established in ordinary houses in ordinary neighborhoods, where their more- and less-abled residents can care for each other in intimate but not isolated contexts. Both Braley and Idler discuss the concept of subsidiarity, a Roman Catholic social teaching that the functions of the society should always be carried out at the most local level possible. In the examples found in these chapters, the wisdom of promoting local control over resources and increasing local knowledge—in other words, growing the social capital of communities—shines through again and again.

Perhaps the most important shared characteristic of chapters in Part IV, however, is the vision of what religious institutions bring to the concept of public health itself. ARHAP, in a village-by-village mapping project in Zambia and Lesotho funded by the WHO, documented religious health assets such as primary care clinics, traditional or indigenous healers, local midwives, and informal care groups in numbers that far exceeded other such enumeration attempts. In doing so, ARHAP developed the concept of "healthworlds"—an enlarged understanding of health as a characteristic of a community and the lifeworlds of the people within it.

The institutions described in these chapters build on what people know, have, and can do and not on what they are in need of. They seek to develop the capabilities of individuals and the social circles that they are a part of while recognizing and respecting the strengths that are already there. In these accounts, we see the social capital of villages, neighborhoods, and communities as a characteristic of the public health of those societies. Religions around the world have been incubators for many of these institutions. Their daily work to improve the health of their communities—health in the broadest sense—shows us yet another way in which religion is a social determinant of public health.

20 | Religion and Global Health

PETER J. BROWN

A CCORDING TO SOME SCHOLARS AND activists at Harvard University, global health is the major social movement of the twenty-first century.[1] Like the anti-slavery movement of the nineteenth century and the civil rights movements of the twentieth century, the international struggle for improved global health is linked to discourses of morality, social justice, ethical responsibility, and human rights. Yet the connection between contemporary global health and religion—including religious institutions, motivations, and activities—remains generally unexplored.

On the surface, global health may seem to be an entirely secular field related to public health, medicine, and economic development. But this is not the case. As this volume demonstrates, religion and religious institutions are significant but hidden determinants of both individual and population health. This chapter provides an interdisciplinary review of the relationship between religion, religion-based institutions, and the contemporary field of global health; the focus is primarily on Christian entities and in low- and middle-income countries. Some sections of this chapter that examine cross-national data may seem to argue against the primary message of this volume because poverty and poor population health are correlated with the level of religiosity of a society. On the other hand, the chapter provides very strong evidence that the religious motivations of individuals and institutions have played and continue to play an important role in the supply of clinical health care in poor countries, particularly in Africa.

The Origins of Global Health

Global health is a fast-growing area of research, program development, and teaching in public health and medicine. The term "global health" originated in the early 1990s at the beginning of the era of globalization that was also marked by the emergence of the HIV/AIDS pandemic.[2] Koplan and colleagues have recently proposed a general definition of global health as "an area for study, research, and practice that places a priority on improving health and achieving health equity for all people worldwide,"[3] although this definition has generated debate.[4] However it is defined, the contemporary field of global health has evolved from earlier iterations. During the Cold War, the field was known as "international health"; at that time it emphasized bilateral governmental technical assistance between developing countries (the "Third World") and the two superpowers—the United States and the USSR.[5] During the eras of imperialism and colonialism before the Second World War, when medical missionaries played a role in the colonial enterprise, the field was often called tropical medicine. Continuities can be seen in the ways in which faith-based organizations (FBOs) have been involved in contemporary global health efforts across these periods.[6]

The new label represents more than just a discursive shift. In general, global health is different from previous iterations for at least five reasons:

1. It places a new emphasis on nonpaternalistic partnerships between local recipients/communities and international donors.
2. It posits an increased role for nongovernmental organizations (NGOs) and less control by international organizations such as the World Health Organization (WHO).
3. It is supported by significant funding for biomedical research for the development of new technologies to address the "neglected" health problems of poor countries.
4. It emerges from a recognition that, in a time of rapid travel and high levels of migration, health problems transcend national boundaries.
5. It finds support both from political conservatives concerned with biosecurity and from political progressives interested in social justice and human rights[7].

Global Health, Global Poverty, and the Millennium Development Goals

The growth of the field of global health reflects increased public awareness of some dangerous and disturbing consequences of globalization in the contemporary world. Significant media coverage has brought worldwide attention to issues such as the extreme disparities in health and wealth between nations and within societies, the threat of disastrous global pandemics from novel and incurable infectious diseases, the threat of bioterrorism, the suffering caused by the HIV/AIDS epidemic and the lack of access to antiretroviral drugs in poor countries, the conditions of refugees in international emergencies, and the burden of extreme poverty and underdevelopment on an interdependent global economy. This increased awareness has given rise to a new generation of students and activists committed to global health, development, and social justice.[8] Through the media, these social activists have pressured world leaders to commit to programs to alleviate extreme poverty and deplorable levels of health.[9]

This activism has had significant results. At the beginning of the twenty-first century, world leaders agreed upon eight common goals for the global community—the UN Millennium Development Goals. Based on a recognition that poverty and poor health are inseparable, most of the Millennium Development Goals focused on health-related challenges, either directly or indirectly. These included eradicating extreme poverty and hunger; reducing child mortality; improving maternal health; and reducing the prevalence of HIV/AIDS, tuberculosis, and malaria. The ambitious roadmap includes detailed targets, strategies, benchmarks, and timetables for reaching targeted improvements in health measures, compared to 1990 levels, by 2015. In general, progress reports on the goals have been encouraging. In 2013, Ban Ki-Moon, Secretary-General of the UN, declared that the Millennium Development Goal effort has been the "the most successful global anti-poverty push in history."[10] Improvements in some arenas, such as the reduction of extreme poverty and expansion of primary education, have been remarkable, largely because of progress in Asia. Despite these advancements, however, the gaps remain huge, especially in sub-Saharan Africa. Furthermore, the global economic recession of 2008 has threatened the political and financial commitment to global health efforts, so that sustaining the progress is fragile.[11]

New Funding for Global Health

The expansion of global health has also been fueled by previously unimaginable increases in funding—from both government sources and private philanthropy—some of it associated with the HIV/AIDS epidemic. Development assistance for health has increased from $6.6 billion in 2000 to $19.9 billion in 2009.[12] The three largest global health institutions (World Bank, the US government, and the Global Fund) have total annual global health disbursements of approximately $8 billion,[13] 98 percent of which is for health service delivery.[14] In terms of private philanthropy, two of the richest men in the United States (Bill Gates and Warren Buffett) have pledged their personal fortunes to global health. The Bill and Melinda Gates Foundation, founded in 1998, has awarded $26.1 billion in grants, mostly to support global health research projects with technological orientations.[15]

Government funding, particularly from the United States, has seen similar growth. Under the politically conservative President George W. Bush, US funding for international health work grew enormously through programs such as the Presidents' Emergency Plan for AIDS Relief (PEPFAR) and the Presidents' Malaria Initiative. Begun in 2003, PEPFAR has provided approximately $46 billion to bilateral HIV/AIDS programs and to the Global Fund to Fight HIV/AIDS, Tuberculosis, and Malaria.[16] PEPFAR is responsible for remarkable numbers: 5.1 million people placed on antiretroviral treatment (up from 1.7 million in 2008), HIV testing and counseling provided to 46.5 million, and prophylactic antiretroviral treatment for 11 million pregnant women.[17] It has been called the largest healthcare program ever initiated by a single government.

Global health governance and financing, however, is provided by an uncoordinated patchwork of donors, UN agencies, governments, civil-society organizations, and private-sector actors. PEPFAR funds as well as global health funds from international sources are awarded to local agencies for specific on-the-ground interventions. Most of these agencies are international NGOs with local partners. Furthermore, the explosion of funding has resulted in a proliferation of NGOs working in poor countries, particularly in Africa. This growth in the sheer number of organizations involved has made it extremely difficult to coordinate efforts on the ground. Given the number and diversity of institutional actors, it is likely that the field of global health will remain "fragmented, complicated, messy and inadequately tracked."[18]

HIV/AIDS, PEPFAR, and Faith-Based Organizations

The George W. Bush administration also saw an expansion in the participation of FBOs in US-funded programs in health, development, and social welfare. On the international front, FBO participation in global health activities became recognized and funded in relation to the HIV/AIDS pandemic. An FBO has been defined as an "organization that is influenced by stated religious or spiritual beliefs in its mission, history, and/or work."[19] The term generally includes three types of organizations: faith communities (for instance, local churches) or religious orders (for instance, Sisters of Charity), faith-based NGOs (for example, Catholic Relief Services), and networks of FBOs working under a shared organizational structure (such as the Christian Medical Commission, discussed in chapter 21). The FBOs examined in this chapter primarily fit the third category. In terms of on-the-ground activities such as disaster relief, it is very difficult to distinguish between FBOs and "humanitarian" agencies.[20] FBOs have properties that make them uniquely able to deliver health care, health education, and other services, including well-established health service-delivery networks and infrastructures, histories of clear commitments to local communities, the trust of local communities, and a capacity to mobilize volunteers.[21]

FBOs have become a standard part of the US Agency for International Development (USAID) procedures and a special office to assist them in contract procurement was established in 2002.[22] The incorporation of FBOs into PEPFAR and USAID programs has drawn both praise and criticism. The most obvious source of praise is the recognition that FBOs have been necessary partners in the scale-up of antiretroviral therapy distribution in the early 2000s. For example, Jim Kim's ambitious UNAIDS "3 by 5" program, with its goal to put 3 million HIV-positive people on antiretroviral treatment by 2005, singled out FBOs as essential partners for mobilizing communities.[23] FBOs have also earned special recognition for their role in providing hospice and palliative care at the beginning of the AIDS epidemic in Africa. On a completely different global health challenge—controlling tobacco use to prevent cancers—the work of FBOs has been praised by the WHO.[24]

On the other hand, politically powerful evangelical Christians and FBOs have been criticized for the way in which their fundamentalist religious ideologies have shaped PEPFAR and USAID policies. For example, PEPFAR originally required that 33 percent of all HIV prevention programs be spent on "abstinence only" education, which neglects critical information on condoms, safe sex, and family planning.[25] HIV testing and counseling sessions were not permitted to include education about family planning and abortion. Critics have argued that teaching only abstinence was a counterproductive waste of money that undermined rights-based approaches to reproductive health.[26] Another result of this influence, some have asserted, was an emphasis on the scale-up of antiretroviral treatment for people with HIV/AIDs at the expense of efforts to prevent the spread of the virus. The shift from prevention to treatment is sometimes considered to be a product of the influence of pharmaceutical companies, but the political pressure placed on Congress and USAID by religious conservatives and FBOs may have been more important.[27] Ultimately the prevention/treatment controversy seemed to be partly resolved when a World Bank report showed that antiretroviral treatment improves prevention because HIV-positive people treated with antiretrovirals have lower viral loads and are therefore less infective.[28] Finally, critics have also pointed out that some evangelical FBOs that procured PEPFAR funding had little or no experience in global health, particularly in Africa.

Both critics and advocates agree that the participation of FBOs in global health activities accelerated with American PEPFAR funding and the scale-up of antiretroviral treatment. Yet, in part because of the influence of FBOs in formulating its policies, PEPFAR was also an emergency program that did not grapple with the contexts of global poverty and global health underlying the emergency.

Correlations between Religiosity, Poverty, and Poor Health

It is a fundamental fact of global health that poor health and poverty are intertwined; stated more simply, wealth makes health. According to WHO, approximately 1.2 billion people in the world live in extreme poverty, surviving on less than one dollar per day. Poverty creates ill health because it forces people to live in environments that make them sick, without decent shelter, clean water, adequate sanitation, or access to health care.[29] In low-income countries, there is a very strong relationship between income and longevity up to a per capita income level of about $3,000 to $7,000; then the life expectancy curve levels off at around age 70 (Figure 20.1).[30] However, comparison of the highest-income countries alone shows no correlation between income and life expectancy; the United States has relatively poor health and relatively high rates of infant mortality. Wilkinson and Pickett have demonstrated that the reason for this phenomenon among

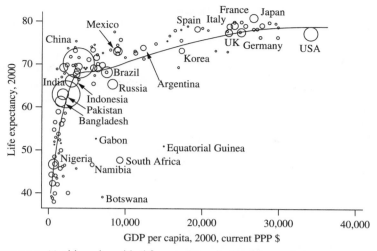

FIGURE 20.1 Health and wealth (life expectancy by GNP per capita).

SOURCE: Angus Deaton, "Health, Inequality and Economic Development," *Journal of Economic Literature* 41 (2003): 117.

high-income countries is the predictive power of income inequality.[31] They argue that any society that tolerates a high level of income inequality simply cannot achieve high levels of population health or low levels of social problems, such as violence, that affect population health.

According to data from the Pew Foundation, there is a strong *inverse* correlation between religiosity and income.[32] Examining forty-seven countries with per capita annual incomes ranging from less than $500 to over $40,000 and using an index of religiosity, the Pew survey found that populations characterized by strong religious beliefs and practices are among the poorest in the world (Figure 20.2).[33] Similarly, national surveys showed an inverse correlation between purchasing power and agreement with the statement "religion is very important." The obvious exception to this pattern is the United States, which is generally rich but religious; the most common explanation for this phenomenon is the extremely high level of income inequality in the United States, reflected in the relationship between the frequency of prayer and income inequality in a cross-national sample (Figure 20.3).[34]

One conclusion of the Pew/Templeton Foundation's Global Religious Futures project was that Africa south of the Sahara is "the most religious place on earth."[35] The most religious continent, then, is also the poorest and least healthy. This reflects a number of factors that influence both health and religious belief. Technological advancement, including biomedical technologies, and economic growth generally make societies

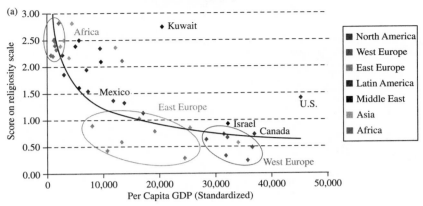

Wealth and Religiosity

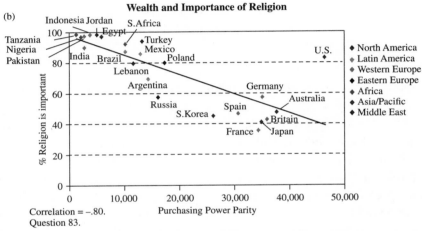

Wealth and Importance of Religion

Correlation = –.80.
Question 83.

FIGURE 20.2 Panel A. Religiosity index by GDP per Capita. Panel B. Importance of religion by purchasing power.

SOURCE: A) Pew Foundation Global Attitudes Project, "Chapter 2: Religiosity," *Unfavorable Views of Jews and Muslims on the Increase in Europe*, September 17, 2008, http://www.pewglobal.org/2008/09/17/chapter-2-religiosity/; B) Pew Foundation, "Chapter 4: Values and American Exceptionalism," *World Publics Welcome Global Trade—But Not Immigration*, October 4, 2007, http://www.pewglobal.org/2007/10/04/chapter-4-values-and-american-exceptionalism/.

more secular. Science and technology may also provide answers about causes of disease and death, lessening the need for the cognitive mechanisms religion provides for explaining such things. Traditional religions also provide ethnomedical systems of disease prevention and cure; healing rituals are a central part of shamanistic systems. However, the power of this last should not be overestimated. Traditional folk medicine and faith healers are used not only because they are culturally consonant and

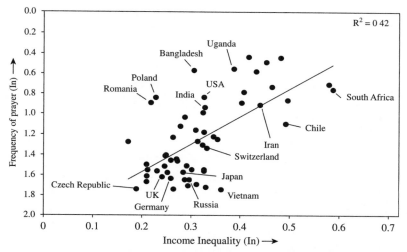

FIGURE 20.3 Frequency of Prayer by Gini Coefficient, Non-Muslim Countries.

SOURCE: Tomas James Rees, "Is Personal Insecurity a Cause of Cross-National Differences in the Intensity of Religious Belief?," *Journal of Religion and Society* 11 (2009): 7.

psychosocially useful but also because they are relatively inexpensive and accessible. Ethnomedical treatments have been shown to have some limited efficacy—explained in the biomedical perspective by the placebo effect (also known as the meaning effect) or simply "miracles"[36]—but they are not comparable to scientific biomedical treatments, particularly for the infectious diseases that burden low-income countries. Given a choice, the poor prefer modern medicine.

There is, however, a long history of programs designed to incorporate traditional healers into health programs because of inadequate numbers of biomedical practitioners and because of the success of traditional healers in dealing with mental health problems.[37] Medical anthropologists, particularly Edward Green, have been involved in programs that incorporate traditional healers into AIDS and STD prevention campaigns.[38] The inclusion of these traditional practitioners in the African Religious Health Assets Programme's (ARHAP) conceptualization of religious health assets is also worth noting.[39] It is valuable to recognize that, particularly in Africa, "traditional" religions can no longer be recognized in any pure precolonial form. Official religion on the continent is primarily either Christian or Muslim, and most people self-identify in one of these ways. However, Africa-based Christian churches frequently reflect a syncretism between mainstream beliefs and practices and older traditional religion,[40] and traditional beliefs in witchcraft and spiritual entities persist—in fact, these increased at the beginning of the AIDS epidemic[41]—and traditional healers using spiritually based etiological theories and therapies are still very important.

Global Public Health versus Health Care in Low-Resource Settings

When looking at a global scale, then, the connections between poverty, poor health, and religiosity are clear. There are two fundamental distinctions that are essential for understanding religion as a social determinant of health. First, religion per se must be distinguished from religious institutions. Second, public health is very different from medicine and clinical health care. In rich societies, there is a widespread tendency to confuse health and medical care, based on a popular belief that modern scientific biomedicine is the primary reason for improved levels of population health.[42] Both historical and global health data demonstrate that this is not the case. The classic analysis by McKeown[43] demonstrated that the historical decline in mortality in England occurred *before* the invention of modern biomedical technologies such as antibiotics. Rather, clean water, sanitation, quality diet, and housing have been the primary physical determinants of population health. Access to effective primary health care—particularly vaccinations, oral rehydration therapy, and treatment of respiratory infections—is extremely important, but in relative terms, clinical health care is far less important to population health than changes in living conditions and lifestyle.

Medicine and public health intersect in the realm of prevention. Medical health care can be preventive, curative, or palliative. Primary prevention—efforts to keep disease from occurring in the first place—is the realm of public health, while curative and palliative treatments are the bailiwick of medicine. Secondary prevention—efforts to keep a health condition from progressing—fall between the two fields. For example, providing antiretroviral drug therapy for people with HIV is secondary prevention; it does not cure HIV but rather delays the onset of full-blown AIDS.

Historically, global health policy has vacillated between emphases on the control of specific diseases (for instance, malaria, smallpox, yellow fever) and the improvement of health care on a local level. The first approach stressed science, technology, and cost effectiveness while the second emphasized immediate action to reduce suffering. Public health disease-control programs have typically been secular whereas medical care has been characterized by a more spiritual ethos based on concepts of mercy and obligations to relieve the suffering of the poor. The crucial shift in global health policy from disease control and eradication to primary health care in the late 1970s was driven by the Christian Medical Commission (CMC). As Matthew Bersagel Braley describes in chapter 23 of this volume, the CMC led the way in transforming Western-designed hospitals that had been linked to missions and serving primarily the privileged few into "people-controlled" health systems with the goal of "Health for All."

Religious Belief and Health in the Global Context

On an individual level, religious beliefs and behaviors can have effects in the realms of primary prevention and health maintenance. Part I of this volume offers detailed descriptions of religiously dictated practices and traditions that may help to maintain health and prevent disease. Such behaviors are what medical anthropologists would label "cultural adaptations"[44] because they have latent health-enhancing effects despite being performed for different reasons. Religious belief may also influence health in other ways. Medical sociologists have demonstrated how religious motivations and traditions can play important roles in health maintenance by providing social support and coping during times of stress. Religious beliefs can also enhance mental health by supplying meaning and answers to existential dilemmas.[45] These important contributions are generally not recognized by global public health researchers and practitioners.

Religious beliefs and ritual practices are also linked to health care and healing more directly through a number of conduits. For instance, various types of faith healing thrive in most cultures today. In Africa, the growth of evangelical churches—particularly those based on the "prosperity gospel"—has been remarkable, and those churches that regularly offer ritualized healing services are among the fastest growing.[46] Faith healing may well come into play when the folk etiology of an illness has a spiritual basis, as in spirit possession, sorcery, evil eye, or divine retribution for sin. Religion is also extremely important in creating an atmosphere of trust between healer and patient in what has been called the "shamanistic complex."[47] The process of becoming a healer—whether a folk healer or a medical doctor—follows culturally mandated ritualized procedures, and many healers consider their vocation a religious calling. As such, the personal religious motivations of biomedical practitioners—doctors, nurses, and medical assistants—would seem to be critical in the recruitment and retention of healthcare personnel. This is especially the case for practitioners who choose to work in FBO facilities in low-resource settings.

Obviously, religion can also have negative effects on health. Religious beliefs can hasten disease processes and death, an occurrence referred to as the *nocebo phenomenon*.[48] In regard to the HIV/AIDS pandemic, religious beliefs have often increased suffering by creating social stigma (as detailed in chapter 24). Religious ideologies like the Catholic Church's opposition to condoms and birth control have hampered public health efforts for STD prevention, family planning, and reproductive health. Religious belief may also affect health by inciting violence; religious motivations have historically been given for war, persecution, and acts of terrorism; this has been the case in the past and continues today, for instance, in the violence between Sunni and Shia Muslims in Iraq and Syria and the work of suicide bombers around the world.

Global Health and Faith-Based Organizations

It is difficult to know how many FBOs are currently involved in global health work.[49] A complete catalog of FBOs working in global health has not been compiled, but the list is obviously long. The *Mission Handbook* of North American Protestant ministries overseas lists thirty-five FBOs involved in the delivery of medical supplies and eighty-six religious entities involved in the delivery of medical, dental, and public health services.[50]

FBO-run facilities such as hospitals, clinics, and hospices play a major role in global health; FBOs are also important in supplying an expatriate healthcare workforce and medical supplies as well as training local personnel. Many of these organizations have had a continuing presence in Africa for over 150 years; they are linked to the activities of Christian missionaries of the colonial period. Manji and O'Coill, who have shown how these FBOs transformed themselves into actors in the "development industry" in the post-colonial period,[51] distinguish between two categories of NGOs based on different historical origins. The first group consists of overseas missionary societies and charitable bodies that were present in the African colonies before independence. Christian Aid, a network of forty Protestant churches in the United Kingdom, evolved in this way. The second group is typified by organizations like Oxfam, CARE, Save the Children, and Plan International, which had no direct involvement in the colonies. These organizations were "war charities," established to deal with the human consequences of conflict in Europe, that moved into Africa in the post-colonial period.

In terms of contemporary activities, proposals to funding agencies, and so forth, many scholars argue that it is difficult to make a clear distinction between FBOs and humanitarian NGOs.[52] In addition, some Europe-based health and development organizations have clear origins in religious institutions that later partnered with government-run overseas aid agencies. One example is Holland, where the government jointly funds two such groups—ICCO, an alliance of Protestant churches, and CORDAID, a Catholic network of 890 partner organizations in twenty-eight countries.[53] The medical activities of many of these entities may be small, but the net effect is big.

FBOs deliver an incredible amount of health care in the developing world. In many nations, FBOs contribute as much to the healthcare system as do government ministries of health (Figure 20.4).[54] For example, ARHAP estimates that in Tanzania and Kenya, FBOs provide more than 40 percent and 60 percent of healthcare services, respectively.[55] The Catholic Church, one of the biggest global healthcare providers, operates 5,246 hospitals, 17,530 dispensaries, 577 leprosy clinics, and 15,208 houses for the chronically ill and handicapped worldwide.[56] Birn and colleagues studied eleven exclusively religious global health entities.[57] The largest of these is World Vision, a network of evangelical Protestant churches and charities working in ninety-seven countries; its 2011 budget was $2.79

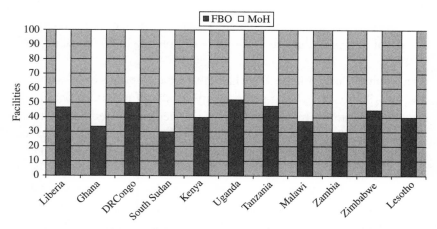

FIGURE 20.4 Contribution of FBOs to Availability of Health Facilities in African Nations.

SOURCE: S. Mwenda, "The Africa Christian Health Associations Platform: Showcasing the Contributions of CHAs," *Contact* 190 (2011): 2.

billion.[58] Another network of global health and development FBOs, called Action by Churches Together for Development, includes 130 affiliated NGOs and approximately 25,000 people working in the field; the core of this network is the World Council of Churches and the Lutheran World Federation.

There is also a significant history of FBOs being involved in the supply or recycling of pharmaceuticals and medical supplies to health facilities in low-income countries. The Catholic Medical Mission Board (CMMB) was founded in New York in 1912 by a physician who later worked in a "leper colony" in Haiti.[59] Supported by the Archdiocese of New York, the CMMB not only recruited volunteer medical practitioners but also specialized in procuring pharmaceuticals and medical supplies for mission hospitals; in its first fifty years, it sent 38 million pounds of supplies to more than five thousand overseas hospitals.[60] CMMB is one of the fifteen faith-based drug supply organizations operating in ten African nations that were evaluated by Banda and colleagues for the Ecumenical Pharmaceutical Network (EPN) and the WHO.[61] The study found that:

- An average of 43 percent of the populations in these countries were served by the organizations, indicating that the public drug supply system was insufficient and needed supplementation.
- Half of the participating organizations received donated drugs that were distributed to customers free of charge.
- Donated drugs could create serious problems in terms of expiration dates and appropriateness for local needs.
- The entire system required better communication between donors and local clinics so that the FBOs were responding to real local needs[62].

As a result of this work, the EPN has shifted the emphasis of its work from drug distribution to training and capacity building for African pharmacists and administrators. This move is part of a larger trend; over the past twenty years, nearly all FBOs working in the global health field have hired local nationals to take over the administration and daily operations of their facilities and organizations. Thus, the EPN's shift toward local capacity building reflects a wider change from the charity model of international health to the partnership and empowerment model of contemporary global health.

However, FBOs still face tension between their religious foundations and their financial requirements, particularly with regard to hospital care, of which they are major providers. Public funding for health facilities is insufficient, and FBOs have filled the gap in clinical medicine in the post-colonial period. However, as private hospitals without government support, FBO hospitals must charge for their health services. But user fees, even minimal ones, can make medical care inaccessible to the poorest people. Some critics say that it is wrong for private charitable hospitals to charge fees, thus catering to the relatively wealthier urban populations. On the other hand, without user fees, these facilities are financially unsustainable. On another level, some critics say that the presence of these hospitals perpetuates injustice; in this perspective, the continuation of foreign-funded charitable hospitals lets national ministries of health "off the hook" and encourages the perpetuation of dependency and underdevelopment. Moreover, it allows those nations to invest resources in military rather than social goals.

Medical Missionaries: Past and Present

The terms "mission" and "missionaries" have been repeatedly raised in this discussion. Mission, used in religious, military, medical, and diplomatic contexts, suggests the act of sending a group to another place to accomplish a specific, self-imposed purpose. A missionary is a member of a religious group sent into an area to evangelize or offer service, such as health care, economic development, education, or social justice. The term primarily refers to a Christian tradition of proselytizing and converting nonbelievers, but other religions may also have missionaries.[63]

These terms warrant analysis because of the differences between the historical and contemporary contexts of their usage. For example, there is a difference between missionary medicine and medical missionaries. There can be individuals whose missionary zeal is primarily to spread the ideas of science and biomedical technology. Cueto refers to the Rockefeller International Health Foundation as "missionaries of science."[64] Similarly, the contemporary context includes the phenomenon of short-term medical missions that did not exist in the past.

During the sixteenth-century Age of Exploration, Catholic missionaries from a variety of orders were sent to North America, South Asia, and Africa; these efforts continue today. The heyday of Protestant missionaries was in the nineteenth and early twentieth centuries. Like other pioneers, missionaries intended to stay indefinitely, and they built permanent outposts to "serve the natives" in a complete way—body, mind, and soul. Missionaries (and mission societies) established churches, hospitals, and schools. Lindland describes the famous mission station Livingstonia (in what was then

Zambia), founded in 1874 by the Free Church of Scotland. The mission was inspired by the call of David Livingstone, a heroic explorer and medical doctor, to bring "Christianity, commerce and civilization" to southeast Africa.[65] From the very beginning of the mission movement, the delivery of Western medicine was an important part of the effort. At Livingstonia, Lindland states, "The medical missionaries . . . conceived of their work as not only curative, but also evangelical and educational. They justified it as a means to relieve physical suffering among members of the local population, but also as a witness to the love of God, and as a demonstration of the superiority of Western Christian society, culture and science."[66] The clinics at Livingstonia had a limited biomedical scope and nonphysician missionaries emphasized the original historical function of a *hospitium*—a place for the old, sick, neglected, and injured to either recover or die with dignity. The ideal purpose of the hospital was to demonstrate Christian kindness and mercy, an exercise that was spiritually beneficial to the missionaries themselves. This tradition is an antecedent of the FBO-based hospice care that characterized the beginning of the HIV/AIDS epidemic.

Missionary doctors were responsible for the health of the European missionaries themselves, but they also were pioneers of modern biomedicine and surgery who saw a staggering number of patients. Dr. Robert Laws, for example, did the first surgery in Africa using chloroform anesthesia in 1876, only fifteen years after the discovery of anesthesia in Britain.[67] By 1897, he had treated nine thousand patients, of whom seven thousand received surgery. Between 1903 and 1905, the Livingstonia mission built thirteen hospitals and sixteen dispensaries; these facilities treated more than eighty thousand patients.[68] From the start, these medical activities allowed the overall mission at Livingstonia to flourish; clearly, the power of Western medicine was attractive.

Albert Schweitzer followed in Livingstonia's model with his mission hospital in Lambarene, in the west African colony of France now known as Gabon, founded in 1913 with a plan to spread the Gospel through the Christian labor of healing rather than through the verbal process of preaching.[69] Schweitzer worked at Lambarene for several three-year missions between 1913 and 1947, spending a total of twenty years in the field. During periods in Europe, although he published volumes on the historical Jesus and a philosophy of civilization, he was obliged to spend a great deal of time raising money for the hospital, giving illustrated lectures and organ recitals to church groups.[70] Like the physicians at Livingstonia, he emphasized in these talks the surgeries that he did and the large number of patients seen at his facilities.

In many ways, Schweitzer was the heroic epitome of a medical missionary of the colonial age; however, he also epitomized some of the darker elements of the medical missionary movement. Although he was an outspoken critic of the injustices, cruelties, and land grabs of colonialism, he was also observed to be very patronizing to local peoples, and his hospital was operated at questionable standards.[71]

While historical missions were associated with imperialism and oppression, some contemporary missionary work, particularly by Catholics working in Latin America, has been engaged with an explicit consciousness of social justice issues and the dangers of cultural imperialism or economic exploitation disguised as religious conversion. Of particular note is the adoption of liberation theology and advocacy for the poor, which has been interpreted as political, even revolutionary, by people in power. Advocacy for the poor and dispossessed who have little access to medical care is an attribute of contemporary leaders in global health like Paul Farmer in Haiti[72] and Caroll Berhorst, who worked with the Maya-Kaqchikel of Guatemala.[73] These individuals and the healthcare systems that they have created fit all of the criteria of medical missionaries without the outward signs of religious faith.[74]

On the other hand, there has been another recent development in missionary activity that is quite different—short-term missions. A reported 1.6 million Americans participate in short-term mission trips each year, in an expansion that has been characterized as an "explosion."[75] Many of these trips are organized for teenage youth groups from white evangelical Protestant congregations who visit North American missionaries in Latin America or the Caribbean for an average of ten days, through organizations such as Youth with a Mission. Short-term missions are often engaged in construction activities or proselytizing through "vacation bible schools."[76] While short-term mission participants describe their experiences as "life changing," research has not been able to document such positive outcomes.

Indeed, researchers have offered a number of critiques of short-term missions. The seven basic criticisms are:

1. Much of the construction is unnecessary and expensive and displaces local employment.
2. Most of the money spent goes to airlines, tour organizers, and missionaries, while almost nothing reaches the local communities.
3. Participants' preexisting ideas that the poor are personally responsible for their economic circumstances are reinforced.
4. Participants have very little interaction with the local community.

5. Previous levels of ethnocentrism are increased.
6. Local people are romanticized as being more spiritually pure and happy because of their poverty, which unburdens them from the distractions of the material world.
7. Participants are no more likely to become missionaries or contribute to missionary efforts than those who have not experienced a short-term mission.[77]

Despite these problems, it appears that short-term missions are an indication of the growing popular interest of young Americans in issues of economic underdevelopment and global health inequalities. This interest, of course, is also seen in universities developing global health institutes, global health curricula, and faculty research.[78]

Short-term medical missions are also a relatively new phenomenon, although some describe the history of medical missionaries as medical volunteerism.[79] Short-term volunteer medical missions are best known in the context of specific surgical procedures such as the repair of cleft palates (SmileTrain) or the removal of cataracts (Unite for Sight). Medical educators have described the benefits of a variety of programs for medical students to participate in time-limited overseas medical programs.[80] However, although these surgical efforts are popular with donors, there has been considerable criticism of them within the medical community in terms of effectiveness, neglect of training of local medical personnel, and medical error.[81]

These programs also carry some dark resonances with historical missionary efforts. The emphasis on the large numbers of patients seen in the programs is reminiscent of the reports of early medical missionaries. Furthermore, some of these short-term missions seem to reflect a paternalism reminiscent of colonial-era missions in that unqualified students are allowed to gain clinical experience on the bodies of the poor. One study of participants in a short-term medical mission in rural Nepal, "Paul Farmer Made Me Do It!," analyzes the ethical complications and religious motivations of volunteers.[82]

Conclusion: Global Health's Wariness of Religion

While global health is a rapidly growing field and FBOs supply an extraordinary amount of healthcare in low- and middle-income countries, a certain wariness and skepticism of religion and religious institutions remains in the minds of global health researchers and practitioners. The topic of religion is seldom discussed in textbooks for global health courses; when religious institutions are mentioned, there is frequently a negative tone to the discussion. Within schools of public health, discussions of religion are rare, despite the fact that many students are motivated by both religious and humanitarian concerns.[83] It seems that there is a conflict of cultures between global health and religion. There may be two reasons for this suspicion and conflict. First, there is a legacy of missionaries as supporters of colonial or totalitarian regimes. FBOs' own discourse and self-presentation tends to create distance between the contemporary institutions and their historical antecedents. NGO alliances of FBOs and secular humanitarian organizations also obscure this connection. Second, there is the difference between public health as a field and clinical health care. Global public health is closely linked with economic development and movements for social justice; this is somewhat distant from hospital-based health care in the minds of many practitioners.

Global health, as a social movement of the twenty-first century, can only be strengthened by a greater recognition of and alliance with religion and religious institutions. Such an alliance requires not only mutual respect but also the effort of both sides to learn the terminologies and epistemologies of the other. Common understandings and cooperative research can be enhanced by dialogue. People in religious studies must be tolerant of public health researchers' need to simplify and quantify variables capturing complex human behavior. They must also recognize that religious health assets have utilitarian value for on-the-ground interventions and that collaboration can be mutually beneficial. At the same time, public health practitioners must show respect for the complexity and indeterminate nature of human behavior, beliefs, and motivations and become more sophisticated about variations of religious activities and the role of religion in community organization. They should acknowledge that religious beliefs may not be measureable, but that does not diminish their importance. Finally, public health practitioners would benefit from not viewing religion as an obstacle to health. Global health and religion have many common goals; an alliance will create synergies that may help improve health throughout the globe.

Notes

1. Paul Farmer, Arthur Kleinman, Jim Yong Kim, and Matthew Basilico, eds., *Reimagining Global Health: An Introduction*, California Series in Public Anthropology (Berkeley: University of California Press, 2013).

2. In fact, the historian Alan Brandt has argued that the origin of the field of global health can be tied to the HIV/AIDS pandemic. Alan M. Brandt, "How AIDS Invented Global Health," *New England Journal of Medicine* 368, no. 23 (2013): 2149–2152.

3. J. P. Koplan, T. C. Bond, M. H. Merson, K. S. Reddy, M.H. Rodriguez, N. K. Sewankambo et al., "Towards a Common Definition of Global Health," *The Lancet* 373, no. 9679 (2009): 1993.

4. R. Beaglehole and R. Bonita, "What is Global Health?," *Global Health Action* 3(2010): 5142.

5. T. M. Brown, M. Cueto, and E. Fee, "The World Health Organization and the Transition from 'International' to 'Global' Public Health," *American Journal of Public Health* 96, no. 1 (2006): 62–72.

6. Terminologies for organizations or institutions that are simultaneously religious and health oriented are not fixed. The term "faith-based organization" is an American neologism. "Religious health assets," a term developed by ARHAP, is more general.

7. A. Lakoff, "Two Regimes of Global Health," *Humanity: An International Journal of Human Rights, Humanitarianism, and Development* 1, no. 1 (2010): 59–79.

8. R. Handler, "Disciplinary Adaptation and Undergraduate Desire: Anthropology and Global Development Studies in the Liberal Arts Curriculum," *Cultural Anthropology* 28, no. 2 (2013): 181–203.

9. For example, through the 2003 Live Eight Concerts and the celebrity-driven "Make Poverty History" and "One" campaigns.

10. United Nations, *The Millennium Development Goals Report 2013* (New York: United Nations, 2013), http://www.undp.org/content/undp/en/home/librarypage/mdg/the-millennium-development-goals-report-2013/.

11. Pew Foundation, *World Publics Welcome Global Trade—But Not Immigration: Global Attitudes Survey* (Washington, DC: Pew Foundation, October 2007), http://www.pewglobal.org/2007/10/04/world-publics-welcome-global-trade-but-not-immigration/.

12. Karen A. Grépin, Katherine Leach-Kemon, Matthew Schneider, and Devi Sridhar, "How to Do (Or Not to Do) . . . Tracking Data on Development Assistance for Health," *Health Policy and Planning* 27, no. 6 (2012): 527–534.

13. This might not be an extraordinary sum in relative terms; the United States spends approximately $689 billion per year on defense.

14. D. Sridhar and R. Batniji, "Misfinancing Global Health: A Case for Transparency in Disbursements and Decision Making," *The Lancet* 372, no. 9644 (2008): 1185–1191.

15. Bill and Melinda Gates Foundation, "Who We Are: History," http://www.gatesfoundation.org/Who-We-Are/General-Information/History.

16. Cumulative budget as of FY2012.

17. US President's Emergency Plan for AIDS Relief (PEPFAR), "Working Toward an AIDS Free Generation: Latest PEPFAR Funding," April 2013, http://www.pepfar.gov/documents/organization/189671.pdf.

18. David McCoy, Sudip Chand, and Devi Sridhar, "Global Health Funding: How Much, Where It Comes From and Where It Goes," *Health Policy and Planning* 24, no. 6 (2010): 415.

19. PEPFAR and Interfaith Health Program, Emory University, *A Firm Foundation: The PEPFAR Consultation on the Role of Faith-Based Organizations in Sustaining Community and Country Leadership in the Response to HIV/AIDS* (Washington, DC: US Department of State, 2012), http://www.pepfar.gov/documents/organization/195614.pdf.

20. Humanitarianism is a belief system based on secular nonreligious principles, although some argue that humanitarianism is a religion; see B. Taithe, "Reinventing (French) Universalism: Religion, Humanitarianism and the 'French Doctors,'" *Modern & Contemporary France* 12, no. 2 (2004): 147–158.

21. PEPFAR, *A Firm Foundation*.

22. USAID and CapacityPlus, "Faith-Based Organizations," Issue Brief no. 4, February 2012, http://www.capacityplus.org/files/resources/Issue-Brief-4-FBOs.pdf.

23. World Health Organization, 3 by 5 Initiative, "Mobilizing Communities to Achieve 3 by 5," WHO/HIV 2003.15 (Geneva: World Health Organization, 2003), http://www.who.int/3by5/publications/briefs/communities/en/; D. E. Messer, *Breaking the Conspiracy of Silence: Christian Churches and the Global AIDS Crisis* (Minneapolis: Augsburg Fortress, 2004).

24. F. El Awa, "The Role of Religion in Tobacco Control Interventions," *Bulletin of the World Health Organization* 82, no. 12 (2004): 894.

25. J. Santelli, M. A. Ott, M. Lyon, J. Rogers, D. Summers, and R. Schleifer, "Abstinence and Abstinence-Only Education: A Review of US Policies and Programs," *Journal of Adolescent Health* 38, no. 1 (2006): 72–81; Rosemary Morgan, Andrew Green, and Erica Gadsby, "Religion and HIV/AIDS Policy in Faith-Based NGOs," paper presented at ARHAP Conference: When Religion and Health Align—Mobilizing Religious Health Assets for Transformation, Cape Town, South Africa, July 13–16, 2009.

26. PEPFAR Watch, "Abstinence & Fidelity," 2013, http://www.pepfarwatch.org/the_issues/abstinence_and_fidelity/.

27. C. W. Shin, "Are Culture Wars Over? U.S. Evangelicals and the Global AIDS Crisis," (Syracuse, NY: Luce Project in Religion, Media, and International Relations, 2009); PEPFAR, *A Firm Foundation*.

28. E. C. Green, *Faith-Based Organizations: Contributions to HIV Prevention*, The Synergy Project no. 1701 (Washington, DC: USAID, 2003).

29. World Health Organization, "Poverty and Health," http://www.who.int/hdp/poverty/en/.

30. Purchasing power parity is a standard econometric measure that standardizes monetary values or exchange rates based on nation-specific consumer prices. The graph of this relationship becomes clearer when a logarithmic scale is used for income.

31. R. G. Wilkinson and K. E. Pickett, "Income Inequality and Population Health: A Review and Explanation of the Evidence," *Social Science & Medicine* 62, no. 7 (2006): 1768–1784.

32. Pew Foundation, *World Publics Welcome Global Trade*.

33. Religiosity was measured using a three-item cumulative index ranging from zero to 3, with 3 representing the most religious position. Respondents were given 1 point each for affirmative answers to questions about "believing that faith in God is necessary for morality," "religion is very important in their lives," and "praying at least once a day."

34. K. Pickett and R. Wilkinson, *The Spirit Level: Why Greater Equality Makes Societies Stronger* (New York: Bloomsbury Press, 2010).

35. Pew-Templeton Foundation, Global Religious Futures Project, http://www.globalreligiousfutures.org/.

36. D. E. Moerman, and W. B. Jonas, "Deconstructing the Placebo Effect and Finding the Meaning Response," *Annals of Internal Medicine* 136, no. 6 (2002): 471–476.

37. D. W. Dunlop, "Alternatives to 'Modern' Health Delivery Systems in Africa: Public Policy Issues of Traditional Health Systems," *Social Science & Medicine (1967)* 9, no. 11 (1975): 581–586; M. Freeman and M. Motsei, "Planning Health Care in South Africa—Is There a Role for Traditional Healers?," *Social Science & Medicine* 34, no. 11 (1992): 1183–1190.

38. E. C. Green, "Can Collaborative Programs between Biomedical and African Indigenous Health Practitioners Succeed?," *Social Science & Medicine* 27, no. 11 (1988): 1125–1130; E. C. Green, B. Zokwe, and J. D. Dupree, "The Experience of an AIDS Prevention Program Focused on South African Traditional Healers," *Social Science & Medicine* 40, no. 4 (1995): 503–515.

39. Miriam Kiser, Deborah L. Jones, and Gary R. Gunderson, "Faith and Health: Leadership Aliging Assets to Transform Communities," *International Review of Mission* 95, no. 376–377 (2006): 50–58.

40. E. Lindland, "Crossroads of Culture: Religion, Therapy and Personhood in Northern Malawi," PhD Dissertation, Emory University, 2005.

41. A. Ashforth, "An Epidemic of Witchcraft? The Implications of AIDS for the Post-Apartheid State," *African Studies* 61, no. 1 (2002): 121–143.

42. Another reason for the confusion of public health with medicine is that "public health" is sometimes used colloquially to refer to publicly funded medical care (for instance, in public clinics) as opposed to privately funded treatment facilities.

43. T. McKeown, *The Role of Medicine: Dream, Mirage, or Nemesis?* (London: Blackwell, 1979).

44. A. Alland, "Medical Anthropology and the Study of Biological and Cultural Adaptation," *American Anthropologist* 68, no. 1 (1966): 40–51.

45. L. M. Chatters, "Religion and Health: Public Health Research and Practice," *Annual Review of Public Health* 21, no. 1 (2000): 335–367.

46. J. Trinitapoli and A. Weinreb, *Religion and AIDS in Africa* (Oxford: Oxford University Press, 2012).

47. J. Neu, "Levi-Strauss on Shamanism," *Man* 10, no. 2 (1975): 285–292.

48. K. I. Pargament, H. G. Koenig, N. Tarakeshwar, and J. Hahn, "Religious Struggle as a Predictor of Mortality among Medically Ill Elderly Patients: A 2-Year Longitudinal Study," *Archives of Internal Medicine* 161, no. 15 (2001): 1881–1885.

49. The number of NGOs is unknown, in part because there is no standard definition or registration. Estimates include 1.5 million in the United States, 3.3 million in India, and 275,000 in Russia ("Fact Sheet: Non-Governmental Organizations (NGOs) in the United States «". Humanrights.gov.;. Doh, J.P., Teegen, H (2003) Globalization and NGOs: Transforming Business, Government, and Society . NY: Greenwood Publishing Group, p. 3

It should also be noted that, although they are repeatedly found in the literature, the origins of the reported proportions of health services offered by FBOs versus ministries of health are unclear.

50. D. Welliver and M. Northcutt, *Mission Handbook—US and Canadian Protestant Ministries Overseas, 2004–2006*, Wheaton, IL: EMIS/Billy Graham Center, 2004.

51. F. Manji and C. O'Coill, "The Missionary Position: NGOs and Development in Africa," *International Affairs* 78, no. 3 (2002): 567–583.

52. Y.-W. Cheung and P. New, "Toward a Typology of Missionary Medicine: A Comparison of Three Canadian Medical Missions in China Before 1937," *Culture: Canadian Ethnology Society Outremont* 3, no. 2 (1983): 31–45; Helen Rose Ebaugh, Paula F. Pipes, Janet Slatzman Chafetz, and Martha Daniels, "Where's the Religion? Distinguishing Faith-Based from Secular Social Service Agencies," *Journal for the Scientific Study of Religion* 42, no. 3 (2003): 411–426.

53. Birn, Pillay, and Holtz, *Textbook of International Health*.

54. S. Mwenda, "The Africa Christian Health Associations Platform: Showcasing the Contributions of CHAs," *Contact* 190, P. 2–3 (2011).

55. PEPFAR and Interfaith Health Program, *A Firm Foundation*.

56. Caritas, "Our Work: HIV and AIDS," http://www.caritas.org/activities/hiv_aids/index.html.

57. Anne-Emanuelle Birn, Yogan Pillay, and Timothy H. Holtz, *Textbook of International Health: Global Health in a Dynamic World* (Oxford: Oxford University Press, 2009). They studied the Mennonite Central Committee, Lutheran World Relief, Adventist Development and Relief Agency, American Friends Service Committee, World Vision, Catholic Relief Services, Comité Catholique, Hadassah, Muslim Aid, Islamic World Relief, and American Jewish World Service.

58. World Vision, *2012 Annual Review* (Federal Way, WA: World Vision, 2012), http://www.worldvision.org/content.nsf/about/ar-financials.

59. The special relationship between Catholic institutions and the stigmatized disease of leprosy (Hansen's disease) is noteworthy. CMMB has a long-standing relationship with Haiti. This is one reason why it received the largest USAID grant awarded to an NGO after the Haitian earthquake of 2010.

60. Catholic Medical Mission Board, "CMMB History: 100 Years of Healing and Hope," http://www.cmmb.org/cmmb-history.

61. Marlon Banda, Eva Ombaka, and Sophie Logez, *Multi-Country Study of Medicine Supply and Distribution Activities of Faith-Based Organizations in Sub-Saharan African Countries* (Geneva: World Health Organization, 2006), http://www.who.int/medicines/areas/access/EN_EPNstudy.pdf.

62. For a detailed explanation of these problems, see E. Kawasaki and J. Patten, *Drug Supply Systems of Missionary Organizations. Identifying Factors Affecting Expansion and Efficiency: Case Studies from Uganda And Kenya* (Geneva: World Health Organization, 2002).

63. A limitation of this chapter is its exclusive focus on Christian institutions. Both Islamic and Jewish charitable organizations, it appears, may be oriented more toward the problems of their own communities. There is no tradition of missionization in these religions as there is in Christianity. This area requires more research.

64. M. Cueto, ed., *Missionaries of Science: The Rockefeller Foundation and Latin America* (Bloomington: Indiana University Press, 1994). See also E. R. Brown, *Rockefeller Medicine Men: Medicine and Capitalism in America* (Berkeley: University of California Press, 1979).

65. Lindland, "Crossroads of Culture."

66. Lindland, "Crossroads of Culture," 150.

67. M. King and E. King, *The Story of Medicine and Disease in Malawi: 130 Years since Livingstone* (Blantyre, Malawi: Montfort Press, 1992).

68. M. Gelfand, *Lakeside Pioneers: A Socio-Medical Study of Nyasaland (1875–1920)* (Oxford: Basil Blackwell, 1964).

69. A. Schweitzer and C. T. Campion, *On the Edge of the Primeval Forest: Experiences and Observations of a Doctor in Equatorial Africa* (London: Black, 1922).

70. A. P. Polednak, "Albert Schweitzer and International Health," *Journal of Religion and Health* 28, no. 4 (1989): 323–329.

71. J. Cameron, *Point of Departure: An Attempt at Autobiography* (New York: McGraw-Hill, 1967).

72. T. Kidder, *Mountains Beyond Mountains: The Quest of Dr. Paul Farmer, a Man Who Would Cure the World* (New York: Random House Digital, 2009).

73. R. Luecke, *A New Dawn in Guatemala: Toward a Worldwide Health Vision* (Long Grove, IL: Waveland Press, 1993).

74. Privately, both Farmer and Behrhorst are religious individuals, but these beliefs are purposefully excluded from their social presentation of self.

75. R. J. Priest, T. Dischinger, S. Rasmussen, and C. M. Brown, "Researching the Short-Term Mission Movement," *Missiology: An International Review* 34, no. 4 (2006): 431–450; B. M. Howell, *Short-Term Mission: An Ethnography of Christian Travel Narrative and Experience* (Downers Grove, IL: InterVarsity Press, 2012).

76. W. V. Taylor, "Short-Term Missions: Reinforcing Beliefs and Legitimating Poverty," MA Thesis, Department of Sociology, University of Tennessee–Knoxville, 2012.

77. J. A. Van Engen, "The Cost of Short-Term Missions," *The Other Side* 36, no. 1 (2000): 20–23; K. Birth, "What Is Your Mission Here? A Trinidadian Perspective on Visits from the 'Church of Disneyworld,'" *Missiology: An International Review* 34, no. 4 (2006): 497–508; K. A. Ver Beek, "The Impact of Short-Term Missions: A Case Study of House Construction in Honduras after Hurricane Mitch," *Missiology* 34, no. 4 (2006): 477–495; K. Beyerlein, J. Trinitapoli, and G. Adler, "The Effect of Religious Short-Term Mission Trips on Youth Civic Engagement," *Journal for the Scientific Study of Religion* 50, no. 4 (2011): 780–795.

78. Consortium of Universities for Global Health, "Background," http://www.cugh.org/about-us/background; Handler, "Disciplinary Adaptation and Undergraduate Desire."

79. O. Olakanmi and P. A. Perry, "Medical Volunteerism in Africa: An Historical Sketch," *Virtual Mentor* 8, no. 12 (2006): 863–870.

80. M. P. Alcauskas, "From Medical School to Mission: The Ethics of International Medical Volunteerism," *Virtual Mentor* 8, no. 12 (2006): 797–800; K. Parsi and J. List, "Preparing Medical Students for the World: Service Learning and Global Health Justice," *Medscape Journal of Medicine* 10, no. 11 (2008): 268.

81. L. M. Montgomery, "Short-Term Medical Missions: Enhancing or Eroding Health?," *Missiology: An International Review* 21, no. 3 (1993): 333–341; E. L. Hoover, G. Cole-Hoover, P. K. Berry, E. T. Hoover, B. Harris, D. Rageh, and W. L. Weaver, "Private Volunteer Medical Organizations: How Effective Are They?," *Journal of the National Medical Association* 97, no. 2 (2005): 270–275; A. J. Wolfberg, "Volunteering Overseas: Lessons from Surgical Brigades," *New England Journal of Medi-*

cine 354, no. 5 (2006): 443–445; M. Decamp, "Scrutinizing Global Short-Term Medical Outreach," *Hastings Center Report* 37, no. 6 (2007): 21–23.

82. D. M. Citrin, "'Paul Farmer Made Me Do It': A Qualitative Study of Short-Term Medical Volunteer Work in Remote Nepal," Master's Thesis, School of Public Health University of Washington, 2011.

83. The Rollins School of Public Health at Emory University may be an exception. Nevertheless, a certain skepticism has been expressed by faculty members in discussions of curricula related to religion and health. I would like to thank Ellen Idler for her leadership in this seminar as well as for her great patience.

21 | The Christian Medical Commission and the World Health Organization

MATTHEW BERSAGEL BRALEY

God is watching. The people are waiting. You are commissioned to go to wipe the tears away from all faces and bring forth lives filled with strength, and purpose which will make for peace.

Archbishop Desmond Tutu[1]

O N MAY 20, 2008, ARCHBISHOP Desmond Tutu of South Africa ascended a plenary dais to address the sixty-first annual meeting of the World Health Assembly, the governing body of the World Health Organization (WHO). While the WHO's definition of health does not include spiritual well-being, Tutu reminded the gathering of scientists, program specialists, and health ministers who set the global health agenda for the twenty-first century that "faith and health have been together a very long time."[2]

In the Christian tradition that formed Bishop Tutu, faith and health have, indeed, been together a long time. The story of Christianity and health care dates back to the early church, as Jesus' disciples preached and practiced his distinctive healing ministry.[3] Over the centuries, this healing ministry has assumed diverse forms. As Tutu concluded his remarks to the World Health Assembly, he offered a brief history lesson to highlight one of these forms and the integral role it played in the institutional history of the WHO:

It is a godly coincidence that nearby the World Council of Churches (WCC) is also celebrating its 60th year. Together WHO and WCC share a common mission to the world, protecting and restoring body, mind, and spirit. It is important that this is also the 40th anniversary of the Christian Medical Commission, whose values and experience in primary health care, informed and shaped the 1974 WHO Guidelines for Primary Health Care, which were reaffirmed at Alma-Ata.[4]

This chapter focuses on the "godly coincidence" that brought the WHO and the Christian Medical Commission (CMC) together in the late twentieth century, as the CMC sought to reinterpret the healing ministry of Jesus for an increasingly globalized world defined, in large part, by unequal access to health care.

The Healing Church or the Priesthood of All Healers

While Tutu was correct that faith and health had a long history, the nature of the relationship was rapidly changing in the twentieth century as the cognitive revolution of Western medicine took increasingly powerful institutional forms and political revolutions challenged assumptions about who should control those institutions. It was in the midst of these changes that the members of the Christian ecumenical consultation in Tübingen, Germany, in 1964 sought to discern the appropriate role of Christian medical missions and, in the process, "rediscovered" what they believed to be the distinctive, enduring witness of Jesus's healing ministry for the modern world.[5]

Two years earlier, the Lutheran World Federation and the WCC's Division of World Mission and Evangelism initiated a joint study on the "essential issues" of medical missions.[6] Keeping the study intentionally modest in scope, the two bodies sought the advice of a small group, constituted primarily of medical doctors, on the appropriate role of the Lutheran World Federation and the WCC in responding to the perceived challenges facing medical missions. Preparatory papers focused on different conceptions of and contexts for healing, from the pre-scientific to modern medicine and from the congregation to the mission field. The gathering in Tübingen was the culmination of this work. By the end of the week together, the members of the consultation, much to both their own surprise and that of the planners, had moved—or, to echo the tenor of the participants, had been moved—from reflection to proclamation.

The findings of the consultation found expression in a "Statement on the Christian Concept of the Healing Ministry of the Church," understood by participants and subsequent generations of Christian health workers as a fundamental challenge to what was traditionally understood as the two-fold task of medical missions: meeting physical needs and preaching the Gospel.[7] The statement reconfirmed in language both theological and practical that the Christian Church has a distinctive role to play in healing. While acknowledging that Christians involved in health work express similar ethical commitments as non-Christians—to compassion and a concern for the dignity of individuals—the statement makes explicit the relationship between healing and the Christian drama of salvation history.

Theologically, healing bears witness to the "breaking into human life of the powers of the Kingdom of God, and of the dethroning of the powers of evil."[8] Such an incarnational view of healing is intended as an invitation for the "priesthood of all believers" to become a priesthood of all *healers*, actively responding to the spiritual as well as the physical dimensions of suffering. In the older, Enlightenment-inflected formulation, curative medical practices were a jumping-off point for proselytizing, but physical healing was neither the means to nor evidence of salvation; rather— consistent with Cartesian ontology—care for the body and care for the soul were seen as distinctive activities.

The incarnational theology articulated at Tübingen presented both epistemological and eschatological challenges to this distinction. Epistemologically, the consensus that emerged in this first gathering at Tübingen (later called Tübingen I) sided with nascent liberation theologies that legitimized knowledge generated outside of the professional medical establishment. Knowledge of the body—more specifically, one's own body— was not the exclusive domain of medical doctors and researchers. In the medical missionary encounter, these theologies noted, knowledge of the body was more accurately described as an amalgamation of Western science, traditional medicines, culturally specific anthropologies (theological or otherwise), and experience.

This is not to say that the participants at Tübingen I had embraced cultural relativism.[9] Rather, Tübingen I interpreted disease within the framework of Christian eschatology or the vision of a future world in which humanity is reconciled fully with God. According to this interpretation, disease is a "sign for a world awaiting salvation" and "healing represents the defeat of transpersonal evil that contradicts the original good intention of God for all human beings."[10] The eschatological frame describes a shift in emphasis from "broken" individuals in need of fixing to a broken world in need of healing—physically as well as spiritually. Practically, this is embodied by a medical missionary who sees his or her role not as the primary vessel through which individuals are saved but as a witness to a Christian theological understanding of history in which the dialectic between sin and salvation finds this-worldly expression in the breaking and healing of relationships—with God, with others, and with one's self.

Health itself is understood as an eschatological concept. It is never achieved, but as David Jenkins, one of the key interlocutors in the CMC's early discussions, describes, it is "what God promises and offers in the end . . . what is available now both in foretastes and as the aim and ideal which judges our current activities and structures while at the same time provoking us to more healthy responses."[11] The work of Jenkins and James McGilvray to develop an eschatological idea of health reclaimed medicine as a service profession that should be "more widely and directly available to all suffering human beings."[12] As such, it was a call for reorientation, not rejection, of Western medicine, an invitation to think of health as a "vision of possibilities" that cannot be reduced to the "possibilities or failures of medicine."[13]

The concern for a Christian understanding of healing at Tübingen I could, if taken in certain other-worldly directions, call into question the grounds on which hospitals and clinics were deemed necessary. But the participants at Tübingen I, most of whom were medical professionals and not theologians, advocated a less radical reform of medical mission that sought to reintegrate (rather than excommunicate) the professional medical worker into the wider healing church and to supplement medical skills with "practical acts of love and service . . . sanctified by the ministry of the word, prayer and the sacraments."[14] In this commitment to reconnecting medical missionaries to the corporate life of Christian fellowship, Tübingen I offered a new ecclesiology, a new vision of the purpose of the church.

The church as healing community was a correction to what was identified by participants as one of the critical issues in medical missions: the increasing power, specialization, and professionalization of medicine. Specialized medical practice and the institutions in which it was practiced, even if nominally Christian, had become, they argued, disengaged from the life of the congregation. This had an effect not only on the practice of medicine but also on how Christians understood their own capacity to be agents of healing. In a health worldview described largely in the language of professional medicine—that is, health understood as the absence of disease—the authority of the Great Physician to heal is masked by the proliferation of pretty good physicians who can diagnose, treat, and, in some cases, cure the physical ills that humans suffer. One of the fundamental claims of Tübingen I, however, was that "all healing is of God."[15]

As members of healing communities, they argued, Christians must recognize their theologically rooted moral obligations to accompany others at every stage of their health journey, especially those stages not recognized or adequately addressed by the hospital-based system. In effect, Tübingen participants exhorted Christians to reclaim their capacity to heal by recognizing both the theological grounds of healing and the multidimensional reality of health. This multidimensional view of healing affords multiple entry points for persons with diverse talents to participate in healing processes and thus decenters the medical professional without necessarily rejecting its contribution.

Tübingen I urged the church not "to surrender its responsibility in the field of healing to other agencies," since Christianity is understood as offering a distinctive approach to health and healing that is derivative of the Gospel's emphasis on wholeness and the reconciliation of human relationships with one another and with God. For the participants at Tübingen, the healing church offered a vision of a transformed community that took seriously its unique responsibility to be a place of refuge from both the existential anxiety and the physical illnesses that plagued the modern world.

Reflecting on the consultation nearly two decades later, James McGilvray offered this assessment of the epiphany at Tübingen I:

> Their original intention had been to address themselves to the problems of their service and to discover a cogent rationale for the churches' involvement in medical care. Yet, in every case, they found themselves concluding that the church had somehow lost its capacity to heal partly because it had chosen to define this role too narrowly in terms of medical practice, addressed especially to those in sore need, and, partly because it had lost its sense of corporateness and community through a pre-occupation with individual salvation. In this sense, the church suffered the same imbalance as medicine which was most frequently practiced on a one to one relationship between physician and the individual patient.[16]

According to this line of thinking, the Enlightenment and the development of modern medicine in its wake effectively ruptured the intrinsic connection between the Gospel and health, first by separating out the constitutive parts of the human (mind, body, spirit), and second by transferring the authority to heal to institutions and technologies driven by the logic of scientific positivism. The upshot, in Christian theological terms, is that modern medicine could not account for the paradoxical place of suffering in the Christian tradition. Healing or salvation in medical terms was preoccupied with the total removal of illness; health was negatively defined as the absence of disease. Modern medicine did not offer a satisfactory soteriology or account of salvation and healing to persons who experienced illness and suffering as more than physical.

The problems with medical missionary work had been identified and a general reorientation articulated at Tübingen, but what that actually meant going forward remained undecided. Despite drawing such a stark contrast between the logic and practices of Western medicine and a theology of Christian healing—perhaps, as the quote from McGilvray suggests, humbled by the church's own failure to walk the talk—the participants at Tübingen I left open the question of whether to fulfill this "responsibility in the field of healing" through the maintenance of separate Christian health facilities or through the participation of individual Christians in secular agencies.[17] Any answer to this question would, of course, need to be consistent with the theology of health and healing rediscovered at Tübingen I, but it would also have to account for the radical historical transformations in which this rediscovery was taking place.

Medical Missions in a Postcolonial Context

The new ecclesiology may have found theological justification in a recovery of earlier Christian conceptions of healing, but it was the profound political and social upheaval of the independence movements throughout the European colonies that served as the catalyst for rethinking the relationships between the institutional legacy of the medical mission model (that is, hospital-based curative care centers) and the emerging nation-states of Africa, Asia, and the Americas. With independence, nations were beginning to develop their own public health systems and in the process were calling into question the working relationships between church hospitals and colonial administrators. As Christoph Benn and Erlinda Senturias observe in their historical review of the ecumenical discussion of health and healing, "The churches had to face the issue of whether or not there was a specific Christian ministry of healing and how to define this ministry. They also had to articulate the differences between a government and a church hospital."[18]

Politically, church hospitals were associated with the colonial regimes and thus were suspect, an impediment to complete liberation. Practically, however, church-supported health care made up a significant amount of the total health care available in these newly independent countries.

Governments responded in various ways: by building new government hospitals, by nationalizing mission hospitals, and by allowing the hospitals to continue operating under the auspices of emerging independent national churches (for instance, the Evangelical Lutheran Church of Tanzania). Yet, all of these responses confronted the problem of financing. The practical (and urgent) problem of financing a new health system can be seen as one of both revenue generation and escalating healthcare costs. The former is part of the larger array of challenges facing governments in transition, including the necessity of establishing a tax structure capable of providing revenue to fund the health budget. The latter problem, however, was not unique to new nations, though it had a disproportionate effect on them. Rising healthcare costs were associated not with particular political events but with expensive new technologies and a growing emphasis on specialized curative services delivered by tertiary institutions.

The Tübingen consultation had been convened around the essential issues facing medical missions and the church's role in healing. But as the participants articulated a renewed vision for the church's role in healing—a response motivated by political and economic considerations as much as by theological reflection—the very model of medical missions was called into question. Political changes had raised questions about the legitimacy and purpose of the medical mission enterprise, financial considerations at the local and denominational level had forced questions about its viability and sustainability, and theological questions had surfaced a Christ-informed holistic understanding of health and human being that challenged the positivism and individualism of the predominant medical mission model.

Here Is the Healing Church, Here Is Its Steeple, Open It Up and . . . ?

Something happened at the first Tübingen conference. A healing church was, if not born, at least conceived. Tübingen I identified a distinctive identity for Christian communities, yet in so doing it made explicit the gap between Christian understandings of health and healing on the one hand and Western biomedical explanations of illness and health on the other. In attempting to "discover a cogent rationale for the churches' involvement in medical care," participants at Tübingen I called into question the premises of medical care itself, at least as practiced in the West and among medical missionaries.

The take-home message from Tübingen I was that medical accounts of health are insufficient without insights from Christian theology, especially insights about salvation. But this message left open two important questions: Would "the theologian's view of salvation . . . be complete and sufficient without the contribution of the scientist?"[19] And what would a healing church actually look like in practice?

These questions formed the basis for a second consultation at Tübingen in 1967, three years after the initial gathering. By this time, efforts were under way to look for examples of the healing church in the world. The WCC's Committee for Specialized Assistance to Social Projects had fielded surveys with the intention of eliciting the scope and role of "church-related medical programs" in the context of emerging independent states.[20] The results of these surveys, which informed the discussions of Tübingen II, offered specific evidence of the ways in which the medical missionary model failed to meet the health needs of the vulnerable persons whom it was intended to serve. Echoing concerns about the disproportionate emphasis on curative care, surveys found that 95 percent of church-related health programs focused on curative rather than promotive or preventive medicine. Moreover, as governments in newly independent states rushed to modernize, they, too, placed an emphasis on curative services. As a result of this narrower emphasis and the legacy of colonial disregard for a comprehensive health system, it was estimated that only 20 percent of vulnerable populations had access to modern medical care—either government or church provided. Even with access to care, the curative care focus contributed to a rise in operational costs for hospitals (for instance, the expense of upgrading diagnostic technologies). Higher fees for services, implemented to offset these additional costs, further restricted the potential clientele to those who could afford to pay the higher fees.

The postcolonial era underscored two additional findings of the surveys. First, locations of health services tended to follow identifiable patterns left over from colonial rule. The placement of hospitals and clinics was largely a function of strategic decisions on the part of colonial administrators and missionary churches rather than a response to the specific health needs of the colonized. As a result, the health system inherited by new leaders in sub-Saharan Africa was a patchwork of various colonial and denominational interests incompatible with a planned, comprehensive national health system. The church-related hospitals and clinics dotting the landscape in the former colonies did not reflect a coordinated effort to provide medical care across localities.

Second, the surveys showed that the actual and potential contribution of churches to healthcare services in postcolonial Africa was largely ignored by the leaders of newly independent states, in part because the lack of co-ordination within and across denominations prevented the emergence of a coherent church voice in debates about how to address the health needs of all citizens.[21] Given this environment, examples of what the healing church might look like were hard to find, especially when the search was conducted within the amalgam of existing church-related health programs.

Still, the concept of the healing church served to disrupt the dominance of biomedical frameworks for health that had relegated religious leaders to the role of "reactors,"[22] uncritically adopting the language and approach of Western biomedicine. Medical-speak had increasingly become the default language for articulating the fundamental questions of human suffering as well as the responses that they evoke—questions Tübingen participants recognized as central to the Christian story. At the same time they sought to disrupt that framework, however, participants at the first Tübingen consultation attempted to reclaim elements of the Christian healing tradition without retreating to premodern understandings of healing (for instance, healing as miracle) or reverting to a narrow view of medical mission as primarily a means of proselytizing, or saving bodies to save souls.

The reassertion of the priority of healing in the Christian tradition was intended as a constructive critique, animated by an impulse to reform rather than reject the assumptions of Western medicine, a corrective to what James McGilvray lamented as the "idolatry of the problem-solving powers of science."[23] McGilvray sees the consequences of such idolatry as a form of hubris: "What is wrong is not the 'medical model' but the human tendency to invest too much in valuable human powers and discoveries so that, first, idols are produced and then there is nowhere to turn when both their tyranny and inadequacy (on their own) begin to be obvious."[24] Indeed, for Robert Lambourne, whose book *Community, Church, and Healing* (1963) emerged as one of the core texts at Tübingen II, recognition of the tyranny and inadequacy of the medical model had become increasingly obvious even within the profession of medicine:

Recent years have seen a revival of interest within Medicine and Church in the possibility of co-operation with each other. There is now amongst the majority of men and women working in the medical and social services, some sympathy with church and religion. This is something new, for before two world wars shook man's confidence in his ability to master the world and himself, a mood of atheism or condescending agnosticism was dominant in Medicine. One sign of these new times is that universities and hospitals founded at the end of the last century without a chapel are now building chapels and appointing chaplains. Another is the growing emphasis amongst doctors upon a holistic approach to medicine. This holistic approach respects the fact of the psychosomatic unity of the person. As a consequence the clinician, whatever his personal position in matters of faith, now recognises ideally that no case history is complete which does not record some understanding of the patient's thoughts and feelings about his place and purpose in the universe. This understanding is not, of course, necessarily communicated in religious language.[25]

In the mid-twentieth-century interest in holistic health, the psychosomatic unity of the person, or what might be described as the phenomenon of human being appeared widespread.[26] For those at Tübingen II, this interest raised questions about the capacity of both science (that is, medicine) and Christian theology, in and of themselves, to articulate a comprehensive understanding of the multiple and interlocking dimensions of healing. Tübingen I had proposed the healing church as a corrective to the limits of the dominant medical view of health, but Tübingen II was forced to confront the limits of the healing church.

Of immediate concern was the practical implications of the healing church model for the ongoing provision of medical care in developing countries. Did the epiphany at Tübingen I imply that government or other nonreligious healthcare providers would always fall short of the vision of health made possible by a Christian framework of salvation history? If so, did that provide a mandate for Christian healthcare providers to resist the increasing intrusion of secular health care into what was understood to be the rightful domain of churches?

Reflecting on the criticisms of Tübingen I and the clarifying work undertaken at Tübingen II, Benn and Senturias suggest that the healing church was never intended as a substitute for other healthcare institutions. Drawing on notions of subsidiarity as well as the financial and professional impracticality of the church as health system, they underscore the idea that the "primary responsibility for the health care of people remains with the government of nations." The churches should "try to complement government services when these cannot fulfill their commitments or when there are particularly disadvantaged people for whom nobody cares." To task the church with the maintenance of a national health system "would be a misunderstanding of the church's mission."[27] The healing church as manifest in actual institutions on the ground stands in society's gaps and in so doing provides a witness to the specific ways national health systems fail to meet the health needs of their citizens (for instance, by discriminating against certain populations).

In addition to practical concerns, the vision of the healing church raised theological concerns. If healing is linked to salvation as a sign of the coming kingdom of God, to borrow from Tübingen I, what does that mean for those who do not experience healing, for example, those with chronic diseases? The theological vision that gave rise to the notion of the healing church risked falling into Christian triumphalism ("healing as a sign of the beginning of the kingdom of God and of the dethroning of the powers of evil"[28]) or fatalism associated with concepts of double predestination (the idea that whether a person is healed provides direct knowledge of his or her state of grace or damnation). Yet, the fundamental insight that "all healing is from God" was intended neither as an abdication of human responsibility to provide medical care to those in need nor as a rationale for not seeking this-worldly healing. Rather, it was a call for all members of the church to participate as healers according to their particular gifts and in the process transform congregations into healing communities. In this way, the theological vision of the healing church might be translated into an ecclesial and social reality with the power to impact the varied dimensions of suffering in this world.

The holistic understanding of health and the priesthood of all healers that it created space for was not, in the end, a denial of the critical role of medical professionals in church-related health programs. Indeed, the epiphany of Tübingen II was that understanding the implications of the healing church required an intimate and ongoing conversation between the disciplines of theology and medicine, among others. The key question of whether theology and medicine could speak coherently to one another about the phenomena of health or, more broadly, about what it was to be human remained open.

Tübingen II did not provide definitive answers to the questions of "whether the physician's view of health is complete and sufficient without a contribution from Christian theology, and whether the theologian's view of salvation would be complete and sufficient without the contribution of scientists."[29] Instead, the second consultation ended with a deeper awareness of the challenges that would need to be overcome in order to move the healing church from vision to reality. The bold call for a healing church announced in 1964 (Tübingen I) as a corrective to trends in Western medicine by 1967 (Tübingen II) gave way to a kind of epistemic humility that recognized the partiality of all disciplines—including theology—for comprehending fully the phenomenon of healthy human being. Tübingen II ended with a greater resolve to address these challenges with the full resources of the larger ecumenical movement. This resolve eventually found expression in a new institution, the CMC.

The Christian Medical Commission: An Institutional History

Established by a mandate of the WCC in 1968, the CMC was "charged with the responsibility to promote the coordination of national church-related medical programmes, and to engage in study and research into the most appropriate ways in which the churches might express their concern for total health care."[30] The mandate emphasized the practical tasks of the CMC even as it implied the theological dimensions of the new approach to medical missions articulated in the Tübingen consultations.

Surveys conducted prior to 1968 revealed that member churches of the WCC were affiliated with 1,200 hospitals worldwide, but the growing role of government in public health combined with an increase in costs as a result of both technological advances and aging institutions required a re-evaluation of church-related health programs.[31] As Gillian Patterson recounts, the CMC was set up as "an enabling and supporting organization. When the Commission identified an innovative programme, it would use the Commission's contacts to get funding for its work, and put its organizers in touch with people doing similar work elsewhere."[32] But as James McGilvray, the CMC's first director, noted at the inaugural annual meeting, the mapping of these innovative programs had a "theological flavour."[33]

Documenting church-affiliated healthcare programs provided answers to the descriptive question, what are churches doing? But analysis of the programs, especially in relation to other nonchurch health services, offered a starting point for answering theological questions about the distinctive contribution of church-affiliated services as well. Recalling the emphasis on salvation history and wholeness that permeated the Tübingen discussions, McGilvray declared, "The Church is not simply another service agency or an ecclesiastical foreign aid programme."[34] After Tübingen, the church was not simply the church anymore. It had become the healing church, leading some observers to suggest that "healing considered as the responsibility of the entire community may be precisely one of those gaps into which Christian congregations should do pioneering work."[35]

The initial mandate from the WCC located the CMC within its Division on World Mission and Evangelism and affiliated it with its Division of

Inter-Church Aid, Refugee, and World Service. The commission's twenty-five members included the chairs of these two divisions as well as the general secretary of the WCC. Though a priority was placed on selecting healthcare and community development professionals, representatives with theological and mission interests were also included.[36] The bylaws required that at least ten members come from non-Western countries, defined as *not* North America, Australasia, or Europe.

The mandate divided the commission's work into two stages. Stage 1 (1968–1971) was concerned with establishing the evidence base: "For a period of three years it shall be primarily engaged in surveys, the collection of data on existing institutions, investigation of more adequate forms of administrative relationships and research into the most appropriate ways of delivering health services."[37] It was also to be a period for promoting cooperation on global health issues among national, regional, and international organizations. Stage 2 was conceived of as the application phase. Based on the evidence from Stage 1, the commission would begin dispersing financial support to supplement existing or initiate new programs consistent with the CMC's commitments to "comprehensive and promotive heath."[38] Programs funded by the commission would have to demonstrate "a reasonable amount of local support" such that their reliance on commission funding would not exceed five years.[39]

The CMC, echoing the theological and institutional concerns of Tübingen, was interested in models of comprehensive primary health care, that is, programs that balanced preventive, promotive, and curative health care. Hospital-based care should, the CMC contended, remain a vital component of medical missions, but the near-exclusive emphasis on hospitals in medical mission activities to that point was problematic for two reasons in addition to the financial and infrastructure challenges. First, hospitals serve only those who come through their doors. Second, curative treatment is only one part of health and healing. In other words, hospital-based care is inherently exclusive and, by implication, is at odds with a Christian gospel that emphasizes inclusivity.

Central to the CMC story is the fact that its activities and priorities were influenced not only by the pendulum swing of public health strategies, emerging methodologies, and increasingly sophisticated data sets but also by a theological understanding of the world in which healing itself was a process through which God breaks into human lives. That the stories of this "in-breaking" presence could be narrated in diverse modes—for instance, as successful vaccination campaigns or as faith healings—and by an infinite number of voices was, as noted above, an invitation to think of health as a "vision of possibilities" that could not be reduced to the "possibilities or failures of medicine" or public health for that matter.[40]

Thus a significant part of the task of the CMC during its initial years was to bear witness to this "vision of possibilities" as embodied in the variety of church-affiliated (and many nonchurch-affiliated) health programs throughout the world. One of the primary forms this bearing witness took was the popular and widely disseminated *Contact* magazine, which became the public forum for theological and philosophical debates about the contours and content of primary health care as well as a repository of practical examples of how the tenets of primary health care were being enacted around the globe.

Health for All! For a Moment, Anyway

Despite divergent interpretations of the approach, the basic commitments of primary health care found widespread consensus in the mid-1970s. At its core, primary health care was about increasing equality throughout health systems and protecting the dignity of patients.[41] Though the two aims are not automatically mutually exclusive, the emphasis on equality placed the burden on health system administrators to justify resource allocations that resulted in disparities between urban and rural populations, rich and poor, racial or ethnic subpopulations, and types of disease burden. Protecting the dignity of patients, often referred to as patient-centered care, involved, among other things, increasing the participation of patients in defining health needs at the individual and systems level, striving for transparency with regards to treatment options, and generally acknowledging the patient as an equal partner in the healing process.

In 1975, the WHO gave formal expression to these commitments in its seven principles of primary health care, eventually articulated in the 1978 Declaration of Alma-Ata. These principles, in turn, set the stage for the unveiling of the ambitious slogan "Health for All by 2000" at the World Health Assembly in 1977 and the subsequent consensus document, the Declaration on Primary Health Care, drafted at Alma-Ata a year later. The principles emphasized the health (i) *ecology* of a community; (ii) *integration* of primary health care with the various components of the health system; (iii) *intersectoral* cooperation; (iv) *participatory* planning; (v) *practicability* in terms of cost and existing community assets; (vi) *complementarity* among promotive, preventive, and curative health approaches; and (vii) a form of *subsidiarity* linking health interventions to the appropriate providers.

Since its earliest days, the CMC made equality and patient dignity part of its core commitments. But the primary healthcare movement was more than just a growing consensus on its definitional attributes. Commitments to primary health care had found expression in the primary healthcare practices of communities throughout the world.[42] Charles Elliott, a development economist and Anglican priest, writing for *Contact*, identified five trends that suggested a growing appreciation for the effectiveness of strategies consistent with the primary healthcare approach:

1. The increasing reliance on paraprofessionals (often referred to as community health workers) as frontline workers;
2. The addition of preventive medicine to curative approaches;
3. A noticeable shift from vertical, disease-specific global health initiatives (for instance, the campaign to eradicate malaria) to integrated, intersectoral programs;
4. A willingness to challenge the dominant cost-effectiveness analysis, particularly as it was used to justify a disproportionate distribution of healthcare resources for urban areas; and,
5. A heightened sensitivity to the practices of traditional healing as complementary rather than contradictory to the dominant Western medical model.[43]

The work of the CMC as documentarian, disseminator, and definer of these trends was well respected by the WHO leadership in the 1970s. The close relationships between then WHO director Halfdan Mahler and CMC director James McGilvray and the proximity of the two organizations in Geneva played a role in the frequency of contact between the two organizations, whether in formal consultations or simply as observers at various high-level meetings. Though many factors led to the Declaration of Primary Health Care, recent historical scholarship emphasizes the important role of the CMC in preparing global health actors for the policy-level paradigm shift to primary health care.[44] The degree to which the Declaration reflects the initial commitments of the commission provides further confirmation of this cross-pollination—though it does not necessarily establish the direction of causal arrows—between the two organizations.[45]

In its first decade, the CMC played a significant role in framing the concept of primary health care that would eventually be adopted by the WHO at the Alma-Ata Conference. By the 1980s, however, *selective* primary health care (SPHC) had become the buzzword among donors and international institutions seeking to quantify progress in global health according to a standardized set of measurable health outcomes.[46] Criticizing the comprehensive primary health care call at Alma-Ata as too idealistic and vague, SPHC advocates sought to bring order and clarity to the concept of primary health care, though critics contend that in its selectivity SPHC effectively rolled back the conceptual advances that had been made in linking health and socioeconomic development or what is now referred to as the social determinants of health approach. While SPHC was donor friendly, critics argued that the measures on which it relied did not address the structural problems that could have a bigger impact on sustaining global health improvements. As Kenneth Newell, a prominent WHO staff member and pivotal figure in the move toward intersectoral approaches to global health, argued, SPHC was a "counter-revolution" because it prioritized short-term goals at the expense of sustained change over time.[47]

As SPHC became the program of choice in global health circles in the 1980s, CMC's leadership role on the global health agenda became more limited. The CMC found it increasingly difficult to find a sympathetic hearing for its comprehensive, theo-ethical vision of health and human flourishing, a vision grounded in both the practices of community health and the concept of the church as a healing community.

Though the work of the CMC continues, its organizational structure and programmatic priorities reflect shifts in the global health landscape since Alma-Ata. For example, in the 1980s the CMC, in conjunction with other humanitarian organizations, articulated the first guidelines for drug donations, guidelines that would eventually be institutionalized in 1990 in the WHO Action Programme on Essential Drugs. During this period, the CMC continued to try to understand the practical implications of its vision of the healing church, coordinating regional meetings to elicit feedback on how the healing church is expressed organizationally, liturgically, and in its financial priorities.[48] In the 1990s, the CMC (or CMC-Churches' Action for Health, as it came to be called) became active in the response to HIV, coordinating consultative processes throughout the world and helping to spur the development of the International Christian AIDS Network.[49]

Eventually, in 1998, the formal organization of the CMC dissolved, though its work has been taken up by various other parts of the WCC. For example, the highly respected *Contact* magazine continues to be published under the auspices of various regional bodies of the WCC. Recent issue themes show the extent to which the original intentions of the CMC continue to find expression in responses to contemporary global health concerns such as HIV and health system strengthening.[50]

Faith and Health—Now More than Ever?

Despite the initial international (and ecumenical) consensus on the concept of primary health care, the effort never really got off the ground, or rather it never got on the ground after Alma-Ata, at least not in formal global health policy, priorities, and programs. Yet, in 2008, a decade after the CMC dissolved and amid global health commemorations of the thirtieth anniversary of Alma-Ata, the WHO resurrected primary health care, touting it as an urgent priority with particular relevance for the scale-up of access to antiretroviral treatment for persons infected with HIV.[51]

Seen against the backdrop of Alma-Ata, the current emphasis on primary health care and social determinants reflect the letter but perhaps not the spirit of the CMC's work. The emphasis in this chapter on the theological backstory of the primary healthcare movement illustrates one way in which this spirit proved catalytic for new programs and policies that promote health and human flourishing. The visibility of the CMC in the global health public square was due in large part to the connective practices that it encouraged, many of which were initiated prior to its formal collaboration with the WHO in the 1970s. Yet, those connective practices grew directly out of the theological reflection on the healing ministry of the church. For example, theological reflection on the communal dimensions of healing oriented efforts to connect communities to the best community-oriented primary healthcare approaches and the resources required to implement these approaches. Similarly, the CMC's theological sensitivity to health as a social justice issue—that is, sensitivity to human suffering and the social conditions that give rise to it—found expression in the many consultative sessions designed to generate new ties and strengthen existing ones among organizations committed to bringing about greater access to health care.

For many global health leaders, the take-home message from the CMC story appears to be that religious entities, properly trained and with technical support from global health institutions, can serve as a para-health workforce, extending the reach and accelerating the scale-up of global health priorities. This message, however, fails to appreciate what former WHO director Halfdan Mahler called the "transcendental beauty and significance" of the WHO's definition of health.[52] That the CMC and the WHO in the 1970s recognized and worked so hard to realize this transcendental beauty and significance cannot be fully grasped without understanding something of the processes of theological reflection that infused the primary healthcare movement with its sense of moral urgency.

In the twenty-first century, global health has become one of the primary arenas in which fundamental questions about human being and human flourishing are being contested. The history of the CMC and the primary healthcare movement suggests that global health policies have, in the past, stimulated mutually generative encounters between theologians and global health leaders—encounters that more accurately reflect the dialogical relationship between scientific descriptions of the determinants of human health and normative arguments about what constitutes human flourishing. Although this chapter highlights the particular theological commitments that gave rise to the CMC, the intention is not to suggest that theology or a particular theology provides the ground for global health. Rather, the theologically resonant history of the primary healthcare movement is a reminder that definitions of health and conceptions of human flourishing that orient global health priorities and drive flows of resources are arguments about what it means to be human. As such, these arguments require attention to the question, why *this* particular vision of human flourishing? Answers to this question are always provisional, revisited by each generation as it seeks to integrate advances in human knowledge with both shared and contested visions of human being.

Bishop Tutu's exhortation to the members of the World Health Assembly serves as a fitting reminder that, nearly a half century later, religious and global health leaders hold in trust—amid the shared *and* contested visions of human flourishing—the legacy of the CMC's theo-ethical commitment to health for all:

> You are the guardians of the dream of "Health for All." You have the opportunity and responsibility to lead the world into a healthy place. You are the enactors of justice: justice in the distribution of a country's wealth for health; justice to meet the Millennium Development Goals; justice to save the lives of your people and enable them to prosper and build healthy nations! God is watching. The people are waiting. You are commissioned to go to wipe the tears away from all faces and bring forth lives filled with strength, and purpose which will make for peace.[53]

Notes

1. Desmond Mpilo Tutu, "Address to the 61st World Health Assembly," Geneva, May 20, 2008, http://www.who.int/mediacentre/events/2008/wha61/desmond_mpilo_tutu_speech/en/index.html.
2. Tutu, "Address to the 61st World Health Assembly."

3. Hector Avalos, *Health Care and the Rise of Christianity* (Peabody, MA.: Hendrickson, 1999); James C. McGilvray, *The Quest for Health and Wholeness* (Tübingen: German Institute for Medical Missions, 1981), especially 2–3.

4. Tutu, "Address to the 61st World Health Assembly."

5. This consultation was not the first attempt to bring theologians and medical personnel together in the hope of clarifying what, if anything, a Christian conception of healing offered to a modern world increasingly characterized by institutional differentiation and the privatization of religion, but earlier attempts failed to get off the ground. See McGilvray, *The Quest for Health and Wholeness*.

6. World Council of Churches, *The Healing Church: The Tübingen Consultation, 1964,* ed. Lesslie Newbigin (Geneva: World Council of Churches, 1965), 5.

7. World Council of Churches, *The Healing Church*, 34.

8. World Council of Churches, *The Healing Church*, 35.

9. The salvation history in which those gathered at Tübingen located healing was unapologetically Christian and could easily be perceived as triumphalist or predestinarian (that is, healing is only possible for the elect). However, Benn and Senturias point out that such triumphalism is mitigated in Tübingen I by an approach to healing that is both holistic and eschatological. Christoph Benn and Erlinda Senturias, "Health, Healing and Wholeness in the Ecumenical Discussion," *International Review of Mission* 90, no. 356–357 (2001): 7–25.

10. Benn and Senturias, "Health, Healing and Wholeness," 12.

11. David Jenkins, "Foreword," in McGilvray, *The Quest for Health and Wholeness*, xiii.

12. Jenkins, "Foreword," xiii.

13. Jenkins, "Foreword," xiii.

14. McGilvray, *The Quest for Health and Wholeness*, 15–16.

15. World Council of Churches, *The Healing Church*, 47.

16. McGilvray, *The Quest for Health and Wholeness*, 21.

17. World Council of Churches, *The Healing Church*, 35.

18. Benn and Senturias, "Health, Healing and Wholeness," 9.

19. McGilvray, *The Quest for Health and Wholeness*, 23.

20. McGilvray, *The Quest for Health and Wholeness*, 15.

21. McGilvray, *The Quest for Health and Wholeness*, 40–41.

22. McGilvray, *The Quest for Health and Wholeness*, 31.

23. McGilvray, *The Quest for Health and Wholeness*, 100.

24. McGilvray, *The Quest for Health and Wholeness*, 101.

25. R. A. Lambourne, *Community, Church and Healing: A Study of Some of the Corporate Aspects of the Church's Ministry to the Sick* (London: Darton, Longman & Todd, 1963), vi.

26. For a general overview of this interest and its historical relation to the religion and psychology conversation, see James M. Nelson, *Psychology, Religion and Spirituality* (New York: Springer, 2009).

27. Benn and Senturias, "Health, Healing and Wholeness," 12.

28. Benn and Senturias, "Health, Healing and Wholeness," 12.

29. McGilvray, *The Quest for Health and Wholeness*, 23.

30. Gillian Patterson, "The CMC Story: 1968–1998," *Contact* 161–162 (1998), 3. See also Christian Medical Commission and World Council of Churches, *First Annual Meeting* (Geneva: World Council of Churches, 1968), 2–3.

31. Based on a sample of twenty-five hospitals in twenty different countries, costs had increased 100 percent to 150 percent between 1958 and 1968. James C. McGilvray, "The Historical Perspective: Our Inheritance," in Christian Medical Commission and World Council of Churches, *First Annual Meeting*, 25.

32. Patterson, "The CMC Story," 8.

33. Christian Medical Commission and World Council of Churches, *First Annual Meeting*, 1.

34. Christian Medical Commission and World Council of Churches, *First Annual Meeting*, 1. For a powerful restatement of this declaration in the context of the HIV pandemic forty years later, see African Christian Health Associations' Technical Working Group on Human Resources for Health, "Letter to Mubashar Sheikh, Executive Director, Global Health Workforce Alliance," August 26, 2008, http://ccih. org/pipermail/news_ccih.org/2008-September/000183.html.

35. Jacques Rossel, "On the Threshold of New Development," in Christian Medical Commission and World Council of Churches, *First Annual Meeting*, 10. Rossel was the former chair of the Specialized Assistance to Social Projects division, one of the WCC divisions to which the CMC reported.

36. Of the twenty-four commission members present at the first meeting, nine can be reasonably identified as representing theological, missionary, or church service interests, for example, persons identified as Reverend, Archbishop, or representatives of church agencies. Christian Medical Commission and World Council of Churches, *First Annual Meeting*.

37. Christian Medical Commission and World Council of Churches, *First Annual Meeting*, 4.

38. Christian Medical Commission and World Council of Churches, *First Annual Meeting*, 2.

39. Christian Medical Commission and World Council of Churches, *First Annual Meeting*, 4.

40. McGilvray, *The Quest for Health and Wholeness*.

41. Alberta W. Parker, Jane M. Walsh, and Merl Coon, "A Normative Approach to the Definition of Primary Health Care," *The Milbank Memorial Fund Quarterly, Health and Society* 54, no. 4 (1976): 415–438.

42. For documentation of various communities committed to primary healthcare approaches, see Kenneth W. Newell, ed., *Health by the People* (Geneva: World Health Organization, 1975).

43. Charles Elliott, "Is Primary Health Care the New Priority? Yes, But . . ." *Contact* 28 (1975): 3–4.

44. For the most explicit examination of the link between the CMC and the WHO's primary healthcare approach, including the personal relationships animating these links, see Socrates Litsios, "The Christian Medical Commission and the Development of the World Health Organization's Primary Health Care Approach," *American Journal of Public Health* 94, no. 13 (2004): 1884–1893, and "The Long and Difficult Road to Alma-Ata: A Personal Reflection," *International Journal of Health Services* 32, no. 4 (2002): 709–732.

45. Indeed, the difficulty in distinguishing whether the CMC influenced the WHO or was simply reflecting trends already developing at the WHO lend credibility to argu-

ments that see the close relationship between the two organizations, especially its leadership, as a relatively short-lived historical anomaly.

46. SPHC advocates emphasized growth monitoring, oral rehydration, breastfeeding, and immunizations as four measures of global health that could be readily operationalized and reported out to various donors. Marcos Cueto, "The Origins of Primary Health Care and Selective Primary Health Care," *American Journal of Public Health* 94, no. 11 (2004), 1869.

47. Kenneth Newell, "Selective Primary Health Care: The Counter Revolution," *Social Science & Medicine* 26, no. 9 (1988): 903–906.

48. Christian Medical Commission, *Healing and Wholeness: The Churches' Role in Health*, (Geneva: World Council of Churches, 1990).

49. Patterson, "The CMC Story," 34. Patterson notes that one of the primary ways the CMC has continued to impact global health is by helping to set up other organizations, such as ICAN.

50. See especially *Contact* nos. 177–178 and 185 for CMC and HIV; for a focus on health system strengthening, see *Contact* no. 189.

51. World Health Organization, *The World Health Report 2008—Primary Health Care (Now More Than Ever)* (Geneva: World Health Organization, 2008).

52. Halfdan Mahler, "Address to the 61st World Health Assembly," Geneva, May 20, 2008, http://www.who.int/mediacentre/events/2008/wha61/hafdan_mahler_speech/en/index.html.

53. Tutu, "Address to the 61st World Health Assembly."

22 | Ingenious Institutions: Religious Origins of Health and Development Organizations

ELLEN IDLER

R ELIGIOUS INSTITUTIONS HAVE LONG AFFECTED the health of populations around the globe through the direct provision of medical care. Christianity in particular has been associated with the founding and support of hospitals, medical and nursing schools, and other institutions of Western medicine in countries around the globe. But changes in population and public health at the end of the twentieth and into the twenty-first century—the decline in fertility, the shift in the causes of mortality from infectious to chronic disease, the rapid aging of the world's populations, and the rise of new infectious diseases—created distinct new problems that have challenged traditional medical models and that call for new solutions. In this chapter, we examine a series of ingenious institutions in religion and public health—new organizations founded in response to emerging public health needs, with religious inspiration at their core and with material help from existing religious institutions. These are institutions that began with a novel idea and the support to make it reality.

Traditionally, we think of social institutions as groups of individuals organized in structured roles to take care of the human needs that are found in all societies—illness, crime, or the raising of children. They are regular solutions to recurring human problems—no society can do without some form of family support, schools, governments, or care for the sick. The abstract sociological concept of an educational, political, religious, or healthcare institution is realized in everyday life as a specific hospital, school, government, or congregation. Such local institutions often have long histories that predate the lives of their members, and they resemble other, similar institutions in how they are organized and what they do. Their functions are simply taken for granted because they are so much a part of our daily lives. It is not often that truly new institutions—with novel structures, functions, or both—arise in society.

However, a number of ingenious, radically innovative social institutions have emerged to serve the health and development needs of large and small populations, young and old, in the world's rich and poor countries. In those we highlight here, the religious origins of the groups and their founders provide a formative influence. Sometimes, there is a clear example of an ancient inspirational text or story that provides a model for solving a modern problem. In other cases, there is a devoutly religious, charismatic founding figure who had a new approach and made it work. In most of these organizations, established religious institutions played a material role in assisting the fledgling organization to get started. Some of the institutions feature their religious origins in their present identity; others do not. But all exhibit a spark of creative genius in responding to a public health need in a way no one had conceived of before, and none would have taken the same shape without the religious idea at its core. The fires ignited by these sparks of genius are social institutions born in our time that did something new and did it in a new way.

The La Leche League

On a hot, sunny summer afternoon in 1956, in the Chicago suburb of Franklin Park, Illinois, two mothers attending a church picnic sat under a tree breastfeeding their infants. The two women, Mary White and Marian Tompson, were both members of the Christian Family Movement, a Roman Catholic group that had organized the picnic. They noticed that some of their friends at the outing were struggling to keep bottled milk cold so it would be safe and then to warm it so the baby would be comfortable feeding. Other mothers there that afternoon spoke to them about the advantages of breastfeeding compared with bottle feeding, but some said they had had difficulties in initiating nursing, or they had been discouraged by their pediatricians from even trying to breastfeed. Indeed, breastfeeding had become a relatively rare practice; by the mid-1950s, barely 20 percent of US mothers were nursing their infants.

Mary White and Marian Thompson decided that could help other mothers successfully nurse their infants. They invited five friends—Mary Ann Cahill, Edwina Froehlich, Mary Ann Kerwin, Viola Lennon, and Betty

Wagner—to join them in the effort. Despite having been actively discouraged—Edwina Froehlich was told by her doctor that, at 36, she was "too old" to breastfeed[1]—all had been successful at nursing healthy babies, and they were convinced that no one could better help new mothers than those who had had actual experience of nursing.

Their first formal meeting, held in October 1956, was attended by the seven women and five pregnant friends.[2] But this was not an organization that struggled long in obscurity. Their second meeting drew thirty women, and the third brought so many that they could not crowd into the room. Clearly, a need and a solution had been identified simultaneously.

The first La Leche League group outside the United States was founded in Quebec in 1960, and in 1964 the La Leche League International held its first conference in Chicago, where it welcomed members from groups in Canada, Mexico, and New Zealand. The organization was granted consultative status with the UN Children's Fund (UNICEF) in 1981, and today there are affiliated La Leche League International groups in more than seventy countries, with more than seven thousand leaders trained to provide free breastfeeding support to new mothers.[3] Their website offers many online resources and a directory to facilitate local contacts for new mothers.

The growth of the La Leche League and the turn of the tide in infant feeding took place together. In 1956, barely 20 percent—one in five—of infants born in the United States was breastfed; a continuous climb began in the 1970s, and in 2007, 75 percent—three out of every four—US children were breastfed.[4] Trends in other countries have also generally improved from the 1990s on.[5] At the same time, research evidence for the positive impact of breastfeeding on infants'—and mothers'—health continues to grow.[6] In developing countries where clean water and refrigeration are often not easily available, the health benefits for infants are even more critical.

The religious origins of the La Leche League are multiple and defining. The leaders named their new organization after a shrine in Florida dedicated to "Nuestra Señora de la Leche y Buen Parto" (Our Lady of Milk and Good Delivery). The image of Mary the mother of Christ has been a powerful symbol of motherhood for Roman Catholics through the centuries (note again the names of the founders). But only in the mid-twentieth century, when bottle-feeding became the norm, would an image of Mary nursing Jesus be seen as an extraordinary act of nurturing; for centuries, nursing was a routine part of motherhood, the only adequate method of infant feeding available for most. Another important influence was the practical help of the Christian Family Movement (CFM), a post-World War II Catholic social movement that had emerged from Young Christian Workers and Young Christian Students, groups that came to the United States from Europe in the 1930s.[7] CFM was a widespread movement, with a US membership of 30,000 couples in 1958; CFM members were active in civil rights, social justice, and international issues, providing a strong contrast to the conservative, anti-Communist tenor of the time. The CFM connection provided the La Leche League leaders (all of them members of CFM[8]) with a shared theological foundation in Catholic moral teaching and the practical skills to organize meetings, create publications, and serve ever-larger numbers of members. Canon Joseph Cardijn, the Belgian priest who founded the Young Christian Workers, taught what he called a "like-to-like" ministry, enacted through small "cells" or groups that used a social inquiry method called observe—judge—act.[9] The idea of mothers teaching mothers was a natural extension of this method, although likely not one that Canon Cardijn could have foreseen.

Ingenious Institutions

In the founding of the La Leche League, we have the origination of an entirely new social institution. It was created against countervailing cultural trends out of a conviction that breastfeeding was best for babies and that breastfeeding mothers were best able to teach other mothers to do it. These convictions were shared by women who knew each other through their membership in a Roman Catholic social movement and who shared a religious view of family life. Their membership in a Roman Catholic community afforded them the social networks and social capital to nurture their small, profoundly intimate model and then to scale it up to the respected, influential international organization it is today. Both the function (to teach new mothers to breastfeed their infants) and the structure (from local chapters where the like-to-like ministry could take place to regional, national, and international councils) of this social institution were created where nothing remotely like it existed. The La Leche League is just the first of our examples of such ingenious institutions.

Although the La Leche League had its origins in Roman Catholicism, it is today a fully secular institution dedicated to the single purpose of increasing breastfeeding worldwide. Not all of the institutions we review in this chapter have taken a secular course; some have retained their religious identities as central to their mission. But all of them began as religious responses to public health needs, and all of them have made a difference.

Heifer International

One day in 1936, in the midst of the Spanish Civil War, an American named Dan West was sitting under an almond tree in Spain. He was a member of the Church of the Brethren; after serving as a conscientious objector in World War I, he had volunteered as a relief worker for Spanish citizens, especially children, affected by the fighting. That day he was thinking about milk. As a relief worker distributing too few rations to too many hungry children, he thought, wouldn't it be better to give these children cows than to ship them milk that was gone as soon as they drank it? If the cow was soon to give birth, he thought, the family receiving the cow would be able to pass the calf on to another family, who could eventually pass it on again and again. He returned to the United States determined to pursue his idea. With the support of the Church of the Brethren, he was able to raise funds to make a first shipment of seventeen heifers (young, female cows) from York, Pennsylvania, to Puerto Rico in 1944.[10]

Following World War II, the Heifer Project shipped hundreds of cows and horses to Europe and thousands of goats to Japan. By the 1950s, it had shipped over ten thousand cows to families around the world. In the 1960s, Heifer began to work with the Peace Corps in Central and South America and started work in Africa. Today, Heifer International has given more than twelve million cows, water buffalo, chickens, goats, sheep, llamas, rabbits, and pigs to families living in poverty and to those who have suffered from natural disasters or war, without regard to their religion. These families promise to pass on the offspring of their Heifer gifts and teach the receiving family the animal husbandry skills that they need to care for the animals. To support this work, Heifer International raises funds from individuals with its popular gift catalog, through which shoppers make donations by buying "gifts" of animals for those on their list. Heifer also has particular outreach to congregations and other religious organizations. Its work has been recognized countless times by national and international agencies and foundations.[11]

From the start, the organization's concept was to build the capacities of individuals, families, and communities and to turn them quickly from recipients to givers who offered not only goods (the young animal) but also expertise (the skills to care for it). In the 1990s, Heifer International developed the Cornerstones Model to build the capacity of rural, community-based organizations to plan and manage their own livestock resources. The Cornerstones Model is a positive-vision model rather than a problem-solving one; the four corners include:

1. Defining the situation;
2. Envisioning the future;
3. Planning for reaching the goal; and
4. Implementing, monitoring, and evaluating the plan.[12]

Some aspects of the Heifer model have been questioned. For sustainability reasons, the animals are required to "zero graze"—in other words, to have food brought to them. This method requires much less land than grazing animals would, and it allows the collection of the animal's dung, which can be used for fuel. But it necessitates that some family member remain at home to care for the animal, preventing that person from seeking outside employment. Some modest investment may also be required if the family does not have a suitable shelter for the animal. These requirements prevent the very poorest families with no land at all from participating. One study of Heifer projects in Uganda found that the beneficiaries tended to be members of the community who were somewhat less poor than the very neediest.[13]

However, the Heifer approach does produce results. Another evaluation found that heifer recipients in Uganda had per capita incomes five times the national average, largely due to daily milk sales.[14] A primary use of these families' additional funds was for school fees. The women in the study reported that they had invested their profits, often in poultry, that their families were healthier, and that they were now practicing inter-cropping and other new agricultural methods that they had learned while participating in the program.[15]

Heifer International's religious origins are, like the La Leche League's, multiple and foundational. Dan West's conscientious objector status was a consequence of the pacifist, separatist beliefs of his church, the Church of the Brethren, which originated in eighteenth-century German Pietism and Anabaptism. When he returned from Spain, the Church of the Brethren supported his idea by forming the Heifer Relief Committee and funding the first shipment of cows about to give birth. Judeo-Christian references are common throughout the Heifer gift catalog: there are descriptions of congregational study tours and mission trips and materials to help synagogues or church congregations organize a $5,000 "Fill the Ark" fundraising drive. The catalog also offers tailored materials for faith communities, including the Animal Crackers curriculum for Jewish and Christian children's education. The story of Noah's ark, with its saving stock of animals who went forth following the flood to be fruitful and multiply, is a powerful reference of promise and hope. Heifer International receives the bulk of its donations during the religious holiday and gift-giving season of December, when crèches with farm animals decorate many Christian homes. But if Heifer seeks donations especially from Judeo-Christians, it does not discriminate in its giving; it has many successful projects in countries where there are few if any Christians, and it does not limit in any way the passing on of the gift from the first family.

Faith-Based Organizations in Health and Development

Consideration of the faith-based sector in health and development has increased in recent years, partly in recognition of the role that these organizations are already playing in meeting the UN's Millennium Development Goals.[16] Harper and colleagues[17] define a faith-based development agency as one that shares many if not all of the following characteristics: it was started by a temple, church, or other religious institution or a religiously inspired individual; it works closely with other religious institutions in its community; and it raises most of its funds from individuals and institutions of the same faith. At the same time, these faith-based organizations do not limit their benefits or services to those of the same faith as the founders and at least some of the staff may also be of a different faith.

Some but not all of the examples to which we draw attention in this chapter belong to this group of faith-based development organizations, for whom such attention in scholarship and policy is overdue. One difference is that while all of our ingenious institutions had their origins in religious teachings or models, some have since developed into secular organizations, as the La Leche League has done. Others have retained their faith-based ties and supports, as Heifer has done, even as it has grown far beyond the small Protestant denomination that gave it its start.

What sets our ingenious institutions apart is both their faith origins and their utter originality—their new approach to a problem in health, with new forms and new functions to meet newly emerging public health needs. This is their genius. Each was, in a phrase, created "out of whole cloth"; it may have been a small piece of cloth, but it was one that could be stitched to others in patterns that gave it direction. Like a quilt, a small successful social model can be replicated over and over, by many hands and in many colors, and it can spread in all directions.

Shri Kshetra Dharmasthala Rural Development Programme

In the state of Karnataka in southwest India, near Bangalore, there is a temple that was built in the fifteenth century. Its earliest structure was erected by a farmer named Barmana Heggade, who provided hospitality to two travelers who, the legend says, were in reality angels. After the visit, they returned to him in a dream and asked him to build them a temple where they could live and to offer hospitality to all who came to worship there. Heggade and his many descendants were Jains, an ancient Indian religion that is related to Hinduism but does not recognize castes. Over the centuries, this temple has been a site of pilgrimage for Jains and Hindus and also a gathering place for the very poor, who receive alms from the pilgrims.[18] The Heggade family, to this day, owns and maintains the Dharmasthala temple, which has grown into a large and beautiful complex that thousands visit each year.

Twenty-year-old Veerendra Heggade became the head of the family and therefore holder of the hereditary position as head of the temple in 1968 when his father died unexpectedly. The son completed a project that his father had begun before his death, the erection of a giant statue to Bahubali, a spiritual leader of the Jains, intended to symbolize the renunciation of desire and the subjugation of the ego. But while carrying out his religious and familial duties, Veerendra Heggade became dissatisfied with the large number of beggars at the temple whose livelihood was made entirely by seeking the alms of pilgrims. He wanted to help them improve their lives and become productive members of society.

In 1982, he organized a development project called the Shri Kshetra Dharmasthala Rural Development Programme (SKDRDP) to help marginal and small farmers in the area around the temple. Community organizers, called *sevanirathas*, worked with small groups of farmers to help them improve their cultivation of rice and other crops. These organized groups then joined together to plant or harvest, working together, in turns, on each other's land.[19]

After several years, as the organization spread to more areas around the temple, SKDRDP registered as a charitable society in 1991. Indeed, there was a notable increase in the profitability of the small farms and the income of the farmers. But these initial steps toward economic development were being wiped out by a new social problem that arose as the farmers' incomes increased: alcoholism. So in the early 1990s, the SKDRDP established its anti-alcoholism program, Jana Jagruthi. This program takes the form of one-week residential camps; participants pay the equivalent of $4 to attend if they can afford it, while fees are subsidized for those who cannot pay. Camps are located in the countryside, so the fifty or so men who attend know each other and have likely worked together, and participants continue to monitor each other after their week together through groups called Nava Jeevana Samitis. Religious practices are an important aspect of both the camp and the groups that continue afterward. Local religious leaders, including Christian, Hindu, and Jain priests and Muslim mullahs, speak to the participants; religious songs and prayers are important elements of the program. The families are also involved; they are required to bring meals to the camp each day. This community embeddedness is considered one of the reasons for the success of the program; families maintain oversight of their relatives while they are in the camp, and the participants maintain oversight of each other through the groups. Harper and colleagues report that by 2005, over 150 such camps had been held, and that over two-thirds of the participants have remained free from alcohol.[20]

Several other SKDRDP programs are also relevant to the public health of this area of rural India: The Grama Kalyana Yojane program helps villages build water supply and sanitation systems and operate local milk cooperative societies. The Rudra Bhoomi is a fund from which the SKDRDP gives grants to communities to build or improve cremation facilities. The Jnana Viakasa program provides education to rural women about health, hygiene, and nutrition; this program is especially important because it draws women away from the practice of rolling *beedis* or cigarettes, to which many poor women turn for small income supplements. The Sampoorna Suraksha is a self-help mutual fund scheme, to which all SKDRDP members contribute, that provides financial assistance for the poor who require hospitalization. Today, the SKDRDP promotes community development in 4,739 villages in the state of Karnataka, covering more than 710,000 families.[21]

Although the Shri Kshetra Dharmasthala temple remains a popular destination for pilgrims and tourists, as it has for centuries, the SKDRDP presents itself (online at least) as a secular microfinance and economic development organization; the organization's religious origins are not mentioned in its public representation of its programs. By contrast with this outward face, Harper and colleagues emphasize the importance of the language SKDRDP uses internally to name its programs, groups, and individuals. Derived from Sanskrit,

> [These names] have strong religious connotations, which link the programmes very firmly to Dharmasthala. . . . Most NGOs, and most government programmes, use English words and acronyms even when speaking in Hindi or local vernaculars. They say "IRDP" for the integrated rural development programme, or "SHG" for self-help groups. Terms of this kind are never used in formal discussions or general conversation by SKDRDP. Nobody uses the words "microcredit" or "microfinance," they refer to *Pragathi Nidhi*" [which connotes precious treasure, and refers to wisdom, faith, or other nonmaterial resources][22].

They go on to provide a glossary of the not-easily-translated spiritual meanings of the Sanskrit terms used by SKDRDP. [23]

There are also other important religious aspects to SKDRDP programs. Jana Jagruthi graduates come together once a week for a religious meeting, called a Bhajan Mandali, which includes hymns praising God and expressions of thanks for their new life free of alcohol. Harper and colleagues note that Hindu rituals do not typically include a routine community religious ritual; the Bhajan Mandali observance mirrors Christian and Muslim practices of worship as well as the secular meetings of Alcoholics Anonymous.[24] Thus, in its representation of itself online (presumably for a primarily Western audience), SKDRDP eschews religious language and even distances itself from the temple from which it gets its name. But in actual practice and operation, SKDRDP intentionally maintains traditional (Sanskrit) religious language for everything it is and does and incorporates syncretic religious rituals culled from all of the local faith traditions to promote a sense of belonging and commitment among its members.

Religious Origins

In this chapter, we take note of the religious origins of these ingenious institutions without passing judgment on how those origins are evidenced in the way the organization presents itself today. All of the organizations discussed here offer ongoing, successful models of innovative ways to address public health needs; some of them have found success by maintaining a strong religious identity while others have left their religious origins behind. These organizations serve and are supported by a variety of faith communities, and they do not discriminate among those they serve. They may employ staff who hold diverse religious beliefs or none at all. Smith and colleagues array faith-based groups along a continuum from "faith-saturated" groups to "faith-centred, faith-background, faith-related, and then to 'faith-secular partnerships.'"[25] Some of the organizations that we include would not even fall on this spectrum; their nascent "faith-base" may have been left entirely behind. Our argument, however, is that it *was* necessary for their conception and infancy and that these organizations would not exist were it not for the religious symbols, texts, images, and holy places that sparked the initial idea and the social and sometimes financial capital of religious organizations that supported their beginnings.

Dhaka Ahsania Mission

Khan Bahadur Ahsanullah was born in 1873 in a village named Nalta, in what is now Bangladesh, the only heir of a wealthy, pious Muslim family. He excelled in school from an early age, eventually receiving a master of arts degree from Calcutta University in 1895, after which he joined government service and spent a long and distinguished career in the field of education. He began as a teacher but moved rapidly into administrative positions, which he used to fight discrimination against Muslims and encourage Muslim students to pursue further education. The Dhaka Ahsania Mission website offers a long list of the education reforms instituted by Khan Bahadur Ahsanullah, including instituting blind grading of examinations to avoid (religious) bias, eliminating wage disparities between Muslim teachers and their higher-paid Hindu counterparts, encouraging more students to continue to higher education, establishing scholarships for poor but meritorious students, and founding schools and colleges for female Muslim students.[26] But this illustrious career of service in education was merely the prologue to the work of the second half of his life: the founding of the Ahsania Mission.

Khan Bahadur Ahsanullah had devoted his professional life to improving education for the poor and disadvantaged. In his retirement, he sought to broaden and continue that work, with the twin objectives of providing enlightenment of the soul and social service for the masses. In establishing the mission, he showed his profoundly spiritual motives when he wrote:

> I have set my life's goal to serve people living far away from the cities. The pleasure that offering of service gives, cannot be found in personal aggran-

dizement. Boundless love will not come unless the element of "self" is negated. If there is no love for the creation, there cannot be any love for the Creator. The only aims of my life are to extend brotherhood, [sic] fraternity, and spread the message of peace[27].

He pursued his lifelong goal of increasing access to education and literacy by founding an organization that offered it to the very poorest members of Bangladesh society, especially women. He began in 1935 with a mission in his home village of Nalta to address four interconnected areas: education, livelihood, health care, and human rights and social justice. Today, there are 117 branch Ahsania Missions throughout Bangladesh; the largest is the Ahsania Mission in Dhaka, the capital, founded in 1958. Now one of the leading nongovernmental organizations in Bangladesh, Dhakia Ahsania Mission has consultative status with multiple UN agencies, including UNESCO.[28]

The Dhaka Ahsania Mission carries out its vision through community-based organizations called Ganokendra, These are action groups or "people's centers" that work to improve literacy, alleviate poverty, and empower the poor, especially women.[29] Ganokendra members, particularly the women, are involved in every stage of community projects, from surveying needs and resources to designing and implementing them. The first Ganokendras began in 1992 with about two thousand members; by 2006, there were more than eighty thousand member families in 807 communities. Their primary focus is on literacy; with literacy comes the ability to read newspapers and journals and discuss in Ganokendra meetings new approaches to a range of community problems. The Ganokendras began water and sanitation projects in 1997 and initiated anti-drug and anti-smoking activities in 1998. They promote preventive health care for mothers and infants, family planning services, nutrition, and access to medical services. In January 2011, the Dhaka Ahsania Mission unveiled a new project in partnership with UN-HABITAT and Coca-Cola to provide water and sanitation facilities to sixteen thousand students in twenty-five "ultra-poor" schools in Dhaka and the surrounding areas.[30]

In keeping with its historical emphasis on education, the Dhaka Ahsania Mission is one of the few development organizations in Bangladesh to maintain a research division. Numerous evaluations of its programs are available on its website, including reports on programs on HIV/AIDS, sexual and reproductive health issues among adolescents, and the success of health warning messages on cigarette packets.[31] A 2003 UNESCO report found that in the Ganokendra areas, there was a "spectacular" increase in children's—including girls'—school attendance and that 100 percent of Ganokendra members used sanitary latrines.[32] With the large scale of its programs and its orientation to Western-style evaluation methods, the Dhaka Ahsania Mission has acquired a number of global governmental and nongovernmental partners, and it has won numerous awards from philanthropic organizations for its promotion of literacy, human rights, and development among the very poor.

Yet, with all of this recognition by the secular world of international development, the Dhaka Ahsania Mission retains a strong spiritual message. Its Founding Aims, listed on its website, focus on spiritual goals; the first is "Develop the social and spiritual life of the entire human community," and others focus on cultivating "unity and peace" and enabling participants to recognize the relationships between the Creator and creation and between the Creator and fellow human beings. This is a universal spiritual message; the site also proclaims that no distinctions are made within its organization by religion, political allegiance, ethnicity, or other criteria.

Khan Bahadur Ahsanullah was a prolific author, writing books on Muslim traditions, thoughts on Islam, and biographies of the Prophet Mohammed and a number of Sufi leaders. He is said to have been an extremely pious man who rejected attempts to compare him to a holy person or a saint; he wrote,

> The responsibility of the peer or the saint is to flourish and nurture the spiritual power of his followers. No saint can create spiritual power. He can only bring to surface, the power already bestowed on one by the Almighty. As friction on any iron substances could create fire, the Almighty has given in all human beings, a secret source of His own power. That power has to be attained through love and prayers. And, for this reason, there is the need for good teachers[33].

Ahsanullah clearly saw himself as a vehicle for the actions of a higher power and, despite his inspired leadership, was not building an organization for his own aggrandizement.

The Religious Origins of Ingenious Institutions

Unlike the young mothers of the La Leche League, the young conscientious objector founder of Heifer International, or the young heir to the temple of Dharmasthala, Khan Bahadur Ahsanullah had achieved a great deal in his professional life and had been well rewarded for his substantial contributions to society before he was inspired to start this new organization. He had already recognized the need for schools for the young, but he clearly saw much broader societal needs, particularly for women who had reached adulthood without learning to read. Perhaps he saw that his primary goal of education needed to be undergirded by improved water and sanitation systems, access to health care, and economic development. Perhaps his spiritual insights broadened his vision to encompass a larger view of the needs of the poor. In any case, he was a man with resources of wealth and professional experience that allowed him to build this large, highly successful organization in one of the poorest countries in the world. He was a rich man who devoted his life to the poor because of his religious faith; as he wrote:

> One of the cardinal instructions of Islam is to establish or offer *zakaat*. It is instructed that the rich should help the poor by offering *zakaat* in the rate of 2.5 percent from his fixed income. This will help breed friendship, global fraternity, and along with it promote global peace. Without sacrificing the heads of rich people to the sword or to the destructive powers of atoms, the rich should take the advantage of financially helping the poor and both should join together in harmony to develop this world. This is the aim of the Creator[34].

Khan Bahadur Ahsanullah took this teaching, combined it with his deep knowledge of the importance of education and his love of learning, and produced a new organizational structure that became a model for community organizing throughout Bangladesh.

Despite his high social status, Khan Bahadur Ahsanullah was a layperson in his religious tradition, as were the other founders of our ingenious institutions. All of these lay leaders were deeply pious people, steeped in the literature and teachings of their traditions. Moreover, while each of them may have had some element of charisma, an ability to inspire others with fresh, passionate approaches, they were not rebellious or sectarian in their religious beliefs. Indeed, each received spiritual or material support from these established institutions for as long as and to the extent that he or she found it useful. From the religious institutions' point of view, these laypeople offered no competition; their new institutions were not encroaching on the spiritual territory of the church or temple or mosque. Rather, they were promoting the religious message in groups where there was a need to hear it. These lay leaders, then, were poised to see rising public health needs from a faith-saturated perspective and to address those needs, with the full support of their institutional religious organizations, in a way that might not have been possible from positions of clerical leadership.

L'Arche Communities

Jean Vanier, the last of our inspired lay leaders, was a Roman Catholic born in 1928 in Geneva, Switzerland, to Canadian parents. As a member of a distinguished military family, he traveled around the world while growing up and served as an officer in the Royal Navy (UK) as a young man. He left the Royal Navy in 1950 and eventually came to live in Paris, in a lay community called Eau Vive, made up of students who attempted to "live the gospel in a spirit of poverty."[35] Vanier left Eau Vive to study philosophy at the Institut Catholique in Paris, where he received his PhD in 1962, after which he took a teaching position at St. Michael's College of the University of Toronto. In late 1963, he visited his friend, Père Thomas Philippe, the former director of the Eau Vive community, in the tiny French village where Père Thomas was then living. In Trosly-Breuil Père Thomas served as a chaplain at Val Fleuri, a small institution for men with mental handicaps. Vanier was very moved by the men he met there, by their vulnerability and by their "spiritual openness."[36]

Inspired by the men at Val Fleuri, Vanier visited other institutions and asylums, where he was "struck by the screams and the atmosphere of sadness, but also by a mysterious presence of God"; he resolved to do something to change the lives of the developmentally disabled.[37] With support from his parents, he bought a small, dilapidated house with an outdoor privy and a wood-burning stove in Trosly-Breuil and set about renovating and furnishing it. In August 1964, he brought two men, Philippe Seux and Raphaël Simi, to live with him in a new community founded on the principles of simplicity and poverty. Neighbors brought food and came to spend time there; these were the group's earliest "assistants," abled residents who live alongside those with disabilities, participating fully in the community with them. The house and the little community growing within it were given the name L'Arche shortly after their opening. A friend suggested the name, and Vanier instantly agreed; in his account, Vanier says that he did not realize the full significance of the name until later. He notes that Noah's ark was the vessel of salvation but also that the Ark of the Covenant symbolized God's promise to the Jewish people and that the early church fathers called Mary, the mother of Jesus, the Ark of the Covenant.[38] L'Arche, Vanier said, "was not my project, but God's."[39]

From its small beginning, L'Arche grew quickly. A second house was opened in Trosly in 1966, a third in 1968, and a fourth in 1969. By 1972, there were 126 developmentally disabled people living in sixteen houses in the area of the village with numerous "abled" assistants. L'Arche rapidly became an international movement; communities were founded in Canada and in the United Kingdom in 1969 and 1973. In 2013, there are 137 L'Arche communities in more than forty countries, including India, Spain, Japan, Brazil, Poland, Uganda, and Hungary, and fifteen states in the United States.[40] Jean Vanier's work has been widely recognized; he has been awarded the Companion of the Order of Canada and the French Legion of Honour as well as awards from Christian and Jewish organizations.

L'Arche residents today are men and women with intellectual or developmental disabilities. Like Philippe Seux and Raphaël Simi, the first two residents of the L'Arche home in Trosly-Breuil, many come from large mental institutions where they had lived for years. The small homes, located in the center of their communities, allow these previously isolated, socially marginalized persons to experience a sense of belonging and a set of caring relationships, perhaps for the first time in their lives. L'Arche homes usually have small workshops nearby where residents assemble items such as lamps or tables; the residents also participate in the common chores of cleaning, cooking, and laundry for the community as they are able. Each L'Arche home also has several abled assistants who live in the community, in full relationship with the other residents, temporarily or permanently. These assistants might be viewed as living a life of voluntary service and sacrificial giving, but in his many books, Vanier writes frequently of the gifts of spiritual growth and healing that the assistants receive from the less-abled residents. In *Becoming Human*, Vanier tells the story of Claudia, a blind and autistic child who came from a crowded asylum to live in the L'Arche community in Tegucigalpa, Honduras, and her relationship with Nadine, the community's leader. When she came to the community at age 7, Claudia was given to rages and violent outbursts, but with Nadine's patient "midwifery," she grew to be a peaceful, smiling adult who frequently sang as she worked. Vanier writes of the mutuality of Claudia and Nadine's relationship and its capacity for revelation, forgiveness, understanding, communication, empowerment, communion, and celebration.[41]

The L'Arche movement has a deeply spiritual core. The original L'Arche community in France was Roman Catholic in its orientation, born as it was out of the lay community of Eau Vive and the friendship of Vanier and Père Thomas Philippe. In 1987, L'Arche International held a meeting in Rome; 350 delegates from eighty-two communities around the world met with Mother Theresa and Pope John-Paul II. But L'Arche communities quickly spread to more diverse, ecumenical settings in North America, Asia, and Africa, and in these communities the predominant faith traditions are represented. On its website, L'Arche states:

> Most communities today consider themselves as Christian, some are ecumenical, some identify as Anglican or Protestant, and the majority are Catholic in their practice. The four communities in India and the project in Bangladesh have an interfaith character. All communities of the Federation welcome people of any or no faith and seek to respect and support members in their particular faith choice[42].

Notably, however, religious institutions do not provide material support to the communities. Even in the beginning, in Trosly-Breuil, funds to support the first community came from private donations and government stipends. In European communities, government subsidies continue to provide the main support, while elsewhere in the world, where social programs for the care of the intellectually disabled are less adequate, support comes from members and from the L'Arche Foundation.

From a spiritual model of small, egalitarian Christian communities and from secular sources of material support, Jean Vanier fashioned a new way to provide dignity and permanent care for severely disabled individuals and to do it in a way that allows those individuals to become healers of those whose wounds may be less obvious. In his many writings, Vanier has articulated a vision of the brokenness of humanity and the healing power of community. In his 1992 lectures at the Harvard Divinity School, he said:

> It is people who are weak, rejected, marginalized, counted as useless, who can become a source of life and of salvation for us as individuals as well as for our world. And it is my hope that each one of you may experience the incredible gift of the friendship of people who are poor and weak, that you too may receive life from them. For they call us to love, to communion, to compassion, and to community[43].

L'Arche, like our other ingenious institutions, began with a singular vision of possible human relationships and possible social structures that had not been seen before and the singular energy of an individual who could make the vision real.

Other Ingenious Institutions

The five examples at which we have chosen to look in some depth are only a few of those that could fit our description of ingenious institutions. Table 22.1 offers information on some of these other organizations; the table is organized chronologically in the order in which the organizations were founded.

Some of these organizations have long histories; all of them are still in existence. Many, like the Foulkeways continuing care retirement community, became models for other similar organizations. Early continuing care retirement communities in the United States were all founded by religious groups along the lines of models such as the *kibbutzim* of modern Israel, Roman Catholic religious orders, or the New England Shakers—communal religious institutions where residents make lifelong commitments and give up all claim to private property. Other ingenious institutions, like the La Leche League, Heifer International, and the YMCA, grew and multiplied in a more controlled and centrally directed way. Still others, like Elijah's Promise or Nyumbani Village, are purely local and one of a kind but may in the future provide models for new organizations in other communities.

These organizations frequently address public health needs for individuals at critical turning points in the life course. Particularly for those focused on maternal and child health, the organization could affect the health of individuals for many years of life. Dor Yeshorim, for instance, addresses the needs of a community vulnerable to specific genetic disorders (and opposed to abortion) to prevent these problem pregnancies from occurring in the first place. The La Leche League and the YMCA are focused on the health of infants, children, and youth. At the other end of the life course, hospice care and continuing care retirement communities have provided alternatives to the predominant twentieth-century model of institutionalized care for elderly persons in nursing homes that isolated them from their families and communities. Largely because of the successful models for small-scale, community-based care provided by these organizations, there is today much more focus on innovative ways to improve the quality of life of the aged and dying than there was fifty years ago.

These institutions that we are calling ingenious are original in both their structures and functions, but they are also ingenious in the diversity of the public health problems that they address and in the nimbleness of their

TABLE 22.1 Ingenious institutions in religion and public health

NAME *Place (date) of Founding*	WEBSITE	DESCRIPTION
Young Men's Christian Association (YMCA) *London, England (1844)*	www.ymca.net	Founded by George Williams to provide lodging, facilities for physical activity, and Bible study for young men of all social classes
Ahsania Mission *Nalta, Bangladesh (1935)*	www.ahsaniamission.org.bd	Founded by Khan Bahadur Ahsanullah, a Muslim educator, to improve education, family planning, water, and sanitation for poor communities in Bangladesh
Heifer International *York, Pennsylvania, United States (1944)*	www.heifer.org	Founded by Dan West, Church of the Brethren, to supply productive livestock to poor families in countries around the world
La Leche League International *Franklin Park, Illinois, United States (1956)*	www.llli.org	Founded by seven Roman Catholic women to provide one-on-one instruction and support for nursing mothers and to increase the number of breastfed infants
L'Arche Communities *Trosly-Breuil, France (1964)*	www.larche.org	Founded by Jean Vanier, a Roman Catholic philosopher, to provide small-scale homes for intellectually disabled persons and their assistants
Foulkeways at Gwynedd *Gwynedd, Pennsylvania, United States (1967)*	www.foulkeways.org	Founded by the Friends Meeting of Gwynedd, on land granted to William Penn, to provide all levels of care for older persons and permit older persons to age in place; one of the earliest continuing care retirement communities
St Christopher's Hospice *London, England (1967)*	www.stchristophers.org.uk	Founded by Dr. Cicely Saunders to provide spiritual and clinical care, particularly pain relief, for dying persons and their families, in homes and inpatient facilities

continued

TABLE 22.1 *continued*

NAME	WEBSITE	DESCRIPTION
Comprehensive Rural Development Project *Jamkhed, Maharashtra, India (1970)*	www.crhpjamkhed.org	Founded by Drs. Raj and Mabelle Arole, Christian physicians who developed a pioneering rural health and development program, now providing training in models that emphasize primary care, traditional remedies, and the training of local care providers
Shri Kshetra Dharmasthala Rural Development Programme *Belthangady, India (1982)*	www.skdrdpindia.org	Founded by Veerendra Heggade, hereditary head of a Jain temple, to reduce poverty by developing agriculture, reducing alcoholism, supplying water and sanitation systems, and improving cremation facilities in southwest India
Dor Yeshorim *Brooklyn, New York, United States (1989)*	webexposite.com/preview/dor_yeshorim	Founded by Rabbi Joseph Ekstein to provide anonymous genetic screening to Orthodox Jewish couples to prevent Tay-Sachs and other genetically transmitted diseases prevalent in this group
Elijah's Promise *New Brunswick, New Jersey, United States (1989)*	www.elijahspromise.org	Founded by local Lutheran and Episcopal churches to fight hunger, beginning with a traditional soup kitchen for the homeless and expanding to a culinary school, catering business, and pay-what-you-can cafe
Sister Connection *Burundi, Africa (2004)*	www.sisterconnection.org	Founded by Denise Patch (American) and Joy Buconyori (Burundian) to provide housing and basic daily needs for widows and children who have been victims of violence and civil war in Burundi
Nyumbani Village *Nairobi and rural Kenya (2006)*	www.nyumbani.org	Founded by Rev. Angelo D'Agostino to provide a home for children whose parents had died of HIV/AIDS and their grandmothers, the "left behind" generations

response to emerging conditions in the health of their populations. They have arisen in response to the emerging public health needs of the twentieth and twenty-first centuries. The La Leche League emerged mid-century, in the midst of the United States's post-World War II baby boom. At the end of the century, the rapid aging of populations, not only in Western industrialized societies but in many countries in the developing world as well, continuing care retirement communities responded to the need for new models of care for older persons needing support in the activities of daily living. At the same time, the emergence of the HIV/AIDS epidemic has had a devastating effect on populations worldwide, leaving thousands of orphaned children with their grandparents—the generations at the beginning and end of the life course have lost the middle generation. Kenya's Nyumbani Village, founded in 2006, provides a village community for hundreds of HIV/AIDS orphan children and their grandmothers. The village offers a model for caring for both generations that is far superior to caring for them separately, consigning children to institutional orphanages that do not provide the experience of family or true community.

In this chapter, we are drawing attention to a set of social institutions that have sprung from religious origins to address public health problems. In addition to their novel structures, innovative functions, and origins in one of the world's religious traditions, they also have in common some important underlying insights about what makes an organization successful. The first of these is drawn from the Roman Catholic social teaching of subsidiarity, a principle articulated by Pope Pius XI in his encyclical *Quadragesimo Anno*. This practical social ethic expresses the belief that the functions of a society ought to be performed by the smallest, simplest, most local group that is capable of performing them adequately.[44] The specific meaning of "subsidiarity" is that higher or more centralized social authorities ought to reserve their functions only for those tasks that cannot be performed at the local level. This principle precisely characterizes the working of our ingenious institutions. Be it the "like-to-like" ministry of the La Leche League, the involvement of participants' families in the Jana Jagruthi alcohol de-addiction camps, or the small house-living situations of the L'Arche communities, the idea that face-to-face relationships are fundamental to healthy communities is clearly a part of the wisdom of these institutions. Even if they have grown, as many of them have, into international organizations, the principle of devolving the work of the organization to the local level is characteristic of them all.

The second common underlying insight is a result of the first. When the functions of society are performed on the local level, by people within their own communities, the result is an increase in the human capital—skills and knowledge—in those communities. Philosopher Martha Nussbaum calls this approach to development the "human capabilities approach."[45] Beginning with the questions "What is each person actually able to do and to be?" and "What opportunities are open to him or her?," Nussbaum and economist Amartya Sen have built an alternative vision of the purpose and possibilities of international development, one that focuses on the capacities or capabilities of individuals to live their lives with dignity and creativity. Capabilities are not just abilities residing inside a person, however; the concept implies both the ability within the person and the opportunity afforded by his or her political, social, and economic environment to exercise and increase that capability.

The organizations that we have described in this chapter all enhance individuals' capabilities by increasing skills and knowledge and building environments where those capabilities can be expressed. In fact, an early member of L'Arche used almost exactly these words to describe that organization's work: "The primary task of L'Arche is to help those who live there, first the individuals with developmental disabilities and then the assistants, to achieve the greatest possible human and spiritual progress."[46] The l'Arche communities, like Heifer husbandry training and the like-to-like ministry of the La Leche League, increase skills and build community environments where the practice of those skills is valued.

That local, human capabilities approach can have powerful results. In a book about Jamkhed, a comprehensive rural health project in India, the authors begin with the following story:

May 1988

In a huge conference hall in Washington DC, over a thousand participants listen with rapt attention to Muktabai Pol, a village health worker from Jamkhed, India. The listeners include officials from WHO and UNICEF, ministers of health, health professionals and representatives of universities from many parts of the world. Muktabai shares her experience of providing primary health care in a remote Indian village. She concludes her speech by pointing to the glittering lights in the hall. "This is a beautiful hall and the shining chandeliers are a treat to watch," she says. "One has to travel thousands of miles to come to see their beauty. The doctors are like these chandeliers, beautiful and exquisite, but expensive and inaccessible." She then pulls out two wick lamps from her purse. She lights one. "This lamp is inexpensive and simple, but unlike the chandeliers, it can transfer its light to another lamp." She lights the other wick lamp with the first. Holding up both lamps in her outstretched hands she says, "I am like this lamp, lighting the lamp of better health. Workers like me can light another and another and thus encircle the whole earth. This is **Health for All**."[47]

Passing the light of a lamp is a metaphor for spreading skills, and indeed many of the institutions we have described here have spread their small lights to countries all over the world. But there was a first light from which the others were lit. That first light, that little spark, was set off in the mind of a person who was immersed in a religious tradition and had its wisdom to call on when faced with the public health needs of the community. The founders of these ingenious organizations had their own personal charisma to draw on, but they also frequently received the support of the religious institutions of which they were members. New, successful social institutions do not spring up every day, especially those that take on radically new forms or functions. The intersection of newly arising public health needs and the religious inspiration for ways to address them has been particularly fertile ground for the appearance of social innovations. If we are lucky, there will be more. Finding the common characteristics of ingenious institutions in religion and public health may be the best way to be alert for that next new spark, to provide it with fuel, and other wicks.

Notes

1. Emily Bazelon, "Edwina Froehlich B. 1915," *New York Times Magazine*, December 28, 2008, 22–23.
2. Jule DeJager Ward, *La Leche League: At the Crossroads of Medicine, Feminism, and Religion* (Chapel Hill: University of North Carolina Press, 2000).
3. La Leche League International, *Annual Report, 2009–2010* (Schaumburg, IL: La Leche League International, 2010).
4. US Department of Health and Human Services, *The Surgeon General's Call to Action to Support Breastfeeding* (Washington, DC: US Department of Health and Human Services, Office of the Surgeon General, 2011), http://www.surgeongeneral. gov/library/calls/breastfeeding/calltoactiontosupportbreastfeeding.pdf.
5. UNICEF, "The Breastfeeding Initiatives Exchange: Facts and Figures," http://www. unicef.org/programme/breastfeeding/facts.htm.
6. US Department of Health and Human Services, *The Surgeon General's Call to Action*.
7. Sara Dwyer-McNulty, "Moving Beyond the Home: Women and Catholic Action in Post-World War II America," *US Catholic Historian* 20, no. 1 (2002): 83–97.
8. Lynn Y. Weiner, "Reconstructing Motherhood: The La Leche League in Postwar America," *Journal of American History* 80, no. 4 (1994): 1357–1381.
9. Dwyer-McNulty, "Moving Beyond the Home."
10. Church of the Brethren Network, "Heifer Project International," http://www.cob-net. org/glossary_brethren-h.htm.

11. Heifer International, "Measure of Success," http://www.heifer.org/ourwork/success/awards.

12. Thomas S. Dierolf, Rienzzie Kern, Tim Ogborn, Mark Protti, and Marvin Schwartz, "Heifer International: Growing a Learning Organisation," *Development in Practice* 12, nos. 3–4 (2002): 436–448.

13. Robert Kabumbuli and Jim Phelan, "Heifer-in-Trust Schemes: The Uganda Experience," *Development in Practice* 13, no. 1 (2003): 103–110.

14. Fred M. Ssewamala, "Expanding Women's Opportunities: The Potential of Heifer Projects in Sub-Saharan Africa," *Development in Practice* 14, no. 4 (2004): 550–559.

15. Ssewamala, "Expanding Women's Opportunities."

16. Katherine Marshall and Marisa Bronwyn Van Saanen, *Development and Faith: Where Mind, Heart, and Soul Work Together* (Washington, DC: World Bank Publications, 2007); Center for Interfaith Action on Global Poverty, *Many Faiths, Common Action: Increasing the Impact of the Faith Sector on Health and Development* (Washington DC: Center for Interfaith Action on Global Poverty, 2010).

17. Malcolm Harper, D. S. K. Rao, and Ashis Kumar Sahu, *Development, Divinity and Dharma: The Role of Religion in Development and Microfinance Institutions* (Warwickshire, UK: Practical Action Publishing, 2008).

18. Harper, Rao, and Sahu, *Development, Divinity and Dharma.*

19. Harper, Rao, and Sahu, *Development, Divinity and Dharma.*

20. Harper, Rao, and Sahu, *Development, Divinity and Dharma.*

21. Shri Kshethra Dharmasthala Rural Development Project, *Annual Report, 2011–12* (Dharmasthala, India: Shri Kshethra Dharmasthala Rural Development Project, 2012), http://www.skdrdpindia.org/pdf%20files/Annual%20Report%202011-12.pdf.

22. Harper, Rao, and Sahu, *Development, Divinity and Dharma*, 45.

23. Harper, Rao, and Sahu, *Development, Divinity and Dharma*, 46–56.

24. Harper, Rao, and Sahu, *Development, Divinity and Dharma.*

25. G. Smith et al., *Working Group on Human Needs* (London: University of East London, 2002), quoted in Harper et al., *Development, Divinity and Dharma*, 3.

26. Dhaka Ahsania Mission, "Khan Bahadur Ahsanullah (R.)," http://www.ahsaniamission.com.pk/khan.php.

27. Dhaka Ahsania Mission, *Annual Report 2009–10*, Dhaka Ahsania Mission publication no. 383 (Dhaka, Bangladesh: Dhaka Ahsania Mission, 2010), http://www.ahsaniamission.org.bd/annual_reports/Annual%20Report_2009-2010.pdf.

28. Dhaka Ahsania Mission, "Programmatic Perspective Plan 2006–2015," http://www.ahsaniamission.org.bd/perspectiveplan.doc.

29. Kazi Rafiqul Alam, "Ganokendra: An Innovative Model for Poverty Alleviation in Bangladesh," *International Review of Education* 52, no. 3–4 (2006): 343–352.

30. Dhaka Ahsania Mission, "Safe Water, Hygiene & Sanitation Are Being Formed at Ultra-Poor Urban Area's School," January 17, 2011, http://www.ahsaniamission.org.bd/detail_news.php?id=313.

31. See the "Research" page of the Mission website at http://www.ahsaniamission.org.bd/Research.php.

32. UNESCO, "Literacy in Communities: Village Revolutions," in *The New Courier*, April 2003, quoted in Alam, "Ganokendra: An Innovative Model," 350–351.

33. Dhaka Ahsania Mission, "Khan Bahadur Ahsanullah (R.)."

34. Dhaka Ahsania Mission, "Khan Bahadur Ahsanullah (R.)."
35. B. Clarke, *Enough Room for Joy: Jean Vanier's L'Arche: A Message for Our Time* (New York: BlueBridge, 2006), 37.
36. Jean Vanier, *An Ark for the Poor: The Story of L'Arche* (Toronto: Novalis, 1995), 15.
37. Vanier, *An Ark for the Poor*, 16.
38. Vanier, *An Ark for the Poor*, 21.
39. Vanier, *An Ark for the Poor*, 16.
40. L'Arche International, "Welcome to L'Arche International," http://www.larche.org/home.en-gb.1.0.index.htm.
41. Jean Vanier, *Becoming Human* (Toronto: House of Anansi, 1998), 22.
42. L'Arche International, "FAQ," http://www.larche.org/en/faq.
43. Jean Vanier, *From Brokenness to Community* (New York: Paulist Press, 1992), 10.
44. Franz H. Mueller, "The Principle of Subsidiarity in the Christian Tradition," *American Catholic Sociological Review* 4, no. 3 (1943): 144–157.
45. Martha C. Nussbaum, *Creating Capabilities* (Cambridge, MA: Harvard University Press, 2011).
46. Quoted in Mueller, "The Principle of Subsidiarity," 63.
47. Mabelle Arole and Rajanikant Arole, *Jamkhed: A Comprehensive Rural Health Project* (Maharashtra, India: Comprehensive Rural Health Project, 1994), 1.

23 | Mapping Religious Resources for Health: The African Religious Health Assets Programme

JAMES R. COCHRANE, DEBORAH McFARLAND, AND GARY R. GUNDERSON

We are committed to interventions leading to an epidemic of good health

Bill Foege

O N FEBRUARY, 8, 2007, AN unusual meeting took place in the Washington National Cathedral in Washington, DC, a special event on "what faith-based organizations (FBOs) are actually doing in the fight against AIDS." Sponsored by the World Health Organization (WHO) in collaboration with the Cathedral's Center for Global Justice and Reconciliation, it was based on work carried out by the African Religious Health Assets Programme (ARHAP), an international, multi-institutional team of researchers. The event was unusual because the WHO seldom showcases in this fashion studies commissioned by it but carried out by others. Even more unusually, it had a double connection to religion: For the WHO to commission research overtly dealing with religious phenomena was unprecedented. To hold the event (which was presided over by WHO Executive Director Kevin De Cock) in a religious building, however stately and prestigious, was wholly uncharacteristic and potentially provocative.

That the event was held in Washington, DC, probably had to do with a concern at the time over US foreign policy expressed in the President's Emergency Plan for AIDS Relief that, because the project was a very large unilateral initiative in global public health, it could undermine the intrinsic multilateral nature of the WHO, a UN body. But the issue of interest here is why the WHO even commissioned research into religious entities. This is unexpected, given the general aversion to religion in UN bodies and the many negative experiences that public health and medical professionals have had with religion in the context of HIV and AIDS (where it has been blamed for promoting stigma, entrenching problematic gender ideologies, and so on).

A partial explanation lies in purely pragmatic considerations: the extensive, empirically demonstrated scope and scale of religious or faith-inspired actors in health promotion, prevention, treatment, support, and care. The work of ARHAP presented at the 2007 conference clearly showed that the true scope of faith-based work in public health extends far beyond what many in the international health and development world realize. What religious health assets (RHAs) can offer in the face of stressed or collapsing public health systems is far from inconsequential. Indeed, they are often the only thing left standing in many communities. Partly, too, this meeting had to do with the focus in HIV and AIDS work on universal access, especially regarding the availability and acceptability of treatment and care. Acceptability means paying attention to the intended recipients of a health intervention, and in most contexts one or another religious tradition deeply shapes many, perhaps an overwhelming majority, of people, affecting how they make choices and how they act in response to any intervention.

Ted Karpf, then Partnerships Officer in the WHO's Department of HIV/ AIDS, recognized that the organization knew far too little about religious actors or resources to make any kind of informed, intelligent assessment of who or what there was to work with and how to work with them. Most of what anyone knew was either highly fragmented or merely anecdotal. A fundamental gap in knowledge existed. Hence the commissioning of the research undertaken by ARHAP, an organization founded precisely to establish a framework for systematically mapping religious assets for public health.

ARHAP, in fact, is an intellectual heir, at least in part, of an earlier piece of WHO history of signal importance: the engagement in the late 1960s and early 1970s of the WHO with public health leaders and theological advocates associated with the Christian Medical Commission, established under the auspices of the World Council of Churches. That engagement provided basic ideas for what came to be called primary health care, backed by extensive case studies, many of which were later published by the WHO in *Health by the People*.[1] That story is dealt with elsewhere in this volume,[2] and it points to what still needs to be done. If primary health care as envisaged by the Alma-Ata Declaration failed to achieve those grand hopes,[3] then many churches also failed to grasp its profound challenge, inseparable from questions of justice and equity. At the same time, that history also reflects what collaboration between religious and public health bodies could mean, at a time when the role of FBOs is once more a topic of interest in public health and primary health care has again attracted attention.[4]

This is what Karpf understood in approaching ARHAP, a jointly managed collaborative group of researchers and practitioners spanning three continents and several institutions (including Emory University and the universities of Cape Town, KwaZulu-Natal, and Witwatersrand). Founded by the three authors of this essay and launched in December 2003 in Geneva, Switzerland, it was made up of people who agreed to work together to fulfill a vision none could achieve alone.[5] The organization represents an exercise in structuring the kind of intellectual collaboration capable of treating the interface between religion and public health in its full complexity. In a 2006 publication, ARHAP researchers described its task as probing a "bounded field of unknowing,"[6] a metaphor meant to capture both the paucity of knowledge in the field and the delimitation of that field as quite specific (accessible through multiple disciplinary angles of investigation where some partial insight already existed) as well as its fecundity (richly fertile in the potential for new knowledge).

ARHAP's intellectual heart lay in the direction of what some have defined as transdisciplinarity, as suggested by Jill Olivier's PhD study of ARHAP.[7] Exactly what transdisciplinarity means is still the subject of considerable debate,[8] but it rests on the conviction, as Manfred Max-Neef puts it, that "an integrating synthesis is not achieved through the accumulation of different brains. It must occur inside each of the brains." It must do so in such a way that "it recognizes as simultaneous modes of reasoning, the rational and the relational."[9] More than this, however, ARHAP understood transdisciplinarity in action research terms, a framework that, as Daniel Stokols argues, requires "coordination among . . . different types and levels of collaboration (i.e., among scholars working together on scientific projects; among the members of community coalitions collaborating to improve conditions within their local community; and among the representatives of organizations, agencies, and institutions spanning local, regional, and national levels who coordinate their efforts to implement and evaluate major public health policies and programs)."[10]

This spirit of inquiry was equally reflected in ARHAP's organizational structure, which was often difficult for other, more rigidly institutionalized bodies to grasp. The core management, advisory, and decision-making body was called its Provisional Integration Team. The designation was somewhat tongue-in-cheek, but it accurately reflected the body's purpose. The Provisional Integration Team was meant to be open-ended in its style and in its membership (which came to include, among others, graduate students of its senior members); its primary intentionality and guiding principles were shaped by a commitment to the integration of different fields of thought and practice, and of its own work with that of others in the field; and its modus operandi was to work as a team, facilitating diverse gifts and abilities while supporting new blood. Despite some members (such as the three founders) having particular authority in holding the vision, the purpose, and the people in place, ARHAP in fact had no CEO or director per se. As odd as that sounds, this openness and flexibility was precisely the source of the organization's innovative strength, giving it an ability to think beyond existing disciplinary and practice boundaries. It was a collection, one might say, of what Gary Gunderson has called "boundary leaders."[11]

Thinking about Religious Health Assets

Those who became part of ARHAP were fully aware of the gaps and weaknesses in our knowledge of religion in relation to public health and that this might be a weakness in the goal of extending public health to all. ARHAP was inspired by the work of the Interfaith Health Program, founded in 1991 under the auspices of the Carter Center in Atlanta with Gary Gunderson as its first director. That initiative had the particular interest of William (Bill) Foege, renowned for his key role in the eradication of smallpox. A former director of the Centers for Disease Control and Prevention and first executive director of the Carter Center, Foege was concerned about how people of different faiths might work together toward health as part of a reconfiguration of health itself.

What Foege sought was what he called a "reverse epidemiology": "Where others look for early signs of pathology and the underlying pathogen, we look for effective community building and the underlying dynamic. Where most look for interventions that can stop the spread of disease, we are committed to interventions leading to an epidemic of good health."[12] For Foege, the Interfaith Health Program's innovative mandate was to reverse the order of priority in epidemiology: pay attention first not to the problems (pathologies or liabilities) but to what is life-giving (generativities or assets) and that may be strengthened.

Liabilities or pathologies by no means disappear in this notion of reverse epidemiology. But the point, echoing the WHO's definition of health as more than the absence of disease, is to challenge the regnant reality, in which pathologies absorb the vast bulk of resources and frame what is taken to be normative in understanding health. Informed by a religious imagination that understands the social determinants of health, the Interfaith Health Program sought to "develop conceptual frameworks that illuminate the most effective ways to describe the strengths of the faith community and how they can be aligned with the resources of the health/public health sector to achieve these shared goals."[13] Readily discernible behind this view is the idea of RHAs, a concept reinforced by the work on asset-based community development originating from Northwestern University.[14]

ARHAP, with its hub at the University of Cape Town, was a direct descendant of the Interfaith Health Program's approach. It tapped into a renewed intellectual and strategic interest in the role of religion in public health that had reemerged after a long hiatus, just as global public health faced its own crises of confidence.[15] As formal public health systems struggled to cope with emerging issues, public health leaders were badly in need of guidance in identifying local or community-based resources that might be leveraged for health. While public health officialdom was unaware or distrustful of religion, religious people and entities of various kinds had at no point ceased to engage in relevant health activities.

The two domains of interest—religion and public health—came together in the genesis of ARHAP. The task that it faced was appropriately dual, with two driving impulses: to earn the respect of the large institutions (the WHO, the Global Fund, the Gates Foundation, and the like) so as to have an impact on policy and practice and, simultaneously, to engage the inconvenient complexity at the intersection of faith and health. We needed to help public health actors, often locked into the instrumental purposes of finding and harnessing additional resources to meet the challenges that they faced, to understand the *communicative* rationality that determines much that happens in the sphere of religion. To treat religious constituencies mainly as an avenue for disseminating health messages, for example, underplays the importance of understanding them in their own terms, and of considering the way that their norms and values impact health delivery. It also undermines their possible role as partners in health with a contribution to make that goes beyond service delivery per se. ARHAP has thus been concerned to move from the more common question posed by public health agencies, "What can you do for us?" to the more productive query, "What can we do together?"

We also needed to help religious actors understand the importance of *public* health for their own conceptualization of what they are doing—all too often focused, like much in health care, on the individual (or the family at most) and forgetful of the social or ecological determinants of health. Religious actors usually have close, credible, and often enduring ties to local communities that make them potentially vital mediators in identifying and building upon local strengths and assets with a view to strengthening community-oriented health systems. What's more, the vast majority of faith traditions have some deeply rooted conception of health as intrinsically linked to well-being and the wholeness of life. This should make the intimate connection between a religious vision and the goals of public health obvious.

Re-Membering Religion in Public Health

What, then, set religion and public health apart from each other? The disjunction is relatively new. If, as William Foege has argued, modern public health traces back to the invention of vaccines beginning with Edward Jenner two hundred plus years ago,[16] it is also deeply rooted in a social understanding of health to which religious people and movements contributed considerably during the Industrial Revolution, in their work around polluted water and air, open sewage, impossible working hours, child labor, overcrowding, and the like. Indeed, the seminal nineteenth-century German health reformer Rudolf Virchow held that medicine in its innermost core and being is a social science, and politics nothing more than medicine writ large.[17] This view is comparable to those of Unitarians such as Edwin Chadwick, England's early public health champion; of English Christian Socialists like F. D. Maurice, Charles Kingsley, and Archbishop William Temple; and of Walter Rauschenbusch's social gospel in the United States.[18] All gave impetus to the modern movement for public health, and that same understanding of health is again evident in the vital contribution of the Christian Medical Commission to the genesis of primary health care, captured in the 1978 Alma-Ata Declaration.

Despite this substantive history, the discipline of public health has for the last half century or so largely ignored the potential of religious entities and resources for public health. There are many reasons for this: many key thinkers of the nineteenth and twentieth centuries saw religion as derivative rather than sui generis (Adam Smith, Ludwig Feuerbach, Karl Marx, Sigmund Freud, and Friedrich Nietzsche, for example); the social sciences thus presumed that religion would diminish in importance as secular society gained in strength; scientism, defined by Outhwaite, following Jürgen Habermas, as "the reduction of all knowledge to that furnished by the empirical sciences, where these are conceived as an unproblematic reflection of reality,"[19] increasingly became a kind of religious creed in its own right, supplanting a more hermeneutic or interpretive approach to social reality; and for organizations like the WHO, a multilateral body of the UN, religion was a complicating political factor best sidestepped. As a result, what interest in religion there has been has been largely confined to qualities or practices hypothesized to have an effect on the health of individual persons[20] and dominated by a search for empirical measures (the effect of prayer on recovery times from operations, of meditation on stress levels, and so on). Little literature on religion and public health has been conceived in any other way.[21]

One result is a relatively weak understanding of the role, scope, and scale of religious entities—a term ARHAP uses to describe not just FBOs but also indigenous or traditional healers, care groups, and the like—in the health of communities or populations. Despite attempts by the African Christian Health Associations or Christian Connections for International Health, we do not have any consolidated picture of the scope, scale, or even location of the hundreds, if not thousands, of hospitals, clinics, and dispensaries in the hands of religious organizations in Africa. What data do exist are partial, fragmentary, and often highly superficial. Critically, virtually no one pays attention to the enormous number of informal religious entities engaged in activities directly relevant to community and public health. Often deeply rooted in local communities and enduring over time, they have remained largely invisible to formal public health systems or interventions, probably to the detriment of all.

The gap in knowledge and the invisibility or misalignment of religious health entities on the ground drove ARHAP's establishment and its goal to map the scope, scale, and role of RHAs. For what purpose, however? The central animating motivation of ARHAP's three founders (the authors), who first met at a gathering hosted by the Interfaith Health Program at the Carter Center in Atlanta, aimed at probing the possibility of establishing a global RHAs initiative. They discovered a shared desire to rehabilitate a social vision of the health of the public as expressed in the best of the history and practice of religion and of public health, in a vision of justice and well-being for all. Propitiously, twenty-seven scholars from the Institute for Health and Social Justice and Partners in Health had just produced a provocative, programmatic, and inspirational volume on "global inequality and the health of the poor."[22] That work emphasized the profound, globally relevant, social determinants of health and called for a much more active response to the challenges of inequity and poverty as they impact on health.

When, then, the WHO commissioned ARHAP to map and assess RHAs in two African countries (Zambia and Lesotho) to establish a generalizable foundation for understanding their scope, scale, and character, the ARHAP team determined at the outset that the study had to be more than an exercise in enumeration. It had to find ways of explaining the dynamics that motivated religious entities engaged in health activity, and it had to do so in ways that paid attention to their self-understanding. It had to aim at strengthening and leveraging the assets already there to support a sustainable partnership between formal health systems, religious entities, and community-based initiatives. It had to do so with a view to greater equity and justice as central to the health of all. In its best and deepest sense, the study had to be about "the health of the public."[23]

Who Does the Mapping? Communicative Action versus Instrumental Legibility

Epidemiology serves public health by mapping the distribution and patterns of disease or illness so that one may know what one is dealing with and how one might best intervene. The frightening outbreak of cholera in 1854 from the Broad Street Pump in Soho, London, is the classic case. Its hero is Dr. John Snow, physician to Queen Victoria, inventor of controlled anesthesia, and the "father of modern epidemiology." Less well known, mostly forgotten, is Reverend Henry Whitehead. Yet without him, key information would have remained hidden, and Snow's theory that cholera was carried by "animalculae" in contaminated water rather than bad air (miasma theory) might well have been ignored. This is a story, then, not just of mapping, but of how religion and public health intertwine in ways beneficial to the health of all.

Snow's first "dot map" identified individual deaths from cholera in Broad Street and its surrounds. It suggested that the pump from which people drew their water, at the epicenter of the outbreak, must be implicated, even though it had been known to have the best water in the area.[24] That map helped Snow to persuade the local authorities to allow him to remove the handle from the suspect pump, and the epidemic subsided. But the dominant miasma theory of disease at that time—the belief that foul air was the source of disease—nevertheless held sway, and the authorities were far from convinced about Snow's waterborne theory of cholera. His map, after all, could as easily be interpreted as depicting the source of some airborne contamination emanating from Broad Street. There were also questions about aberrant patterns in the distribution of deaths that he could not answer. More information was needed than Snow could provide.

The person who would gather the evidence to support Snow's theory was Whitehead, the local parish curate. His knowledge of how people lived and actually moved on the real map of Soho was crucial, as was his personal knowledge of many people in his parish, which afforded him a kind of access that Snow could not possibly have had. His initial motivation was to prove Snow wrong. What he found, however, persuaded him that the doctor was right. Whitehead's sleuthing and inside knowledge not only helped explain the aberrations in Snow's map but also established the index case, a baby whose diarrheic discharges were seeping through decayed brick linings from a cesspit into the Broad Street pump well a couple feet away.

Snow spent two days early in the epidemic tracking the deaths; Whitehead spent months following up the clues, ultimately reaching over half of the roughly nine hundred people affected.[25] Because of his local knowledge, his credibility and the access it gave him to the community, and the passion evoked in him by what was happening to people whom he knew personally, Whitehead may be described as a religious health asset. Actually, he was not alone: his work was commissioned by the local Vestry Committee of the Parish, which had brought him and Snow together, thus enabling the partnership.

The story also has another dimension, concerning what is mapped. Identifying the germ that causes cholera and its patterns of infection so that one can prevent it is important. Here the answer was clear: provide clean water safe from contamination—a classic public health intervention. Yet note that such an intervention is not just about a pathology. In effect, it focuses on that which generates and sustains life: safe water. Two sides of the coin, but how one prioritizes them is vital. A different kind of response to cholera might be to invent drugs to treat the infected person. While some may profit from that intervention, public health would gain much less.

This example, simplistic in some ways, nonetheless makes the point that mapping pathologies is only a partial answer to the challenges that confront public health. Identifying generative agents of health is the other, often underplayed, part. So are assets of the kind represented by people like Whitehead. Understanding RHAs means understanding the ways in which religion or faith enter into what motivates people to engage and persist in activities aimed at improving the health of others, what enables them to succeed, what explains their durability over years or even generations—in other words, how they are generative for health rather than only relevant to a pathology.[26]

A century and more after the Broad Street panic, HIV and AIDS tax public health practitioners, researchers, and social systems in ways that once again prompt questions about engaging communities and leveraging assets for health. To confront the complex, multifaceted dimensions of the pandemic, do we not need credible and acceptable access to the communities most affected? Do we not need the energies of trusted people to enable such access, to help support interventions that must endure over time and do for health promotion, prevention, care, and even treatment what state apparatuses and international agencies cannot do? If so, then must we not necessarily engage with what in many parts of the world is most commonly to be found there—faith-based or faith-inspired religious entities?

The question of religion and the health of the public is indeed once more a topic of growing interest among major agencies, such as the WHO, the Centers for Disease Control and Prevention, the Global Health Council, the Global Fund to Fight HIV/AIDS, Malaria and TB, the Bill and Melinda Gates Foundation, and the World Bank. So, too, many religious leaders, bodies, and institutions have retained or are regaining a keen sense of their own visions of the well-being and health of the public. This is the historical conjuncture of ARHAP's work for the WHO.

Yet the situation is still predominantly shaped by a methodological separation of medical science and religion and faith. This has its rationale at one level (empirical, instrumental); it also has its flaws at another (communicative, practical). For ARHAP, then, to map and assess RHAs beyond mere enumeration, new methods and tools had to be invented. To be sure, traditional mapping or assessment also had to be done, first, because the WHO specifically required ARHAP's data to fit its HealthMapper GIS database, which categorizes health facilities of various kinds, and match its Services Availability Mapping tool (SAM; since replaced by the Service Availability and Readiness Assessment tool), which quantifies myriad items related to heathcare services, and, second, because what is not mapped generally does not count for policy or resource allocation decisions.

Still, the quantitative tools mentioned, theoretically speaking, serve an instrumental purpose: they make legible that which is not legible, meeting the requirements for bureaucratic control and manipulation, serving the need to "see like a state."[27] But they cannot serve the purposes of communicative action, an intersubjective process through which action is coordinated by negotiating definitions of a situation and coming to agreement about action. Here, the perspectives of those affected by any action including the norms and values that they hold, become important. Here, trust becomes a key indicator of the success or sustainability of any intervention. As Habermas puts it, "Communicative action is a switching station for the energies of social solidarity."[28] If the WHO's existing methods do not measure quality except via quantity and if they do not allow for an understanding of the human dynamics of health provision or intervention, then ARHAP needed to find ways to do that.

Participatory Mapping and Assessment "of a Special Kind"

As its name indicates, ARHAP began life with an unambiguous commitment to understanding and mobilizing RHAs. Enough publications exist now, including the report produced for the WHO,[29] to explain what we mean by "religious health assets," and why we use this curious term.[30] Here, it suffices to note that the term focuses attention on religious phenomena relevant to health, including formal health facilities (hospitals, clinics, dispensaries) but also the vast range and types of people, groups, organizations, and institutions of a religious- or faith-inspired kind seldom "counted" in public health that nonetheless actively work toward public health. Crucially, the term prioritizes what the religious phenomena hold, either tangibly or intangibly, of value for health ("assets") that may be leveraged for greater health. There is a dual interest here, then: first, in the visibility of such assets and, second, in what they are and how they work.

This has significant implications for mapping RHAs. ARHAP demonstrated in its work for the WHO, which focused on HIV and AIDS, that there are far more assets for public health in or related to local communities than maps of facilities would ever lead one to believe, discerned in a remarkably wide range of activities concerned with prevention, care, treatment, and support outside traditional facility walls. Yet, because they were not formal health facilities or services, they were not counted as part of any health system. In this sense, they were invisible to public health authorities and agencies. Because public attention, allocation of resources, and policy decisions depend upon visibility, that realization is not inconsequential.

ARHAP was also interested in understanding the dynamics, qualities, norms, and values relevant to the strength and durability of such activities.

The research team therefore decided that it was vital to distinguish between tangible and intangible assets. Tangible RHAs—facilities, equipment, transport, chaplains, traditional healers, care groups, donors, and so on—are the easiest to grasp, count, or measure, and that is where most surveys or mapping exercises begin and stop. Intangible RHAs—motivation, trust, vocation, a principled orientation to the suffering, and so on—are harder to count or measure directly, usually requiring proxy indicators. Moreover, they are rooted in dynamic, fluid, durable, and complex patterns of motivations, relations, and behaviors influenced by religious traditions or worldviews that themselves require some understanding. The ARHAP research team, composed of people from multiple disciplines with rich practical experiences in health and fields influenced by religion, knew that it would be possible to fully grasp the potential of RHAs for public health only by getting at some of these intangible phenomena.

How to do so? That was our most important conceptual decision. We were not without appropriate methods and tools from elsewhere, including those associated with asset-based community development, appreciative inquiry,[31] and participatory rural appraisal,[32] allied to the liberative pedagogy of Paulo Freire.[33] The challenge was to find a fitting mix of them and, above all, a clear logic and purpose for their use. By then, we were all too familiar with mapping and assessment enterprises that produce reams of mostly superficial data that no one uses, least of all those whom the data "describes," those who actually live on the map. The fragmented and partial existing data sets about religious health assets that we initially uncovered in preparation for our work fitted that bill, being mostly dry and of little operational use. We hoped to avoid an outcome that did not look much different.

We were aware that our mix of methods, like any technology, offered no magic formula. Any idea that one need only "use the right instruments and all is well" is a chimera, for participatory tools as much as any others.[34] The logic of the toolset that we planned to adopt and adapt had to match its purposes. On the one hand, we were required to harmonize our outcomes with the WHO's SAM tool and HealthMapper databases, both heavily oriented toward facilities and other tangible markers. On the other, these tools could not meet three critical elements that we regarded as central to what needed to be mapped: (i) an assessment of intangible factors that are often vital to successful, durable public health interventions; (ii) a way of determining which, if any, facility was trusted and used by local community members; and (iii) a recognition of any of the multiple local health programs or initiatives not connected to facilities (hospitals, clinics, dispensaries, health posts). All three elements seemed necessary if one was really to grasp the broader nature and significance of RHAs. Another important variable, but one that exceeded the capacities of the ARHAP study, was time: what changes, how it changes, and why it changes over time, what cannot meaningfully be leveraged for greater health because it is here one day and gone the next, and what will make for durable interventions.

Even more critical for us (but entirely secondary to the technical role that the WHO largely sees itself playing), we wanted to know how our research could produce knowledge of value and use to those whom we were researching. Could our work fulfill a social goal? Could it help transform conditions through the empowering of local people by highlighting the assets that they already have, with which they can work, and upon which others can build? Those questions meant that we could not separate knowledge and power in how we conceptualized mapping and assessment.

That, in turn, meant allowing for the subversion of the very thing that we were commissioned to do. Perhaps, as a widespread aphorism has it, it is true that "if you are not on the map, you don't count" (or, in its stronger form, "if you are not at the table, you are on the menu"). But it is also the case that those who have experienced maps as a means of control or worse, have no desire to be visible, no desire to be mapped. Mapping and assessment, even of religious health assets, is implicated in larger power relations that are not necessarily benign to those being mapped. Put differently, the question arises of whether mapping and assessment serves to strengthen the capacity of local communities to enhance their power over their own lives. In this context, any mapping exercise had to be accompanied by a deep understanding of how to engage people across gaps of knowledge and power, gaps in many ways embodied and perhaps entrenched by the researchers themselves. The toolset could not stand on its own without adequate training in understanding its overall purpose and rationale.

Mapping and assessment of this special kind shaped the toolset that we designed, tested, and redesigned—named, a little tongue in cheek, PIRHANA (Participatory Inquiry into Religious Health Assets, Networks and Agency). The logic of the toolset is the critical dimension, viz. the sequence in which different tools or methods (none magical and all invented by others and adapted by ARHAP) are used in the participatory workshops, and the way that they were shaped to generate the kind of data that we needed to collect. Critically, it includes a careful construction of the engagement with participants that, from the outset, grasps the way in which gaps of knowledge and power can marginalize people and maximizes respect for their own knowledge and ways of thinking and being. It cumulatively builds insights as the work moves from tool to tool, developing knowledge in the process itself. The knowledge gained is always transparent to the participants and available for their immediate use, should they so choose. In sum, the toolset sits—and must sit—within a fundamentally communicative rather than an instrumental approach to the research process, even if the tools and methods themselves are instruments toward that end.

A full description of the PIRHANA process and toolset is available elsewhere.[35] Combined with quantitative and qualitative approaches, it invokes the tricky tension between "quants" and "quals." If PIRHANA was designed to empower people at local level, it also had to produce persuasive evidence about the nature, scope, and scale of RHAs. Qualitative methods fit poorly with SAM (or SARA) and HealthMapper criteria for evidence. Moreover, qualitative methods in the field of health as elsewhere have often been used sloppily with poor theoretical underpinnings, reducing the confidence one might have in them.[36] Nonetheless, for PIRHANA to work, it was essential to include qualitative methods. As powerful as quantitative methods may be for some purposes, for others they are wholly inadequate. This includes understanding how people view the health of their communities, what they understand as religion in this regard, when this matters, why it matters, what intangible assets are involved, and what difference this makes to health interventions and their outcomes. Also important is the relationship between health seekers and providers, including what health seekers regard as, in fact, providing health. The latter is not to be taken for granted. For example, in a workshop in a semi-rural area of Lesotho, the health-seekers ranked as most important for health a post office upon which many families are dependent for remittances from migrant workers, for communication with them, and for safely holding their savings. A village without a post office was viewed as seriously deficient in health. Not a superficial judgment, it does confront one again with what one means by health.

The nature of the research data generated was thus strongly dependent upon its participatory, inductive, and nonextractive approach. This had four implications:

1. Understandings of religion and health were largely generated from below by the participants, producing highly context-specific data.
2. The data were thus uneven across different sites, though across multiple sites (rural, peri-urban and urban, in four areas of Zambia, three

of Lesotho) they were extensive and, considered as a whole, evidenced patterns of relevance to health systems.

3. Individual participants sometimes took hold of discussions, to the detriment of other participants, or to the process and purpose of the workshop.

4. Handling this required a discursive context of sharing, debate, and open (managed, friendly) interrogation, balancing sensitive respect for the participants and attention to the stated research goals.

ARHAP's approach thus combined quantitative data on the location, scope, and scale of RHAs (collected using GIS tools, field surveys, and reviews of existing data sets) with qualitative data drawn from health providers and health seekers at local, regional, and national levels. The qualitative data from PIRHANA workshops also produced quantitative data via counting, ranking, and comparative methods to assess how participants evaluated or experienced health provision or RHAs in their own context. The combination of instrumental and communicative approaches was and remains the strength of the approach. What could not be assessed was the extent of any identifiable or enduring impact on where this work was carried out. Though the workshops always ended by having those present engage with each other on possible next steps in their own contexts (for example, establishing a new cooperative arrangement for the provision of health care), we had no way of knowing what transpired thereafter.

A later adaptation of PIRHANA by Methodist Le Bonheur Healthcare in Memphis, Tennessee, further refined for the Hospice Palliative Care Association of South Africa, sought to address this deficit. Elements were added into the workshop itself—still following the basic rationale and logic outlined above—aimed directly, there and then, at initiating partnerships among those present with a view to community health systems strengthening. The toolset was renamed to Community Health Assets Mapping for Partnership (CHAMP), partly to indicate its added thrust and partly to incorporate not just religious entities or initiatives but also others that do not define themselves in religious or faith terms.

This has allowed different kinds of health providers—community-based and formal facilities (a hospital system in Memphis, local hospices in South Africa), for example—to engage with each other in often innovative and even unprecedented ways to build trust and sustainably align their different activities. In Memphis, it has helped to build the Congregational Health Network, now incorporating over five hundred local communities, each developing a relationship to Methodist Le Bonheur Healthcare that is mutually beneficial and formally acknowledged.[37] This model has since gained the attention of the White House and of many other healthcare providers in the United States. For the Hospice Palliative Care Association of South Africa, with the toolset modified to focus on palliative care in the context of HIV and AIDS (now, in principle, chronic rather than terminal), it has meant seeking partnerships with others in local communities whose work is broader than palliative care but necessary to the partnership. The Hospice Palliative Care Association of South Africa now plans to roll the toolset out through affiliates in some two hundred health districts and sub-districts in South Africa as part of a national plan for reengineering primary health care.

Conclusion

Perhaps ARHAP's most critical lesson is this: mapping and assessing RHAs contributes little to health policy or to the strengthening of any health system if it ignores those who inhabit the map—how they construct their own views of reality or how they behave according to what they value and treat as normative for their health. Here, ARHAP's approach begins to dovetail with a human rights perspective on health, insofar as it respects the dignity of persons and aims at creating the social structures that embody that respect.[38]

In most cases, we believe, health delivery or health provision works best and most sustainably when the persons intended as the recipients of an intervention are able to act as citizens in the process and to exercise their citizenship through it. Public health, from this perspective, is also about the health of the public per se and about the freedom that people have, in concert with others (this freedom is indivisible), to express and exercise their own human capabilities to the fullest.[39] Standard mapping or assessment tools are not made redundant or valueless thereby, but they are put in their place. Only then are they likely to be useful for transforming health at population scale.

Health, to the extent that it is a measure of who is healthy (or un-healthy) and why, is a powerful lens on the well-being (or disorder) of society itself and a crucial component of its development. Seen thus, ARHAP's approach to religion and health offers a "model of integral development" through a fivefold framing: an *epistemological commitment* to knowledge drawn from the "underside" (beginning in Africa); a focus on *religious entities in health* beyond FBOs, including tangible and intangible phenomena; a broad view of health, consonant with the best of religion, to do with *comprehensive well-being*; an *asset-based community-oriented approach* that better allows an alignment between communities and formal health systems or actors; and an approach to collaborative, transdisciplinary scholarship that *defines complexity, rather than simplification, as "the real."*[40]

Here, three basic norms are at work: (i) a commitment to a "thick description"[41] of human beings and of life, (ii) a practice that builds on what people have instead of what they do not have, and (iii) the promotion of an enabling environment for the enhancement of their human capabilities. Using these norms as one's guide is more likely to create a balance between instrumental purposes and communicative action in health interventions than many current strategies, which still tend to be heavily oriented toward the instrumental—not least because of donor imperatives and a desire for quick results, governments who must run bureaucracies, scientists who want research monies, international agencies with short attention spans, and corporations who want profit. Simply put, too little attention is still given to the lifeworlds of persons in relation to economy and polity; they are, after all, to be ironic, the software of the process—unpredictable, continually shifting or changing, less amenable to satisfying measurable inputs and outcomes, full of bugs—so that hardware is generally the name of the game.

Why does religion matter in this context? Why consider RHAs? We do not make these assessments because religious initiatives for health are necessarily better than others by most measures—even if one can make a case for certain aspects of religion that may contribute to public health practice and its outcomes.[42] Rather, as ARHAP's work shows, RHAs matter, alongside community health assets more broadly, simply because they are so widely present and, often, so deeply rooted locally. They are assets, and there is a pragmatic or strategic basis for giving them attention. Not to do so is poor science and short-sighted practice.

There is, however, a deeper reason for doing so. As medical anthropologists, sociologists, and many others have argued, public health is irrevocably and unavoidably affected not just by what medical science or management skills might offer but also by how available, affordable, and acceptable any health intervention is. Whereas some aspects of access have to do with technical matters, others—perhaps the most critical ones where population-scale health challenges are most profound—have to do with human beings and how they relate to any particular intervention. That introduces political and rights dimensions into the frame. That, in turn, confronts one with the norms and values that govern both societies and communities. That, again, has to do with worldviews and lifeworlds.

This, far more often than many like to admit, rests on what we can legitimately describe as a religious socialization or commitment. How persons in communities respond to or initiate a health intervention—how they behave and what choices they make—is frequently dependent on the norms and values associated with such religious factors. To use a term invented within ARHAP circles to express this reality, the healthworlds of persons,[43] which encapsulate their orientation to their and others' well-being, are more than incidental to developing deeply rooted and sustainable practices of public health. Religious norms and values, in short, are often key elements in the necessary communicative practice that we advocate as an essential element of mapping and assessing RHAs. To be absolutely clear, this is not to validate everything religious nor to sidestep the necessity of challenging those elements in religion that may be a liability for health. Rather, challenges to any such liabilities are more likely to produce positive results and enduring outcomes when the pertinent healthworld is properly grasped, and the assets that are present are acknowledged, validated, and leveraged for greater health. This is a purpose worth pursuing.

Notes

1. World Health Organization, *Health by the People* (Geneva: World Health Organization, 1975).
2. See chapter 21. See also James C. McGilvray, *The Quest for Health and Wholeness* (Tübingen: German Institute for Medical Mission, 1981); Gillian Paterson, "The CMC Story: 1968–1998," *Contact* 161–162 (1998): 3–52.
3. Marcos Cueto, "The Origins of Primary Health Care and Selective Primary Health Care," *American Journal of Public Health* 94, no. 11 (2004): 1864–1874; John J. Hall and Richard Taylor, "Health for All Beyond 2000: The Demise of the Alma-Ata Declaration and Primary Health Care in Developing Countries," *Medical Journal of Australia* 178 (2003): 17–20.
4. World Health Organization, *The World Health Report 2008: Primary Health Care— Now More Than Ever* (Geneva: World Health Organization, 2008).
5. For a full description of the goals and activities of ARHAP, relaunched in 2012 as the International Religious Health Assets Programme, see www.irhap.uct.ac.za.
6. Jill Olivier, James R. Cochrane, Barbara Schmid, and Lauren Graham, *ARHAP Literature Review: Working in a Bounded Field of Unknowing* (Cape Town, South Africa: ARHAP, 2006).
7. Jill Olivier, "In Search of Common Ground for Interdisciplinary Collaboration and Communication: Mapping the Cultural Politics of Religion and HIV/AIDS in Sub-Saharan Africa," PhD Thesis, University of Cape Town, 2010.

8. See Basarab Nicolescu, ed., *Transdisciplinarity: Theory and Practice* (New York: Hampton Press, 2008).

9. Manfred A. Max-Neef, "Foundations of Transdisciplinarity," *Ecological Economics* 53 (2005): 5, 10.

10. Daniel Stokols, "Toward a Science of Transdisciplinary Action Research," *American Journal of Community Psychology* 38 (2006): 63–77, 64.

11. Gary R. Gunderson, *Boundary Leaders: Leadership Skills for People of Faith* (Minneapolis: Fortress, 2004).

12. "The Task Ahead," in *Faith and Health* (Atlanta: Interfaith Health Program, Carter Center, 1994), 1.

13. Miriam Kiser, Deborah L. Jones, and Gary R. Gunderson, "Faith and Health: Leadership Aligning Assets to Transform Communities," *International Review of Mission* 95, nos. 376–377 (2006): 50–58, 13.

14. John P. Kretzmann and John L. McKnight, *Building Communities from the Inside Out: A Path toward Finding and Mobilizing a Community's Assets* (Chicago: ACTA Publications, 1993). See also Susan Rans and Hilary Altman, *Asset-Based Strategies for Faith Communities* (Evanston, IL: ABCD Institute, Institute for Policy Research, Northwestern University, 2002), http://www.abcdinstitute.org/docs/Asset-Based%20Strategies%20for%20Faith%20Communities-1.pdf.

15. Laurie Garrett, *Betrayal of Trust: The Collapse of Global Public Health* (New York: Hyperion, 2000).

16. William H. Foege, "Keynote Speech," presented at the Thomas Francis Jr. Medal in Global Public Health 50th Anniversary Program, April 12, 2005, Ann Arbor, MI, http://www.francismedal.umich.edu/history/foege.html.

17. "Die Medizin ist eine soziale Wissenschaft, und die Politik ist nichts weiter als Medizin im Großen," quoted in Harro Albrecht, "Rudolf Virchow," *Die Zeit*, December 11, 2009.

18. Paul T. Phillips, *A Kingdom on Earth: Anglo-American Social Christianity, 1880–1940* (University Park: Pennsylvania State University Press, 1996).

19. William Outhwaite, *Habermas: A Critical Introduction* (Cambridge: Polity Press, 2009), 20.

20. See, for example, Harold Koenig, Michael McCullough, and David Larson, *Handbook of Religion and Health* (New York: Oxford University Press, 2000).

21. For some exceptions, see Linda M. Chatters, "Religion and Health: Public Health Research and Practice," *Annual Review of Public Health* 21 (2000): 335–367.

22. Jim Yong Kim, Joyce V. Millen, Alec Irwin, and John Gershman, eds., *Dying for Growth: Global Inequality and the Health of the Poor* (Monroe, ME: Common Courage Press, 2000).

23. The term comes from a later theoretical work, but it accurately reflects ARHAP's original vision, in which "public health," going well beyond any specific discipline, was understood in its broadest, deepest sense; see Gary R. Gunderson and James R. Cochrane, *Religion and the Health of the Public: Shifting the Paradigm* (New York: Palgrave MacMillan, 2012).

24. For a full record, see Steven Johnson, *The Ghost Map: The Story of London's Most Terrifying Epidemic—and How It Changed Science, Cities, and the Modern World* (New York: Riverhead Books, 2006), and S. W. B. Newsom, "Pioneers in Infection

Control: John Snow, Henry Whitehead, the Broad Street Pump, and the Beginnings of Geographical Epidemiology," *Journal of Hospital Infection* 64, no. 6 (2006): 210–221.

25. Henry Whitehead, "Report on the Cholera Outbreak in the Parish of St. James, Westminster, During the Autumn of 1854," July 1855, http://johnsnow.matrix.msu.edu/work.php?id=15-78-AA.

26. Gunderson and Cochrane, *Religion and the Health of the Public*, 60–79; Gary R. Gunderson and Larry Pray, *Leading Causes of Life* (Memphis, TN: Center of Excellence in Faith and Health, Methodist Le Bonheur Healthcare, 2006).

27. James C. Scott, *Seeing Like a State: How Certain Schemes to Improve the Human Condition Have Failed* (New Haven, CT: Yale University Press, 1998).

28. Jürgen Habermas, *Lifeworld and System: A Critique of Functionalist Reason*. Vol. 2, *The Theory of Communicative Action*, trans. Thomas McCarthy (Boston: Beacon Press, 1987), 57.

29. African Religious Health Assets Programme, *Appreciating Assets: The Contribution of Religion to Universal Access in Africa*, Report for the World Health Organization (Cape Town, South Africa: ARHAP, 2006).

30. James R. Cochrane, "Conceptualising Religious Health Assets Redemptively," *Religion and Theology* 13, no. 1 (2006): 107–120; Gunderson and Cochrane, *Religion and the Health of the Public*, 41–59.

31. Charles Elliot, *Locating the Energy for Change: An Introduction to Appreciative Inquiry* (Winnipeg, MB: International Institute for Sustainable Development, 1999).

32. Robert Chambers, *Whose Reality Counts? Putting the First Last* (London: Intermediate Technology Publications, 1997), and "The Origins and Practice of Participatory Rural Appraisal," *World Development* 22, no. 7 (1994): 953–969.

33. Paulo Freire, *Pedagogy of the Oppressed*, trans. Myra Bergman Ramos (New York: Seabury Press-Continuum, 1970), and *Education for Critical Consciousness* (New York: Continuum, 1980).

34. See, for example, Bill Cooke and Uma Kothari, eds., *Participation: The New Tyranny?* (London: Zed Books, 2001).

35. Steve de Gruchy, James R. Cochrane, Jill Olivier, and Sinatra Matimelo, "Participatory Inquiry on the Interface between Religion and Public Health: What Does It Achieve and What Not?," in *When Religion and Health Align: Mobilizing Religious Health Assets for Transformation*, ed. James R. Cochrane, Barbara Schmid, and Teresa Cutts (Pietermaritzburg, South Africa: Cluster Publications, 2011), 43–61.

36. See the potent analysis by E. Murphy and R. Dingwall, *Qualitative Methods and Health Policy Research* (New York: Aldine de Gruyter, 2003).

37. Teresa Cutts, "The Memphis Model: ARHAP Theory Comes to Ground in the Congregational Health Network," in Cochane, Schmid, and Cutts, *When Religion and Health Align*, 193–210.

38. Cordaid, ICCO, and Institute of Social Studies, *Religion: Source for Human Rights and Development Cooperation* (Soesterberg, The Netherlands, September 2005), http://www.religion-and-development.nl/documents/publications/bbo-rapport-180406_def.pdf; Leslie London, "Community Agency: The Key to Making Human Rights Work for Public Health," in *ARHAP International Colloquium* (Cape Town, South Africa: African Religious Health Assets Programme, 2007), 94–100.

39. See, for example, Martha C. Nussbaum, *Women and Human Development: The Capabilities Approach* (Cambridge: Cambridge University Press, 2000); Jocelyn Dejong, "Capabilities, Reproductive Health and Well-Being," *Journal of Development Studies* 42, no. 7 (2006): 1158–1179; and Kelvin Jasek-Rysdahl, "Applying Sen's Capabilities Framework to Neighborhoods: Using Local Asset Maps to Deepen Our Understanding of Well-Being," *Review of Social Economy* 49, no. 3 (2001): 313–329.

40. James R. Cochrane, "A Model of Integral Development: Assessing and Working with Religious Health Assets," in *Religion and Development: Ways of Transforming the World*, ed. Gerrie ter Haar (New York: Columbia University Press, 2011), 231–252.

41. Clifford Geertz, "Thick Description: Toward an Interpretive Theory of Culture," in *The Interpretation of Cultures: Selected Essays* (New York: Basic Books, 1973), 3–30.

42. See, for example, Chatters, "Religion and Health"; P. C. Hill and Kenneth I. Pargament "Advances in the Conceptualization and Measurement of Religion and Spirituality: Implications for Physical and Mental Health Research," *American Psychologist* 58 (2003): 64–74; David R. Kinsley, *Health, Healing and Religion: A Cross Cultural Perspective* (Upper Saddle River, NJ: Prentice Hall, 1995); Bruce Y. Lee and Andrew B. Newberg, "Religion and Health: A Review and Critical Analysis," *Zygon* 40, no. 2 (2005): 443–468; Peter H. Van Ness, "Religion and Public Health," *Journal of Religion and Health* 38, no. 1 (1999): 15–26.

43. Paul Germond and James R. Cochrane, "Healthworlds: Conceptualizing Landscapes of Health and Healing," *Sociology* 44, no. 2 (2010): 307–324.

Religion and Three Public Health Challenges of Our Time

I N PART V, WE address the role of religion in three global epidemics. HIV/AIDS and Alzheimer's disease have already claimed millions of victims around the globe; pandemic influenza, should it break out, could match those numbers. How has religion played a role in confronting these diseases, or how might it play one in the future? We explore religion's role as a factor in determining risk of disease, as a social care resource, and—sometimes—as a barrier to care in these sharply contrasting contemporary public health and healthcare crises.

In chapter 24, Safiya George Dalmida and Sandra Thurman describe the complicated role of religion in the history of the HIV/AIDS epidemic, exploring the radically divergent responses of different religious communities. They discuss both the stigmatizing harm and the supportive care that have come to those with HIV/AIDS and their families from a range of religious groups as well as the healing role that spirituality has played for many with HIV/AIDS. Next, in chapter 25, Mimi Kiser and Scott Santibañez write about the partnerships that have formed between faith-based organizations in the United States and local and federal public health agencies to confront the threat of pandemic influenza. These alliances have produced successful programs to distribute influenza vaccines and increase the rate of vaccination, particularly in impoverished communities with less access to primary health care. Often, however, such programs must overcome suspicion and distrust among community members who may have been misled or even exploited by well-meaning public health workers in the past. Finally, in chapter 26, Kenneth Hepburn and Theodore Johnson examine the role of religion in confronting Alzheimer's disease and discuss both its failures and its potential in dealing with the disease, which is increasingly relevant to religious communities, especially the mainline Protestant churches in the United States and Europe, whose membership is aging.

Although these three diseases carry different risks of mortality, all *can* be fatal. All three are also global epidemics that know no national boundaries. But there are differences, of course. Alzheimer's disease is prevalent in wealthy countries with long life expectancies; it is the ironic result of the success these countries have had in reducing deaths from other causes, particularly cardiovascular disease and stroke. HIV/AIDS is today a disease of the world's poorest countries and the poorest communities in wealthy countries. Influenza risk crosses socioeconomic boundaries. While the progression of Alzheimer's is fairly well documented, it has no known cure and few treatments. Influenza and HIV/AIDS, on the other hand, are both infectious diseases with well-understood mechanisms of transmission and established prevention strategies. Whatever help or harm religious institutions may offer prevention efforts affects communities well beyond the borders of particular religious congregations, for good or ill.

HIV/AIDS and Alzheimer's disease raise particularly complex issues for religion and religious groups. Both diseases raise questions of identity, moral personhood, and threats to the value of the self in ways that few others do. Uncomfortable with these questions, people turn away from victims out of a sense of vulnerability, and social groups, including religious groups, may stigmatize the disease and those who have it. With HIV/AIDS, the stigmatization may be further driven by homophobia—often with religious origins. At the same time, these are both now chronic diseases, at least in the world's wealthy nations—HIV/AIDS because effective treatments have been found and Alzheimer's because it has a long, insidious course. The implication of this chronicity is that the individual with the disease is not alone; the long period of time in which he or she lives with it means that many others are also touched by it and suffer because of it. The social implications of these diseases—effects on families, workplaces, neighborhoods, communities, and in many cases congregations—play out over years. With Alzheimer's, family caregivers who must remain with victims at all times may be neglected or forgotten about by their religious communities, along with those with the disease themselves. Yet, at the same time, religious congregations and faith-based organizations have actively supported people living with HIV/AIDS and Alzheimer's victims and caregivers. There is research evidence, too, of the beneficial role played by religious and spiritual resources in the lives of those living with these illnesses. Religious groups are thus capable of both social harm and social support when illnesses—particularly these very serious and very prevalent illnesses—strike.

Our authors for these chapters come from the fields of epidemiology, nursing, medicine, gerontology, theology, and global health. Together, the accounts in these chapters sketch out the complex relationship of religious institutions to public health institutions when public health crises arise. We see, in these three cases, that the social structures of religion and public health are sometimes in conflict over perceptions, goals, or approaches, but at other times their interests are aligned.

When there is partnership and collaboration, religious institutions bring powerful assets—local knowledge and shared interests—to public health programs. As ongoing and stable social structures in their communities, not only in the midst of a disease outbreak, but long before it and long after it, they can and do lend their social capital—social networks, facilities, communication channels, time, and above all influence—to public health efforts. This is known as "bridging" social capital—capital that links institutions together, especially across sectors of society. A strong bridge, however, requires structural footings in the community on either side, and the respect and mutuality that equal partners can have for each other. Religious institutions and public health institutions both attend to the vulnerable in their communities and thus share the central ethical value of reducing harm and providing care. But while the great potential for partnerships is surely there, it is not often realized. In these chapters, we can see some of the obstacles to such cooperation and some maps for how it has been accomplished.

24 | HIV/AIDS

SAFIYA GEORGE DALMIDA AND SANDRA THURMAN

IV/AIDS HAS BEEN DESCRIBED BY many as the greatest threat to public health in modern times. Since the beginning of the epidemic over three decades ago, more than sixty million people have been infected with the human immunodeficiency virus (HIV) and nearly thirty million have died of HIV-associated acquired immune deficiency syndrome (AIDS). In 2011, approximately thirty-four million people were living with HIV globally,[1] 3.3 million of them children younger than 15 years old.[2] Sub-Saharan Africa has been hardest hit by the pandemic; 69 percent of all people living with HIV are in this region,[3] followed by South and Southeast Asia, Latin America, Eastern Europe and Central Asia, and North America.[4]

Although a significant number of people are still dying of HIV and AIDS-related illness, and there are still issues with access to HIV care and treatment across the globe, the number of people *living* with HIV/AIDS is growing, due to testing and outreach efforts, advances in treatment options, and increased access to free or affordable therapies and care. As a result, HIV is increasingly recognized, in some regions of the world, as a chronic disease rather than a life-threatening illness and attention is now being given to the role of psychosociocultural factors, including religion, in outcomes for people living with HIV and AIDS.

For individuals living with HIV/AIDS or caring for those who have it, religious belief systems influence their interpretations of and responses to illness in general and to HIV infection in particular. At the same time, religious institutions have both worked to influence the societal response to the epidemic and responded directly to individuals, families, and communities affected by it. These responses, which have sometimes been complicated by tensions between religious calls to compassion and beliefs that the disease is a result of sinful or immoral behavior, have shaped the course of the epidemic in ways both positive and negative.

The Religious Community and the HIV/AIDS Epidemic in the United States

The social factors that contributed to the response to HIV and AIDS were already part of the picture when the disease was identified in June 1981. This was particularly true in the United States, as Randy Shilts describes in *And the Band Played On*, his account of the emergence of the epidemic from the perspective of the gay community.[5] Although other risk factors were later identified, at this early stage the major social determinants of HIV/AIDS were linked to sexual behavior, sexual orientation, social networks, and environmental and geographic location (Haiti and Africa and, in the Western world, certain cities and sites such as bath houses). In the United States, the disease emerged first among primarily white homosexual men in urban areas; as a result, it was initially characterized as a "gay disease." Many religious leaders attributed HIV infection to divine cause—seeing it as a punishment from God, a result of karma, or a consequence of witchcraft and describing it as a punishment for the sins of homosexuality, adultery, or premarital or extramarital sex. Some assumed their faith communities were not affected by the disease because—they believed—only promiscuous or socially deviant people were at risk for infection and these people were not part of their congregations.

At the national level, this dynamic was reinforced by the emergence of a new set of political forces. The dawn of AIDS in America coincided with the rise to power of the conservative Christian right under the leadership of Jerry Falwell, whose enthusiastic support of Ronald Reagan had been essential to Reagan's successful bid for the US presidency in 1986.[6] The US government's lack of response to AIDS at the beginning of the epidemic, despite the urgent pleas of the Centers for Disease Control and Prevention, was due in large part to the influence of conservative anti-gay Christians in the Reagan White House and Congress.

Although many religious organizations drew criticism from AIDS activists, healthcare practitioners, and public health officials for their callous and judgmental response to people living with HIV/AIDS and for their limited support of HIV prevention efforts, other religious or religiously affiliated institutions took an early lead in providing care for those affected by the epidemic. Many faith-based hospitals, such as Saint Vincent's in New York, became epicenters for AIDS care and treatment.[7] Elsewhere, congregation-level responses played an early, key role in addressing the epidemic by providing education and services to those with or at risk for HIV/AIDS. All Saints Episcopal Church in Atlanta, for instance, was the first church in the southern United States to organize support groups and establish care teams to support people living with AIDS and their partners and families and openly invite all people living with the disease to come to worship.

Over time, these congregation-level responses cohered into denomination-wide networks and programs. In 1986, the Episcopal Church sponsored the first national, AIDS-related faith gathering in the United States, which drew about three hundred people working in HIV/AIDS ministry to Grace Cathedral in San Francisco. Bruce Garner, a person living with AIDS, activist, and member of All Saints, attended the conference; the experience was transformative, as he told journalist Sharon Sheridan: "We cried for about three days. We found out that we were all doing the same work, but none of us had been aware that the rest of us were doing it, which was the way it was in the early days of the epidemic."[8] The conference, which spurred Garner to increase AIDS ministry in his diocese and beyond, was the genesis of the National Episcopal AIDS Coalition, founded in 1987 to provide a support structure to the growing number of parish-level AIDS programs.[9]

Other nascent, church-based AIDS programs were also gaining strength. Roman Catholic programs united as the Catholic AIDS Network and incorporated, with support from national church structures, in 1989. They were joined by the Lutherans, Disciples of Christ, and others. By the early 1990s, the AIDS National Interfaith Network, created in 1988 to provide support to faith-based AIDS efforts across denominations, had two thousand members. These faith-based programs partnered with local AIDS service organizations, forging strong and visible ties with the gay community in the process. However, by the time most denominations had reached consensus on their AIDS policies, nearly sixty thousand Americans had died from the disease, and AIDS had become the second leading cause of death among US men aged 25–44, surpassing heart disease, cancer, suicide, and homicide. In San Francisco, New York, and Los Angeles, it was the leading cause of death for men in that age group. Even in the face of these numbers, conservative Christians held firm to their anti-gay and anti-AIDS positions. Their rejection of their members affected by HIV/AIDS, particularly in the southern United States, was devastating to people living with the disease. The impact on AIDS funding and policy was equally as damaging.

One area where response was particularly slow to develop was in African American communities; the response to the HIV/AIDS epidemic from African American congregations and religious institutions has historically been lacking for a variety of reasons.[10] Some African American religious leaders cite a lack of knowledge about HIV and concerns about the appropriateness of sexual content in the pulpit as barriers to engaging the religious community in HIV prevention as well as religious controversy around homosexuality.[11] However, African American religious groups have become more active in recent years, initiating HIV ministries or support groups and engaging in partnerships with academic and government institutions to address HIV-related issues, including stigma and prevention.[12] One such partnership is Your Blessed Health, a program in Michigan designed to increase the capacity to address HIV/AIDS with African American congregations by training religious leaders to deliver HIV education sessions to youth and adults.[13] Similarly, Keeping the Faith invited thirty-eight of Philadelphia's most influential African American faith leaders to examine the role of faith-based institutions in HIV prevention.[14] And Project FAITH (Fostering AIDS Initiatives That Heal) funded HIV-related programs and services at twenty-two churches in South Carolina.[15,16,17]

Religious Responses to HIV across the Globe

Unsurprisingly, given the tensions and controversies stirred by the HIV epidemic, religious institutions across the globe have responded to it in various ways and at various levels. Some religious institutions have focused more on care and treatment while others have directed their energies more toward primary or secondary prevention. Comparative case studies have shown that those religious groups that engaged early in the epidemic tended to focus more on care and support for people living with HIV/AIDS, while those that got involved later tended to focus more on prevention and education.[18] For the most part, it appears that it is easier for religious groups to provide pastoral care for people living with HIV/AIDS or work to raise awareness and promote testing than to promote harm reduction activities such as condom use or safe needle use.[19]

Some faith communities have established local HIV/AIDS ministries, outreach programs, and support groups; others have taken a more national perspective. Brazil's National AIDS Program—one of the world's leading HIV prevention and control programs—serves as a great example of a successful partnership between a religious institution (the Roman Catholic Church) and a governmental institution to address the epidemic. Two recent studies of this partnership noted that its most positive aspects centered around treatment and care for people living with the disease, whereas prevention has been the point of most tension, due to conflicting views between the two institutions regarding some prevention strategies.[20] At times, sustaining the partnership has required compromise between the Catholic Church's position on reproductive and sexual practices, including contraception and homosexuality and the government's interest in promoting prevention strategies such as condom use and addressing the needs of heterosexuals and homosexuals alike. The partnership succeeds despite these tensions because the institutions involved maintain a focus on their shared values and the political structures provide incentives for them to work together.[21] The Church has been similarly active in responding to the epidemic in Papua New Guinea, where it invoked a living theology of HIV/AIDS, recognizing HIV/AIDS as an illness in the "body of Christ" and thereby reconstituting individuals through the liturgical practices of baptism and Eucharist and through the theological virtues of faith, hope, and love.[22] Elsewhere, however, conservative forces have prevailed, hampering the response of religious institutions to the epidemic. In South Africa, one of the countries hit hardest by HIV, both secular and religious leaders agree that although faith-based organizations do attempt to address stigma, they also contribute to HIV/AIDS discrimination by continuing to associate the disease with sin and conflating issues of morality and sexuality.[23]

The Role of Religion in the Lives of People Living with HIV/AIDS

In the early years of the epidemic, with no effective treatment, vaccines, or a cure, an AIDS diagnosis was a death sentence. The repercussions of the diagnosis were complicated by the link to homosexuality. For many diagnosed in that period, their diagnosis forced the first open conversation that they had with their parents about their homosexuality. Individuals from more conservative religious traditions sometimes found themselves shunned by family and ejected from their religious homes just as they were dealing with the physical and emotional fallout of HIV/AIDS. The isolation, as Dr. Jesse Peel, a psychiatrist also living with AIDS, remembers, compounded the difficulties of dealing with the disease:

Many people who were diagnosed with AIDS were rejected by their churches, resulting in personal anguish and increased stigma and discrimination against them in their own families and communities. Others left the church fearing the consequences of the revelation of their sexual orientation or HIV status. This became a particular challenge as people began to face grave illness and end of life issues often without the support of family or faith institutions. . . . Most of these young men were raised in fundamentalist churches and as you start to deal with end of life you have got to deal with spiritual issues, the relationship a person has with God. These fellows needed a pastor more than they needed a psychiatrist. (Personal interview, June 18, 2009)

What was notable to many who worked in AIDS organizations at the time was that so many people living with AIDS clung to their religious beliefs. As one former volunteer, a deacon in the Presbyterian Church, said, "The church left them, but they never left the church" (Nancy Paris, personal interview, June 18, 2009).

Religion and spirituality are a central guiding force for many people, and an HIV/AIDS diagnosis doesn't change that fact.[24] A number of studies show a significant increase in religiousness or spirituality after an HIV diagnosis, reflected in an increased use of spiritual complementary therapies,[25] reports of increased feelings of religion or spirituality (despite feelings of alienation that led at least some participants to change places of worship),[26] and reports of feelings that the illness had strengthened participants' faith[27] or brought them closer to God.[28] Overall, these studies show that among people living with HIV/AIDS, self-reported religiousness or spirituality increased after diagnosis for a large proportion of participants.

As in the general population, levels of spirituality or religiosity are not uniform among people with HIV, and neither are increases in these factors. Two of the most consistent findings are that women are more likely than men[29] and people of color more likely than whites[30] to report greater spirituality or religiosity and greater use of spiritual and religious coping after an HIV diagnosis. Residence in the American South has also been associated with higher levels of spirituality, and patients with high school or college degrees reported higher religiousness than those who did not graduate from high school.[31] Research on the use of religion as a complementary therapy shows similar patterns, with white participants less likely than black participants to name religion as a complementary therapy,[32] women more likely than men to use a spiritual care strategy, and nonwhite patients more likely than white patients.[33] People living with HIV also tend to fall into similar patterns in their use of religious and spiritual coping.[34] Tarakeshwar, Hansen, and colleagues found that greater reliance on spiritual coping was associated with being female, being an ethnic minority, having less education, earning lower income, and being heterosexual.[35]

Religion as a Determinant of Health among People Living with HIV/AIDS

Many people believe that religious and spiritual practices and beliefs improve health outcomes, and there is some evidence to support this belief, as reported in chapter 18. With regard to HIV and AIDS, however, the results regarding the association between spirituality or religion and health outcomes is mixed. Researchers have investigated the effects of spiritual or religious coping on a variety of health outcomes for people with HIV, including psychological health, physical health, and health-related quality of life.[36] In a comprehensive literature review, Mueller, Plevak, and Rummans found that most studies identified significant associations between spirituality or religiousness and improved health outcomes, including better coping skills, greater optimism, less depression and suicide ideation, and better health-related quality of life, even during terminal illness.[37] Researchers have identified significant positive associations between religiousness or spiritual coping and a variety of psychological outcomes among people living with HIV/AIDS, including active coping, social support,[38] psychological adaptation,[39] cognitive and psychosocial functioning,[40] optimism and self-esteem.[41] Researchers have also found significant positive associations between spirituality and religiousness, spiritual or religious coping, and overall quality of life among people with HIV.[42]

Religion and spirituality have also been associated with HIV survival and disease progression. Ironson and colleagues found that long-term survivors scored significantly higher than an HIV-positive control group on measures of religiousness and religious behavior.[43] Ironson, Stuetzle, and Fletcher found that increased spirituality was significantly related to disease progression; compared with patients whose spirituality decreased after receiving an HIV diagnosis, people with an increase in spirituality had significantly less loss of T-cells and less increase in viral load over the four years of the study.[44]

Researchers have proposed several mechanisms to explain how spirituality and religion can relate to better health outcomes, including relaxation of the sympathetic and parasympathetic nervous systems through prayer and meditation, social support from fellow congregants, and increased adherence to medical regimens and healthy lifestyles. Researchers have also investigated possible mediators of the effect of religious activity on psychological outcomes, including coping style (active versus avoidant coping) and social support.[45] Some studies have found that religious involvement was directly related to higher levels of active coping and lower levels of avoidant coping, with active coping negatively and avoidant coping positively related to psychological distress.[46] In this way, active and avoidant coping and social support mediated the relationship between religious involvement and psychological distress. However, other findings suggest that social support is less of a mediator of the relationship between spirituality and health and mental health outcomes.[47]

Taken together, these studies demonstrate the current status of our understanding of religion's role in the clinical course of HIV and in psychological, physiological, and quality of life outcomes among people living with the disease.

Religion as a Social Determinant of Health in HIV/AIDS

While religious behavior and religious participation may provide some benefit to people living with HIV/AIDS, religion also has a role to play—both positive and negative—in preventing the spread of the disease. Most religious institutions teach or prescribe some version of safe sex (generally abstinence and monogamy), which may reduce some members' engagement in sexual risk behaviors. Galvan and colleagues found that religiosity was associated with fewer sexual partners and a lower likelihood of high-risk sex, after controlling for religious denomination.[48] However, "abstinence only" messages, although somewhat beneficial, limit the scope of HIV prevention education.[49] Insufficient or incomplete education—especially a lack of information about correct condom use and incomplete details about HIV transmission modes and risks—may increase HIV risk.

Religion may also serve as a barrier to risk reduction in other ways. For instance, in religions where women are seen as subordinate to men, where polygamy is accepted, or where women's reproductive rights are limited, women may lack agency in sexual behavior, limiting their ability to control their exposure to HIV risk. Furthermore, some religious beliefs may prevent those with HIV/AIDS from seeking medical care or encourage a reliance on religious therapies to the exclusion of medical treatments.

Religion and religious institutions may work indirectly to reduce risk via many of the same mechanisms by which religion produces better general health outcomes. The morals and values taught by religion may translate into better decision-making, many religions encourage or require members to make lifestyle choices and engage in behaviors that coincidentally affect HIV susceptibility, and those who are more religious are more likely to engage in healthcare behaviors that affect disease detection, health maintenance, and treatment compliance.[50] Involvement in a religious community also expands a person's social network, with all the health benefits social support brings.

Conclusion

Randy Shilts eloquently ticks off the reasons institutions in the United States took so long to respond to the epidemic:

> AIDS did not just happen to America—it was allowed to happen by an array of institutions, all of which failed to perform their appropriate tasks to safeguard the public's health. . . . People died while Reagan administration officials ignored pleas from government scientists and did not allocate adequate funds for AIDS research. . . . People died while scientists did not at first devote appropriate attention to the epidemic because they perceived little prestige to be gained in studying a homosexual affliction. . . . People died while public health authorities and the political leaders who guided them refused to take the tough measures necessary to curb the epidemic's spread, opting for political expediency over the public health. And people died while gay community leaders played politics with the disease, putting political dogma ahead of the preservation of human life.[51]

While America's governmental, scientific, and religious institutions engaged in systemic denial in the face of HIV/AIDS, however, community leaders organized effective, sustained community responses; their efforts laid the groundwork for networks that continue to offer treatment, prevention, and support services to this day. Some of those leaders were motivated by religious belief and supported by religious institutions that shape both societal responses to and individual experiences of HIV/AIDS—in some cases, the same religious institutions whose stances on homosexuality and other issues led congregants to ostracize members who contracted the disease. In short, the social narrative of religion's effect on HIV/AIDS is complex and contradictory, and it continues to be so.

Notes

1. World Health Organization, "Fact Sheet: HIV/AIDS," Fact Sheet no. 360, October 2013, http://www.who.int/mediacentre/factsheets/fs360/en/.
2. World Health Organization, UNAIDS, and UNICEF, *Progress Report 2011: Global HIV/AIDS Response—Epidemic Update and Health Sector Progress Towards Universal Access* (Geneva: World Health Organization, 2011), http://www.who.int/hiv/pub/progress_report2011/en/.
3. World Health Organization, "Fact Sheet."
4. World Health Organization, UNAIDS, and UNICEF, *Progress Report 2011*.
5. Randy Shilts, *And the Band Played On: People, Politics, and the AIDS Epidemic* (New York: St. Martins, 1987).
6. Shilts, *And the Band Played On.*
7. David France, "The Shrine of St. Vincent's," *New York Magazine*, April 19, 2010, http://nymag.com/news/intelligencer/65370/.
8. Sharon Sheridan, "Episcopal AIDS Ministries Evolve Along with the Epidemic," May 9, 2011, http://library.episcopalchurch.org/article/episcopal-aids-ministries-evolve-along-epidemic.
9. Sheridan, "Episcopal AIDS Ministries Evolve."
10. Amy Nunn, Alexandra Cornwall, Nora Chute, Julia Sanders, Gladys Thomas, George James, Michelle Lally, Stacey Trooskin, and Timothy Flanigan, "Keeping the Faith: African American Faith Leaders' Perspectives and Recommendations for Reducing Racial Disparities in HIV/AIDS Infection," *PloS one* 7, no. 5 (2012): e36172.
11. Shelley A. Francis and Joan Liverpool, "A Review of Faith-Based HIV Prevention Programs," *Journal of Religion and Health* 48, no. 1 (2009): 6–15.
12. Francis and Liverpool, "A Review of Faith-Based HIV Prevention Programs."
13. Latrice C. Pichon, Derek M. Griffith, Bettina Campbell, Julie Ober Allen, Terrinieka T. Williams, and Angela Y. Addo, "Faith Leaders' Comfort Implementing an HIV Prevention Curriculum in a Faith Setting," *Journal of Health Care for the Poor and Underserved* 23, no. 3 (2012): 1253–1265; Derek M. Griffith, Latrice C. Pichon, Bettina Campbell, and Julie Ober Allen, "Your Blessed Health: A Faith-Based CBPR Approach to Addressing HIV/AIDS among African Americans," *AIDS Education and Prevention* 22, no. 3 (2010): 203–217; Derek M. Griffith, Bettina Campbell, Julie Ober Allen, Kevin J. Robinson, and Sarah Kretman Stewart, "Your Blessed Health: An HIV-Prevention Program Bridging Faith and Public Health Communities," *Public Health Reports* 125, Suppl 1 (2010): 4–11.
14. Nunn et al., "Keeping the Faith."
15. Tyrell, Carol O., Susan J. Klein, Susan M. Gieryic, Barbara S. Devore, Jay G. Cooper, and James M. Tesoriero. "Early results of a statewide initiative to involve faith communities in HIV prevention." *Journal of Public Health Management and Practice* 14, no. 5 (2008): 429–436.
16. Coleman, Jason D., Lisa L. Lindley, Lucy Annang, Ruth P. Saunders, and Bambi Gaddist. "Development of a framework for HIV/AIDS prevention programs in African American churches." *AIDS patient care and STDs* 26, no. 2 (2012): 116–124.
17. Lindley, Lisa L., Jason D. Coleman, Bambi W. Gaddist, Jacob White. "Informing faith-based HIV/AIDS interventions: HIV-related knowledge and stigmatizing atti-

tudes at Project FAITH churches in South Carolina." *Public Health Reports* 125, no. Suppl 1 (2010): 12.

18. Kathryn Pitkin Derose, Peter J. Mendel, Kartika Palar, David E. Kanouse, Ricky N. Bluthenthal, Laura Werber Castaneda, Dennis E. Corbin et al. "Religious Congregations' Involvement in HIV: A Case Study Approach," *AIDS and Behavior* 15, no. 6 (2011): 1220–1232.

19. Derose et al., " Religious Congreations' Involvement in HIV."

20. Laura R. Murray, Jonathan Garcia, Miguel Muñoz-Laboy, and Richard G. Parker, "Strange Bedfellows: The Catholic Church and Brazilian National AIDS Program in the Response to HIV/AIDS in Brazil," *Social Science & Medicine* 72, no. 6 (2011): 945–952.

21. Francis and Liverpool, "A Review of Faith-Based HIV Prevention Programs."

22. Angela Kelly, "The Body of Christ Has AIDS: The Catholic Church Responding Faithfully to HIV and AIDS in Papua New Guinea," *Journal of Religion and Health* 48, no. 1 (2009): 16–28.

23. Marisa Casale, Stephanie Nixon, Sarah Flicker, Clara Rubincam, and Angelique Jenney, "Dilemmas and Tensions Facing a Faith-Based Organisation Promoting HIV Prevention Among Young People in South Africa," *African Journal of AIDS Research* 9, no. 2 (2010): 135–145; Erasmus Otolok-Tanga, Lynn Atuyambe, C. K. Murphey, Karin E. Ringheim, and Sara Woldehanna, "Examining the Actions of Faith-Based Organizations and Their Influence on HIV/AIDS-Related Stigma: A Case Study of Uganda," *African Health Sciences* 7, no. 1 (2007): 55–60.

24. Paul S. Mueller, David J. Plevak, and Teresa A. Rummans, "Religious Involvement, Spirituality, and Medicine: Implications for Spiritual Practice," *Mayo Clinic Proceedings* 76, no. 12 (2001): 1225–1235; W. R. Miller and C. E. Thoresen, "Spirituality, Religion, and Health: An Emerging Research Field," *American Psychology* 58, no. 1 (2003): 24–35; Karl A. Lorenz, Ron D. Hays, Martin F. Shapiro, Paul D. Cleary, Steven M. Asch, and Neil S. Wenger, "Religiousness and Spirituality among HIV-Infected Americans," *Journal of Palliative Medicine* (2005): 774–781; Safiya George Dalmida, Marcia McDonnell Holstad, Colleen DiIorio, and Gary Laderman, "Spiritual Well-Being, Depressive Symptoms, and Immune Status among Women Living with HIV/AIDS," *Women & Health* 49, no. 2–3 (2009): 119–143; Safiya George Dalmida, Marcia McDonnell Holstad, Colleen DiIorio, and Gary Laderman, "Spiritual Well-Being and Health-Related Quality of Life among African American Women with HIV/AIDS," *Applied Research in Quality of Life* 6, no. 2 (2011): 139–157.

25. Andrew Sparber, Jacqueline C. Wootton, Larry Bauer, Gregory Curt, David Eisenberg, Tina Levin, and Seth M. Steinberg, "Use of Complementary Medicine by Adult Patients Participating in HIV/AIDS Clinical Trials," *Journal of Alternative and Complementary Medicine* 6, no. 5 (2000): 415–422.

26. Sian Cotton, Joel Tsevat, Magdalena Szaflarski, Ian Kudel, Susan N. Sherman, Judith Feinberg, Anthony C. Leonard, and William C. Holmes, "Changes in Religiousness and Spirituality Attributed to HIV/AIDS," *Journal of General Internal Medicine* 21, no. S5 (2006): S14–S20; Gail Ironson, Rick Stuetzle, and Mary Ann Fletcher, "An Increase in Religiousness/Spirituality Occurs after HIV Diagnosis and Predicts Slower Disease Progression over 4 Years in People with HIV," *Journal of General Internal Medicine* (2006): S62–S68.

27. Sian Cotton, Christina M. Puchalski, Susan N. Sherman, Joseph M. Mrus, Amy H. Peterman, Judith Feinberg, Kenneth I. Pargament, Amy C. Justice, Anthony C. Leonard, and Joel Tsevat, "Spirituality and Religion in Patients with HIV/AIDS," *Journal of General Internal Medicine* 21 (2006): S5–S13.

28. I. E. Plattner and N. Meiring, "Living with HIV: The Psychological Relevance of Meaning Making," *AIDS Care* 18, no. 3 (2006): 241–245.

29. Nalini Tarakeshwar, Nathan Hansen, Arlene Kochman, and Kathleen J. Sikkema, "Gender, Ethnicity and Spiritual Coping among Bereaved HIV-Positive Individuals," *Mental Health, Religion & Culture* 8, no. 2 (2005): 109–125; Fang-Yu Chou, "Testing a Predictive Model of the Use of HIV/AIDS Symptom Self-Care Strategies," *AIDS Patient Care & STDs* 18, no. 2 (2004): 109–117; Armin Bader, Heidemarie Kremer, Isabella Erlich-Trungenberger, Roberto Rojas, Monika Lohmann, Olivia Deobald, Rainer Lochmann, Peter Altmeyer, and Norbert Brockmeyer, "An Adherence Typology: Coping, Quality of Life, and Physical Symptoms of People Living with HIV/AIDS and Their Adherence to Antiretroviral Treatment," *Medical Science Monitor* 12, no. 12 (2006): CR493–500.

30. Linda Pennington Grimsley, "Spirituality and Quality of Life in HIV-Positive Persons," *Journal of Cultural Diversity* 13, no. 2 (2006): 113–118.

31. Lorenz et al., "Religiousness and Spirituality Among HIV-Infected Americans."

32. Betty L. Chang, Gwen Van Servellen, and Emilia Lombardi, "Factors Associated with Complementary Therapy Use in People Living with HIV/AIDS Receiving Antiretroviral Therapy," *Journal of Alternative & Complementary Medicine* 9, no. 5 (2003): 695–710.

33. Chou, "Testing a Predictive Model."

34. Bader et al., "An Adherence Typology."

35. Tarakeshwar et al., "Gender, Ethnicity and Spiritual Coping."

36. Marsha Wiggins Frame, Constance R. Uphold, Constance L. Shehan, and Kimberly J. Reid, "Effects of Spirituality on Health-Related Quality of Life in Men with HIV/AIDS: Implications for Counseling," *Counseling and Values* 50, no. 1 (2005): 5–19; Jane M. Simoni, Maria G. Martone, and Joseph F. Kerwin, "Spirituality and Psychological Adaptation among Women with HIV/AIDS: Implications for Counseling," *Journal of Counseling Psychology* 49, no. 2 (2002): 139; Magdalena Szaflarski, P. Neal Ritchey, Anthony C. Leonard, Joseph M. Mrus, Amy H. Peterman, Christopher G. Ellison, Michael E. McCullough, and Joel Tsevat, "Modeling the Effects of Spirituality/Religion on Patients' Perceptions of Living with HIV/AIDS," *Journal of General Internal Medicine* 21, Suppl. 5 (2006): S28–38; Dalmida et al., "Spiritual Well-Being and Health–Related Quality of Life"; Kathryn E. Weaver, Michael H. Antoni, Suzanne C. Lechner, Ron E. F. Durán, Frank Penedo, M. Isabel Fernandez, Gail Ironson, and Neil Schneiderman, "Perceived Stress Mediates the Effects of Coping on the Quality of Life of HIV-Positive Women on Highly Active Antiretroviral Therapy," *AIDS and Behavior* 8, no. 2 (2004): 175–183.

37. Mueller, Plevak, and Rummans, "Religious Involvement, Spirituality, and Medicine."

38. Guillermo Prado, Daniel J. Feaster, Seth J. Schwartz, Indira Abraham Pratt, and Lila Smith, "Religious Involvement, Coping, Social Support, and Psychological Distress in HIV-Seropositive African American Mothers," *AIDS and Behavior* 8, no. 3 (2004): 221–235; Tarakeshwar et al., "Gender, Ethnicity and Spiritual Coping."

39. Simone, Martone, and Kerwin, "Spirituality and Psychological Adaptation."
40. C. L. Coleman, "Spirituality and Sexual Orientation: Relationship to Mental Well-Being and Functional Health Status," *Journal of Advanced Nursing* 43, no. 5 (2003): 457–464.
41. Cotton, Puchalski et al., "Spirituality and Religion in Patients with HIV/AIDS."
42. Jill E. Bormann, Allen L. Gifford, Martha Shively, Tom L. Smith, Laura Redwine, Ann Kelly, Sheryl Becker, Madeline Gershwin, Patricia Bone, and Wendy Belding, "Effects of Spiritual Mantra Repetition on HIV Outcomes: A Randomized Controlled Trial," *Journal of Behavioral Medicine* 29, no. 5 (2006): 359–376; Frame et al., "Effects of Spirituality on Health-Related Quality of Life"; Grimsley, "Spirituality and Quality of Life in HIV-Positive Persons"; Joseph M. Mrus, Anthony C. Leonard, Michael S. Yi, Susan N. Sherman, Shawn L. Fultz, Amy C. Justice, and Joel Tsevat, "Health-Related Quality of Life in Veterans and Nonveterans with HIV/AIDS," *Journal of General Internal Medicine* (2006): S39; Inez Tuck, Nancy L. McCain, and Ronald K. Elswick Jr., "Spirituality and Psychosocial Factors in Persons Living with HIV," *Journal of Advanced Nursing* 33, no. 6 (2001): 776–783; Coleman, "Spirituality and Sexual Orientation"; Dalmida et al., "Spiritual Well-Being and Health-Related Quality of Life"; Weaver et al., "Perceived Stress Mediates the Effects of Coping."
43. Gail Ironson, George E. Solomon, Elizabeth G. Balbin, Conall O'Cleirigh, Annie George, Mahendra Kumar, David Larson, and Teresa E. Woods, "The Ironson-Woods Spirituality/Religiousness Index Is Associated with Long Survival, Health Behaviors, Less Distress, and Low Cortisol in People with HIV/AIDS," *Annals of Behavioral Medicine* 24, no. 1 (2002): 34–48.
44. Ironson, Stuetzle, and Fletcher, "An Increase in Religiousness/Spirituality."
45. L. Moneyham, C. Murdaugh, K. Phillips, K. Jackson, A. Tavakoli, M. Boyd, N. Jackson, and M. Vyavaharkar, "Patterns of Risk of Depressive Symptoms among HIV-Positive Women in the Southeastern United States," *Journal of the Association of Nurses in AIDS Care* 16, no. 4 (2005): 25–38; Prado et al., "Religious Involvement, Coping, Social Support, and Psychological Distress."
46. Prado et al., "Religious Involvement, Coping, Social Support, and Psychological Distress."
47. Tarakeshwar et al., "Gender, Ethnicity and Spiritual Coping"; Safiya George Dalmida, H. G. Koenig, M. M. Holstad, and M. M. Wirani, "The Psychological Well-Being of People Living with HIV/AIDS and the Role of Religious Coping and Social Support" *International Journal of Psychiatry in Medicine* 46, no. 1 (2013): 57–83.
48. Frank H. Galvan, Rebecca L. Collins, David E. Kanouse, Philip Pantoja, and Daniela Golinelli, "Religiosity, Denominational Affiliation, and Sexual Behaviors among People with HIV in the United States," *Journal of Sex Research* 44, no. 1 (2007): 49–58.
49. Francis and Liverpool, "A Review of Faith-Based HIV Prevention Programs."
50. Harold G. Koenig, Michael E. McCullough, and David B. Larson, *Handbook of Religion and Health* (Oxford: Oxford University Press, 2001).
51. Shilts, *And the Band Played On*, xxii.

25 | Influenza Pandemic

MIMI KISER AND SCOTT SANTIBAÑEZ

THE CHAPEL AT SECOND EBENEZER Baptist Church is packed full. Every seat is taken and people are standing against the wall and all around the edges of the large room. There is a local TV station film crew in the back corner with a camera mounted on a tripod. It is National Influenza Vaccination Week, January 2010. The new Surgeon General, Dr. Regina Benjamin, has just finished speaking about the 2009 H1N1 pandemic as part of a large public campaign to encourage everyone to get vaccinated. She has only been in office a few months, and Detroit is one of her first public site visits. At least one local pastor has gotten a flu shot during this event in a room set up adjacent to and visible from the chapel, to set an example for others. The event has been organized by United Health Organization, a local religious organization well-known in Detroit for conducting prevention education and health screenings in community settings for thousands of uninsured and underinsured persons each year. They have considerable experience bringing together clergy, community leaders and members, advocacy groups, health agency leaders, and the media. This evening is no exception. Ifetayo Johnson, the executive director of United Health Organization walks slowly through the room picking up index cards on which attendees have written questions for Dr. Benjamin.

This scenario occurred as part of Engaging Communities in Response to Pandemic Influenza, a project developed by Emory University's Interfaith Health Program and the US Department of Health and Human Services Center for Faith-Based and Neighborhood Partnerships. United

Health Organization was the lead partner at one of nine participating sites. The kinds of questions being asked at this event are noteworthy. Three months into an extensive national immunization campaign, public health leaders have expressed concerns that the vaccination rates in African American communities are low. The questions posed at this community event, attended largely by African Americans, provide some insights into community concerns. One question was about a rumor that people walk backwards after getting a flu shot. Another was about vaccine safety. If the vaccine was free and perhaps different in the city than the suburbs, attendees wanted to know, could it contain something harmful that could target their community? These myths stick in the minds of people who may mistrust government and science-based efforts to promote health. This scenario raises issues that are critical in pandemic response planning: what kinds of messages and prevention services best reach certain groups? Who is most effective in delivering them and through what kinds of networks?

Introduction

In stark contrast to mid-twentieth-century optimism that infectious diseases were or soon would be a problem of the past,[1] the 2009 H1N1 pandemic was yet another reminder that we must not become complacent about infectious diseases. Religion, likewise, has not gone away as some twentieth-century scholars predicted that it would.[2] Rather, it continues to play an important role in the lives of many people and communities. Academics have a growing appreciation that many people make sense of how sickness and death fit into the larger scheme of life through the lens of their religious beliefs. These beliefs also help people to understand which actions—such as caring for the needy—are moral and which—such as ignoring the needs of others—are immoral.

Astute public health leaders have recognized that religious organizations can play a key role in reaching the most vulnerable, addressing mistrust among minority communities, and increasing access to information and services. Since 1996, the American Public Health Association has had a Caucus on Public Health and the Faith Community devoted to fostering knowledge and practice of effective public health and faith community partnerships. Similarly, the White House Office of Faith-Based and Neighborhood Partnerships, instituted under the George W. Bush administration and continued under the Obama administration, works to assist states and local communities in engaging community-based organizations (CBOs) and faith-based organizations (FBOs) to address the most pressing health and social issues. The Centers for Disease Control and Prevention (CDC) has worked with the Emory Interfaith Health Program since 2001, training seventy-eight teams of community leaders, like Ms. Johnson, to collaborate with public health agencies to eliminate health disparities.

While the 2009 H1N1 pandemic was not as severe as some previous pandemics, such as the 1918 Spanish influenza, it is still estimated to have infected over sixty million people in the United States, leading to more than 270,000 hospitalizations and 12,000 deaths.[3] Equally important, it provided valuable knowledge about the present-day capacity of communities to respond to health emergencies and about communication approaches that do and don't work. The 2009 H1N1 pandemic and the role that FBOs can play in pandemic preparedness and response are best understood in the broader historical context of how religious organizations have viewed and influenced health over time. As this volume indicates, the health challenges in the late twentieth and early twenty-first centuries have already been considerable—from HIV/AIDS to diseases such as Alzheimer's to pandemic influenza. History shows that religious organizations have been both life-saving and sometimes barrier-producing. In this chapter we review:

- *The role of religion as a social determinant of public health in past epidemics.* When catastrophes occur, many people rely on religious narrative to make sense of what is happening.
- *The role of FBOs in the 2009 H1N1 pandemic.* To fully understand national interest in pandemic preparedness, one must first understand the context of the Hurricane Katrina response and national efforts to strengthen the capacity of public health systems to reach vulnerable persons with the aid of faith- and community-based networks.
- *Ways that religion, as a social determinant of health, can be applied to public health practice.* While religious organizations are increasingly included in planning for pandemics and natural disasters, there is often a limited understanding of the distinct contributions FBOs can make. FBOs provide community resilience, function as repositories of social capital, and have the capacity to reach out through trusted networks to deliver targeted messages to communities beyond the usual boundaries of public health.

Religion as a Social Determinant of Public Health in Past Epidemics

When catastrophe occurs, many people rely on religious narrative to make sense of what is life-threatening and seemingly uncontrollable. One context where this can be seen clearly is in apocalyptic ideology. Andrew Cunningham notes how predominantly Christian societies have for many centuries drawn connections between disease outbreaks and apocalyptic ideology. The 1490s, for example, were notable for the emergence of two pandemics in Europe: pox and typhus. Disease outbreaks appeared every few years, killing thousands of people. "All these epidemics and pandemics had significant economic—and sometimes political—effects, and these disruptions of society encouraged the view that people were living in the Last Days."[4] Many European Christians saw connections between religion and disease outbreaks. Obviously God sends disease, they reasoned, and obviously it must be as punishment for sin.

The church served as the center for seeking divine intervention against this divine punishment. Churches called for communal fasts, instituted prayer marathons, and carried relics in processions through the streets, often accompanied by lay or religious flagellants. They called for the expiation of sins and pleaded for mercy. Apocalyptic ideology continues in some forms in the present day. "Some of that apocalyptic hysteria still crops up when we are confronted by a new epidemic or pandemic whose pattern or origin we do not understand," notes Cunningham. "It was the case in 1918 with the Spanish flu, and again the case with AIDS at the end of the last century: scapegoats are sought among minorities in the population."[5]

Religion and religious institutions can also offer more tangible contributions to help deal with an epidemic; they may help care for the sick or work to control the spread of the disease.

Religion's Role in Caring for the Sick

As epidemics take hold in communities stressed by poverty and social inequities, religious institutions can play an important role in caring for the sick and potentially containing outbreaks. Barrett and Brown have examined historical public health events in the United States and other parts of the world, highlighting the many dimensions of vulnerability and how it is enhanced during epidemics.[6] Vulnerability is associated with stigma, marginalization, diminished access to social resources, and mistrust of government and health services. In times of pestilence and plagues, religious organizations can both mitigate and contribute to this vulnerability. When yellow fever swept through Memphis beginning in August 1878, a mass exodus occurred. By September, less than half the population remained in the city. As news of the epidemic spread north, it was primarily nuns and priests that traveled in the reverse direction to Memphis. The central base of their service when they arrived was St. Mary's Cathedral. Here, Reverend George Harris oversaw services for the care of sick persons as well as an orphanage that was home to hundreds of children whose parents died in the epidemic.

Decades after yellow fever devastated Memphis and other port towns, public health infrastructure was still nascent, particularly in the American South. Hence disease control interventions continued to take on innovative, community-based forms. Churches were often a part of that response. At the turn of the century in Atlanta, some of the nurses who visited tuberculosis patients in their homes were employed by churches and loaned to the Associated Charities.[7] Many of the "friendly visitors" who also went to the homes of those with TB were church-based outreach workers, and churchwomen were regularly called upon to collect and provide material resources needed by those coordinating and providing care. In 1910, churches began to hold "Tuberculosis Sundays," when ministers preached about prevention and treatment of TB.[8]

Religion's Role in Reducing the Spread of Disease

Religion plays a complex role in population-based health initiatives. In his recent work, *House on Fire: The Fight to Eradicate Smallpox*, William Foege writes that missionaries provided a critical function in efforts to eradicate smallpox in Nigeria.[9] Dr. Foege utilized missionaries' connectedness within communities and between villages to conduct disease surveillance and map smallpox outbreaks that guided successful containment vaccination strategies. However, when cases began mounting among members of the Faith Tabernacle Church in a particular area, Foege noted the potential role of the church in the outbreak:

> In late 1966, two very important things relating to smallpox happened during my time in eastern Nigeria. One was a mass vaccination program we did in a place called Abakaliki. We were very successful, getting about ninety-three percent of the population vaccinated. We were pleased by this kind of coverage, only to see an outbreak of smallpox a few weeks later in Abakaliki. We didn't think that this should have happened, because we be-

lieved in the idea of herd immunity. What was different about the outbreak was that it occurred in a religious group, Faith Tabernacle Church. All of the cases were in the Faith Tabernacle Church. The members of this church had refused vaccination. The source of the outbreak had probably come from another Faith Tabernacle member outside of Abakaliki. The point is that we found that no level of vaccination in a population was so high that you could exclude the possibility of smallpox.[10]

A well-known global health case in northern Nigeria reveals the complex and challenging role of religion in another infectious disease, polio. In a predominantly Muslim area of the country, a vaccine boycott fueled by political and religious motives and mistrust in government services has led to opposition to vaccination in a number of African countries.[11] In response to this situation, public health organizations have been working with Muslim clerics and traditional chiefs to create a polio vaccine campaign that is more acceptable to the local populations.

The Role of FBOs in the 2009 H1N1 Pandemic

The national interest in pandemic preparedness can only be fully understood in the context of the aftermath of the Hurricane Katrina response, which formed the backdrop for pandemic response planning. This included several years of developing, refining, and exercising response plans at international, federal, state, local, and community levels. Hurricane Katrina, which struck in August 2005, was the most destructive natural disaster in US history. It impacted nearly ninety-three thousand square miles across 138 parishes and counties. Approximately 80 percent of New Orleans was flooded. Levee failures occurred on the 17th Street Canal, the Industrial Canal, and the London Avenue Canal. Towns and cities up and down the Gulf Coast were destroyed or heavily damaged. An estimated 1,330 people died as a result of the storm.[12]

In the aftermath of the hurricane, federal officials sought to identify "lessons learned" that could inform public health preparedness measures such as for a severe influenza pandemic. Among the many outcomes of the Hurricane Katrina response was a renewed focus on reaching vulnerable populations during emergencies. As *The Federal Response to Hurricane Katrina* noted, religious organizations played a central role in meeting people's needs during the Hurricane Katrina response. However, the assessment recognized, "faith-based and non-governmental groups were not adequately integrated into the response effort. These groups often encountered difficulties coordinating their efforts with Federal, State and local governments, due to a failure to adequately address their role in the [National Response Plan]."[13] This awareness would shape government responses to the 2009 H1N1 pandemic.

The first cases of a new influenza virus, 2009 pandemic influenza A (H1N1), were reported in the United States in April 2009. By July 2009, the Advisory Committee on Immunization Practices recommended use of 2009 H1N1 vaccine (officially called the Influenza A [H1N1] 2009 monovalent vaccine) through a program that would ultimately prevent an estimated one million clinical cases, six thousand hospitalizations, and three hundred deaths.[14] Two examples of the renewed focus on reaching vulnerable persons with the aid of faith- and community-based networks shed light on the community resources that CBOs and FBOs are able to mobilize during emergencies and pandemics.

At-Risk Populations Project

The At-Risk Populations Project (ARPP) was developed by the CDC and the Association of State and Territorial Health Officials based on feedback from a series of public engagement meetings in 2008.[15] Consistent with *The Federal Response to Hurricane Katrina*, ARPP recognized that because CBOs and FBOs play a crucial role in ensuring the health of vulnerable populations, they should be integrated into preparedness planning and response and coordinated with federal, state, and local governments. One participant at an ARPP national stakeholder meeting in Washington, DC, noted, "It is as important for public health agencies to develop trust with CBOs and FBOs as with at-risk individuals, because those organizations are best equipped to engage those at risk. Such a process is time-consuming, so outreach and collaboration must begin well before a pandemic" (unpublished data, CDC). *A 10-Step Approach for Health Communications with Community and Faith-Based Organizations during Public Health Emergencies* was one product developed by ARPP to help state, territorial, tribal, and local public health officials to prepare for a pandemic or other public health emergency in cooperation with FBOs and CBOs.[16] This resource emphasized the importance of identifying, engaging, and collaborating with religious organizations that could reach vulnerable populations, incorporating them into an overarching public health strategy, respecting cultural beliefs and practices, working together to develop messages, and maintaining these relationships over time.

Engaging Communities in Response to Pandemic Influenza

Engaging Communities in Response to Pandemic Influenza was a project developed by the Interfaith Health Program at Emory University and the US Department of Health and Human Services Center for Faith-Based and Neighborhood Partnerships with technical assistance from the CDC. The initial purpose of this project was to reach vulnerable populations during the 2009 H1N1 influenza pandemic. Nine faith and public health coalition sites were selected from across the United States (Table 25.1). Selection was based on multisectoral collaborative relationships, links to trusted local networks, and capacity to reach vulnerable populations. Each of the nine sites received a start-up grant, initial training, technical assistance conference calls, and updated 2009 H1N1 information as it became available.

Over a four-month period, the participating sites engaged a total of 4,606 FBOs and CBOs, health institutions and agencies, and networks in on-the-ground outreach efforts. This made it possible to reach nearly 420,000 individuals with training, educational materials, H1N1 guides, and vaccine event and prevention information. A number of the sites were also part of events that administered over seventy-eight thousand 2009 H1N1 vaccines to minority groups and those challenged by language, those without insurance or a medical home, and those with structural challenges such as transportation.

The lead organization for each site was either an FBO or a health organization with a strong faith-based outreach program. All participants had a long history of institutional commitments to eliminate health disparities in their communities and had built significant relationships with others in

TABLE 25.1 Center for faith-based and neighborhood partnerships 2009 H1N1 sites

LOCATION	LEAD ORGANIZATION
Chicago, IL	Center for Faith and Community Health Transformation
Colorado Springs, CO	Penrose-St. Francis Mission Outreach
Detroit, MI	United Health Organization, Project Healthy Living
Los Angeles, CA	Buddhist Tzu Chi Medical Foundation
Lowell, MA	Lowell Community Health Center
Memphis, TN	Methodist LeBonheur Healthcare
Minnesota	Fairview Health Services
Schuylkill County, PA	Schuylkill County VISION
St. Louis, MO	Nurses for Newborns Foundation

their community who shared this kind of commitment. The interface of this capacity with public health was critical to assuring access to populations beyond the usual reach of the pandemic response. The success of the approach was evident in how quickly these networks were able to mobilize their own organizations and many others to provide 2009 H1N1 prevention services for vulnerable populations:

- Methodist LeBonheur Healthcare in Memphis, Tennessee, was able to reach twenty-five thousand people with prevention messages through four hundred churches in their Congregational Health Network located in areas with known health disparities.
- The Center for Faith and Community Health Transformation in Chicago distributed 2,450 flyers with tailored influenza prevention information and county health department clinic information to African American congregations in southwest Chicago.
- The Buddhist Tzu Chi Medical Foundation trained and placed large teams of volunteers at forty-six Los Angeles Public Health Department clinics that provided over seventy-two thousand H1N1 vaccinations. As trusted cultural brokers, they were instrumental in increasing participation of large numbers of Asians without insurance.
- Fairview Health System's Minnesota Immunization Network Initiative reached diverse religious and ethnic populations in the Twin Cities area. During forty-five events held at faith-based settings, they provided more than 4,500 seasonal and 2,000 H1N1 vaccinations during 2009–2010.

This initiative demonstrated the unique capacity of a community's infrastructure to assure reach to vulnerable populations, for sustainable seasonable influenza preparation as well as for pandemic preparedness and response.

Contributions of FBOs to Pandemic Response

Religious organizations are increasingly included in planning for community responses to pandemics and natural disasters but often with limited understanding of the distinct contributions these organizations can make. Religion as a social determinant of public health has unique assets that can be applied to public health practice, especially in two key areas: community resilience and social capital.

Community Resilience

Norris and colleagues define community resilience as "a process linking a set of adaptive capacities to a positive trajectory of functioning and adaptation after a disturbance."[17] This capacity to adapt in the face of external stressors by using networked resources is related to a community's ability to work together to solve problems, make decisions, and take collective action. These "adaptive capacities" are both a core dimension of community resilience and a distinctive characteristic of FBOs. Hurricane Katrina revealed substantial vulnerability in areas with inadequate social resources and infrastructure. In this setting, FBOs were adaptive, agile, and responsive immediately after the storm in ways that government entities were not. For example, the North American Mission Board of the Southern Baptist Convention and other FBOs provided food and shelter to many evacuees and helped them find temporary and permanent housing after Hurricane Katrina.[18] Their efforts to aid Hurricane Katrina victims and evacuees continued throughout the fall of 2005 and beyond.

FBOs were able to work around cumbersome institutional infrastructures, meet needs, and find creative ways to get things done despite many obstacles. Moreover, this adaptability was not limited to the Hurricane Katrina response. FBOs often provide creative, local need-driven services. Many are able to deploy volunteers quickly and engage networks of other organizations with similar commitments and agility. They are a critical component of the social infrastructure.

In our opening story, Ms. Johnson and United Health Organization brought together community groups and health agencies in Detroit on very short notice to communicate vital health information. Their example exemplifies untapped community resilience. Similar stories could be seen around the United States during the 2009 H1N1 response. The Buddhist Tzu Chi Medical Foundation set up large vaccination clinics where needed—in close proximity to migrant farmworker work sites and late at night at homeless shelters. In Minnesota, Fairview Health Services coordinated health professionals who volunteered at flu vaccination clinics held at temples and churches on the weekends. Agility and commitment go hand in hand to form a vital social infrastructure that can contribute to the goal of public health in communities.

Social Capital

Robert Putnam defines social capital as "features of social organization such as networks, norms and trust, that facilitate coordination and cooperation for mutual benefit."[19] While the concept of social capital is contested in some health science literature, Koh and Cadigan find the concept offers "a rich public health lens for analysis," particularly in the context of pandemic planning.[20] Increasing attention is being paid to the importance of trust in risk communication and population-level health interventions, as noted, for example, in the At-Risk Populations Project. Trust is also a central component of social capital.

> Lack of trust can cause health programs to fail with harmful consequences. Measles outbreaks in the United Kingdom and the United States and the spread of polio across Africa from Northern Nigeria underscore the importance of building—and maintaining—public trust in health interventions and in the authorities who provide them. Trust relationships must be built over time so that they become the social framework in which health interventions—and positive health outcomes—can thrive.[21]

The Engaging Communities in Response to Pandemic Influenza project developed by the Emory University Interfaith Health Program mobilized networks of faith-based and community networks alongside public health agencies and healthcare providers. As part of this project, the Nurses for Newborns Foundation, an FBO in St. Louis, conducted outreach and healthcare support to vulnerable and high-risk young mothers—a priority group for the 2009 H1N1 vaccine. Nurses for Newborns organized a network of volunteers to assemble "flu kits" with information for young mothers attending a Healthy Start program for their children. The group also provided free van transportation to a nearby federally qualified health center to receive the influenza vaccines. The Nurses for Newborns Foundation created "connections between local communities and official agencies and building trust between local residents and authorities."[22]

Similarly, United Health Organization in Detroit demonstrated how critical this kind of connecting was to assure that accurate and life-saving information crossed institutional barriers of mistrust. In each of the nine Engaging Communities participating sites, the lead organizations reached out through trusted connections to deliver targeted, relevant messages and link those who had limited access to public health systems with social and health resources. These connections across individuals and community networks that have different values and identities are, in Putnam's terms, "bridging social capital."

Implications: What Is Important for the Future

The 2009 H1N1 pandemic served as yet another reminder that we should not become complacent about infectious diseases. As we have seen, religion also continues to play an important role in many people's lives. Many people rely on religious narrative to make sense of sickness and death in the midst of catastrophe. Religious institutions also provide a venue for caring for the needy. In communities stressed by poverty and social inequities, religious resources can play an important role in containing epidemics. Unfortunately, religion can also sometimes be an impediment to reducing the spread of disease. The gaps identified in the Hurricane Katrina response highlighted the vast resources that FBOs are able to mobilize during emergencies, serving as a catalyst for pandemic preparedness and shaping the 2009 H1N1 response.

A better understanding of religion as a social determinant of public health can contribute to improved public health practice. Public health planners can build on existing community resilience, social capital, and FBOs' adaptability, flexibility, and trusted networks. If these efforts are nurtured and sustained through ongoing seasonal influenza and preparedness activities, they can be a resource when needed. We have provided a few examples that demonstrate how public health and religious organizations are ready and willing to collaborate. Unfortunately, FBOs remain an underdeveloped and often hidden community resource. It is our hope that this brief examination will contribute to understanding and future proactive engagement of FBOs in pandemic planning and response.

Notes

1. A. L. Reingold, "Infectious Disease Epidemiology in the 21st Century: Will It Be Eradicated Or Will It Reemerge?," *Epidemiology Reviews* 22, no. 1 (2000): 57–63.
2. Charles T. Mathewes, "An Interview with Peter Berger," *Hedgehog Review*, June 28, 2007, http://www.iasc-culture.org/THR/archives/AfterSecularization/8.12PBerger. pdf.
3. S. S. Shrestha, D. L. Swerdlow, R. H. Borse, V. S. Prabhu, L. Finelli, C. Y. Atkins, K. Owusu-Edusei et al., "Estimating the Burden of 2009 Pandemic Influenza A (H1N1) in the United States (April 2009–April 2010)," *Clinical Infectious Diseases* 52, Suppl. 1 (2011): S75–S82.
4. Andrew Cunningham, "Epidemics, Pandemics, and the Doomsday Scenario," *Historically Speaking* 9, no. 7 (September/October 2008), 29–37, http://www.bu.edu/ historic/_hs_pdfs/religious_reponses_disease_sept_oct_09.pdf.
5. Cunningham, "Epidemics, Pandemics, and the Doomsday Scenario."

6. Ron Barrett and Peter J. Brown, "Stigma in the Time of Influenza: Social and Institutional Responses to Pandemic Emergencies," *Journal of Infectious Diseases* 197 (2008): S34–S37.

7. Margaret Ellen Kidd Parsons, *White Plague and Double-Barred Cross in Atlanta, 1895–1945* (Atlanta: Emory University, 1985).

8. Parsons, *White Plague and Double-Barred Cross.*

9. William Foege, *House on Fire: The Fight to Eradicate Smallpox* (Berkeley: University of California Press, 2011).

10. Victoria Harden, "Bill Foege Oral History," *Global Health Chronicles*, July 13, 2006, http://www.globalhealthchronicles.com/items/show/3516.

11. Ayodele Samuel Jegede, "What Led to the Nigerian Boycott of the Polio Vaccination Campaign?," *PLOS Medicine* 4, no. 3 (March 2007): 419–422.

12. The White House, "Chapter One: Katrina in Perspective," *The Federal Response to Hurricane Katrina: Lessons Learned*, February 2006, http://georgewbush-whitehouse.archives.gov/reports/katrina-lessons-learned/chapter1.html.

13. The White House, "Chapter Four: A Week of Crisis (August 29–September 5)," *The Federal Response to Hurricane Katrina*, http://georgewbush-whitehouse.archives.gov/reports/katrina-lessons-learned/chapter4.html.

14. R. H. Borse, S. S. Shrestha, A. E. Fiore, C. Y. Atkins, J. A. Singleton, C. Furlow et al., "Effects of Vaccine Program Against Pandemic Influenza A (H1N1), United States, 2009–2010," *Emerging Infectious Diseases* 19, no. 3 (March 2013), http://dx.doi.org/10.3201/eid1903.120394.

15. Project methods included a 2008–2009 literature review and meetings with academics, community organizations, and at-risk populations. For an in-depth description of project methods and recommendations, see www.astho.org.

16. S. Santibañez, A. LaFrance, A. DeBlois Buchanan, and C. Barnhill, "A 10-Step Approach for Health Communications with Community- and Faith-Based Organizations during Public Health Emergencies," in *Health Communication and Faith Communities*, ed. Ann Neville Miller and Donald L. Rubin (New York: Hampton Press, 2011), 29–45.

17. F. H. Norris, S. P. Stevens, B. Pfefferbaum, K. F. Wyche, and R. L. Pfefferbaum, "Community Resilience as a Metaphor, Theory, Set of Capacities, and Strategy for Disaster Readiness," *American Journal of Community Psychology* 41, nos. 1–2 (2008): 130. Other authors provide similar definitions. D. Paton, B. Parkas, M. Daly, and L. Smith, "Fighting the Flu: Developing Sustained Community Resilience and Preparedness," *Health Promotion Practice* 9, no. 4 suppl. (2008): 45S–53S, describe community resilience as a function of people's knowledge, resources, community relationships for providing social support and plans to adapt to the consequences of a pandemic (45S). Anita Chandra, Joie Acosta, Lisa S. Meredith, Katherine Sanches, Stefanie Stern, Lori Uscher-Pines, Malcolm Williams, and Douglas Yeung, *Understanding Community Resilience in the Context of National Health Security: A Literature Review* (Santa Monica, CA: RAND, 2010), http://www.rand.org/pubs/working_papers/WR737.html, define it as "social connectedness for resource exchange, cohesion, response and recovery" (3). Rachel Davis, Danice Cook, and Larry Cohen, "A Community Resilience Approach to Reducing Ethnic and Racial Health Disparities in Health," *American Journal of Public Health* 95, no. 12: 2168–

2173, have employed the concept of community resilience to focus action in "vulnerable environments" using twenty factors in four groups: built environment, social capital, services and institutions, and structural factors.

18. White House, "Chapter Four: A Week of Crisis (August 29–September 5)."
19. Robert Putnam, "Bowling Alone: America's Declining Social Capital," *Journal of Democracy* 6, no. 1 (1995): 66.
20. Howard K. Koh and Rebecca O. Cadigan, "Disaster Preparedness and Social Capital" in *Social Capital and Health*, ed. Ichiro Kawachi, S. V. Subramanian, and Daniel Kim (New York: Springer, 2010), 274.
21. H. J. Larson and D. L. Heymann, "Public Health Response to Influenza A (H1N1) as an Opportunity to Build Public Trust," *JAMA* 303, no. 3 (2010): 271–272.
22. Koh and Cadigan, "Disaster Preparedness and Social Capital," 274.

Disclaimer:
The findings and conclusions in this chapter are those of the authors and do not necessarily represent the official position of the Centers for Disease Control and Prevention (CDC).

Although the focus of this chapter is the role of communities in pandemic preparedness and response, we will not discuss medical or scientific aspects of influenza. Because information about influenza can change rapidly, we encourage interested readers to visit www.flu.gov and www.cdc.gov for the most up-to-date information.

26 | Alzheimer's Disease and Dementias

KENNETH HEPBURN AND THEODORE M. JOHNSON II

ALZHEIMER'S DISEASE AND OTHER DEMENTING conditions affect 5.2 million persons in the United States and 36 million world-wide.[1] The numbers will likely treble over the next forty years.[2] Alzheimer's, the most common type of dementia, is a disease insidious in onset and of long duration (eight to twelve years) that initially affects memory primarily in persons 65 years and older. Alzheimer's progressively erodes cognition and eventually eradicates a person's capacity for self-care and social functioning.[3]

Most with this illness live in community rather than institutional settings; most are sustained in community living through the care provided by family members. Currently in the United States more than fifteen million family members serve as caregivers for those with Alzheimer's, a role that exacts a substantial toll from those who assume it; caregivers typically suffer declines in physical and emotional well-being, experience compromised immune function, and become socially and economically stressed.[4]

Common speech—how family members and clinicians describe what they are seeing and experiencing—typically captures the progression of Alzheimer's as a gradual process of disappearance. Alzheimer's victims are said to fade away, described as no longer there or no longer the people whom they were. They are said to be lost, strangers in a strange, unfamiliar, unnavigable, and threatening universe. This metaphoric speech underscores the alteration in the fabric of things that the disease produces; it also expresses a fundamental discomfort family and friends experience in the presence of the person who is affected. These phrases of otherness and difference may be distancing and stigmatizing; they establish the possibility that the person no longer *is*—that he or she has become an other, a nonperson.

But even as Alzheimer's and related dementias progressively limit function and threaten sufferers' capacities to interact with family, friends, and the broader world, personhood remains. In that context, attention to the *person* is a central care proposition. Religion may enter into the care of persons with Alzheimer's in several ways. First, spiritual and religious history offers a possible pathway to addressing some of the person's emotional and behavioral needs. Second, religious institutions can and have begun to play a meaningful role in the community-based care of persons with dementing illnesses. Finally, the role of family caregiving can have religious or spiritual dimensions.

Personhood

A fundamental question in thinking about people with Alzheimer's is how to consider them as persons throughout the course of their illnesses, up to the point of death. This question shapes relationships with those with Alzheimer's as well as the care that they are given and the care choices made on their behalf. It is complicated by the toll that Alzheimer's and related dementing illnesses, which affect about one in eight older persons, take on the brain. These diseases produce clear and harmful progressive changes in the brain, far beyond that of normal aging. In Alzheimer's, for example, beta-amyloid and hyperphosporylated tau proteins accumulate in the brain in inappropriate amounts and patterns. These processes either mark the destruction of or directly cripple and eventually destroy neurons and neuronal connections and lead to loss of critical key functional areas (the hippocampus and amygdala, for instances).[5] Over time, the accumulation spreads, robbing function as it goes, until only instinctual reactions and autonomic functions remain.

The brain controls our ability to organize day-to-day phenomena into temporal, social, personal, and affective contexts and to respond to them in ways that are socially constructed and interpreted as "appropriate." Alzheimer's can be said to cause the eradication of connections: friendships evaporate, children are forgotten, long-standing relationships may remain locked in the structure of the brain, but they are irretrievable by the person. Some long-term memories of childhood and family may initially be preserved, and patterns of belief and practice set in infancy and adolescence may adhere. But eventually even the intensely close constellation of family begins to disintegrate, losing order, only vaguely recalled and felt only occasionally and fleetingly (but vividly) and with no apparent pattern.

Mastery of daily life deteriorates. The complex and subtle cognitive activities that allow persons to perform individualistically, effectively, and creatively in relationships, social interactions, work, and play yield to increasing amounts of error and randomness. Persons with Alzheimer's become unable to act meaningfully in the world. This loss of personal efficacy—and the confusion and frustration that accompany it—characterizes Alzheimer's, although it is much less widely appreciated than the loss of memory.

Although the disease renders individuals increasingly incapable of linking the parts of their personhood together or of enacting them in socially meaningful ways, the parts appear still to be present. Personal connections seem to persist at some fundamental level. Even those deep into the disease do, by report, retain a patchwork of linkages that eludes characterization—connections, memories, skills, capacities, and emotional ties to their pre-illness lives. They may still tell accurate stories from their youth. Some can complete complicated handwork or sing or play music, even when basic communication may be absent. Small cues can somehow trigger accurate recollections. Of particular note, there are clearly moments of authentic presence. Caregivers and others regularly report "contact" with those they care for, moments when they have felt powerful links with persons apparently deep into dementia, times when they and their persons are "as they once had been."

The assertion of sustained personhood provides a basis for a spiritual and religious response to Alzheimer's and to caregiving. The conversation about religion, religious institutions, and those with Alzheimer's can be framed in a way that at once affirms the continued presence of the person while also acknowledging that the person is increasingly less present. This is the aim of person-centered care.

Person-Centered Care

Those who care for a person with Alzheimer's understand that their basic task is to guide the person through each day with as little upset and as much pleasurable engagement as possible. Savvy caregivers appreciate that persons with Alzheimer's are increasingly unable to create and manage engagements for themselves. These caregivers accept that the rhythm, tone, and outcomes of events and encounters depend on how well they can understand and outmaneuver the effects of the disease on the person.

Evidence-based care of persons with Alzheimer's is predicated on personhood. Care strategies focus on tailoring care around an understanding of who the recipient of care is and assuming responsibility for connecting with him or her and connecting him or her to the flow of daily life. One strategy posits that all Alzheimer's behavior is a form of communication. In this paradigm, the burden of interpreting the message of a behavior falls on caregivers, who must take into account the person's history, current situation, and personality traits to devise approaches and responses designed to guide the person to calmer and more engaged behaviors.[6] Caregivers have to learn to read signs of confusion and discomfort and deploy strategies for moving the person into less stressful situations, promoting greater calm and comfort. These interpretive and responsive strategies must be based on the understanding that there is a disease interfering with the person's abilities. Models that link behavior to interactional and environmental antecedents recognize that stimuli must be controlled to promote the person's well-being.[7] Likewise, a model that identifies lowered stress thresholds as a potential source of behavioral upset recognizes that such thresholds are both individual and elastic, varying according to individual characteristics and retained—and sporadically deployed—capacities.[8]

Family members' experiences of connectedness with the person offer another set of person-centered caregiving strategies. When moments of intense emotional connection occur, spontaneously or as the result of caregiver facilitation, such moments typically appear pleasurable for the person with Alzheimer's, providing moments of peace and calm.[9] Thus, caregivers can use their knowledge of the person's history to support a positive emotional environment. Validation therapy emphasizes identifying and using recalled emotion to help the person maintain connectedness.[10] A question about a long-dead relative can be turned not into a confrontation ("Don't you remember? She died.") but into an opportunity to connect, through viewing photographs or reminiscences, with an authentic feeling that has been triggered about that relative.

The Role of Individual Religious History in Alzheimer's Care

An individual's history of spiritual or religious practice and involvement may offer a pathway to connect with the person and to provide emotional support. Engagement in familiar religious practices or rituals can contribute to a familiar daily structure and provide meaningful avenues for satisfying day-to-day involvement. Religious practices or objects may offer ways steer a person with Alzheimer's away from agitated or disturbing behaviors back to comfortable involvement with familiar, pleasurable activities, thus reestablishing calm and realigning the person to the familiar patterns of the day. To the extent that such activities resonate with the person, time spent listening to religious music, engaging in prayer or worship, or viewing worship services on TV or DVD might contribute to fulfilling days.

Participation in religious practices need not entail a communal setting and can be supported by family caregivers or by visiting faith community leaders or volunteers. All religious traditions incorporate individual religious practices into the expression of belief and membership. Such practices might be "overlearned behaviors" whose familiarity is comforting. The recitation of prayers or chants, the wearing of ritual clothing (shawls or yarmulkes), or the use of certain objects (prayer beads) might all be available to persons with Alzheimer's, even deep into the disease. Other kinds of practices, such as meditative walking (through a labyrinth or following the Stations of the Cross, for instance), may have a comforting and familiar effect. Remarkable stories abound of persons in late-stage Alzheimer's singing remembered hymns in perfect pitch and in apparent connectedness.

We assert that persons with Alzheimer's, at whatever stage of illness, retain the capacity for genuine religious or spiritual experience, although the nature of Alzheimer's makes it practically impossible to prove this claim. However, affirming the personhood of individuals with Alzheimer's affirms the possibility of their connectedness with something larger, including a larger spiritual realm. Building religious or spiritual events into the day and making objects of spiritual significance readily available at least offers ways for persons with Alzheimer's to gain access to a larger spiritual reality.

The Role of Religious Communities in Alzheimer's Care

Religious communities can play a significant role in the lives of individuals with Alzheimer's; arguably, they have an obligation to do so.[11] Care for the sick and respect for elders are basic religious tenets common to nearly all faith traditions. Religious institutions may both affirm the ongoing membership of a person with Alzheimer's and minister to that person and his or her family caregiver in any of several ways.

The presence in their congregations of persons with Alzheimer's provides religious institutions an opportunity to examine the meaning and basis of community membership. In most traditions, congregational membership begins with an acceptance of belief principles and is sustained by codes of moral behavior. Growth in the spiritual life involves a deepening of belief, commitment, and practice, all processes that, at least in part, rely on cognitive abilities and the capacity to act autonomously. How, then, do persons whose illness robs them of these capacities maintain membership in a religious congregation? More practically, how do they continue to take part in the life of that congregation? We believe that an individual's ongoing personhood and history of prior profession establishes full membership; however, it is incumbent on the congregation to provide ways for the person to continue to exercise that membership. As these persons become increasingly unable to enact intentional membership, the community can do so on behalf of those members through various forms of ministry.

Congregations need to identify or create ways that allow the person with Alzheimer's to experience a sense of membership in the religious community. These membership roles or activities must align with the person's retained capacities and need to be changed over time to accommodate the progression of the illness. Active and complex involvements, such as assisting in liturgy or greeting, will need to give way to less complicated activities, such as ushering, and eventually passive participation. An individually tailored sequence of participation maintains involvement; equally important, it keeps alive in the mind of the congregation the personhood and membership of those with Alzheimer's and may also help build support for programs for caregivers. However, in allowing for the participation of persons with Alzheimer's, congregations need to understand the full range of behaviors that might be expected in the course of illness and agree on their tolerance and plan for dealing with potentially disruptive behaviors, such as talking during periods when silence is expected, unexpected or liturgically inappropriate responses, wandering behavior, or incontinence. A charitable tolerance for these behaviors enables ongoing participation for those with Alzheimer's and their caregivers.

Because they can be part of the store of long-term memories that are more readily accessed by persons with Alzheimer's, even in its late stages, rituals are a particularly important part of religious participation for these persons. By intentionally acknowledging the ongoing membership of persons with Alzheimer's, congregations are challenged to find ways to make congregational rituals, such as ceremonies around Eid, Passover, or Christmas, available to them. In every instance, the congregation's expectations for the person's participation in ritual must be scaled to the person's capacities as the disease progresses. To use an example from Christian practice, a person in early Alzheimer's might take part in the Eucharistic service. As the disease progresses and going to the altar becomes difficult, confusing, and potentially disruptive, a minister might deliver communion to the person at his or her seat. Even later, when accepting communion is no longer a familiar gesture (and might be threatening), a minister might come to confer a blessing or a sign of recognition, belonging, and positive regard. This kind of scaling makes ritual available and reinforces for the community the inclusive and embracing meaning of membership.

Communities might also create congregational events specifically for persons with Alzheimer's. The Episcopal Church of the Holy Redeemer in Atlanta, for example, has established services and communal dinners for persons affected with mental disorders, including Alzheimer's. Volunteers from churches in the area help to prepare the dinners and, in so doing, bring back to their congregation an appreciation for the condition of persons with Alzheimer's and a greater understanding of the ways ministry can occur. At these events, too, the world of persons with mental disorders is the norm; those outside that norm—the volunteers preparing and serving the meals—must discover ways to be members of that congregation, offering a path to empathy and a broader appreciation of personhood.

Religious institutions can reach out to persons with Alzheimer's and their caregivers through other forms of ministry as well. Explicit recognition of the trying situation facing a family unit within the community is an important beginning, and many religious congregations have begun to provide education about the illness. Other institutions provide space for services to persons with Alzheimer's or to their caregivers that are provided by their own volunteers or by organizations from the outside. A church in Eagle River, Alaska, for example, provides room for Alzheimer's Resources of Alaska to offer the six-week Savvy Caregiver program to families in the area.[12]

Before religious leaders and congregations can offer relevant ministry, they must first identify when members and their caregivers are encountering difficulties associated with Alzheimer's. Recognition of Alzheimer's and a caregiving situation can then trigger focused responses from the community. The caregiver and the person can both benefit from counseling provided by a religious leader, which can have considerable value for a person (or dyad) with professed attachment to a religious tradition, providing a broader perspective than psychological or social worker counseling, addressing the spiritual and meaning-centered questions facing those involved in this illness. Counseling opportunities can include the person–caregiver dyad's initial adjustment to a diagnosis of dementia, end-of-life decision-making and the establishment of advanced directives, adjustments in the relationship as the disease progresses, execution of end-of-life choices, and formal discussions with the healthcare team. Counseling sessions may promote family communication and collaboration or help caregivers deal with a variety of issues—navigating changing responsibilities and affirming the dignity of the person with Alzheimer's while taking increasing control of day-to-day life, managing feelings of loss and guilt, or dealing with grief and the reestablishment of life when caregiving ends. These conversations have to do with ethical choices (and sometimes dilemmas—what if a spouse caregiver of a person with dementia finds meaning in another relationship?) and questions about the larger meaning of the situation.

Religious communities may also play more practical roles in supporting persons with Alzheimer's and their caregivers. Religious institutions have traditionally excelled at addressing human needs within and beyond their own communities. It is common in many congregations for members to bring meals throughout the week after a member family has a child; a more sustained practice of this sort can alleviate significant stress in an Alzheimer's household. Broader forms of support—transportation, home chores, in-home respite care—can be of great value. What is especially important in religious institutions providing such functional assistance is that the help comes from a trusted source.

Individually or banded together, religions have a greater and more intimate reach and greater capacity of talent and infrastructure than any governmental entity. If harnessed, this reach could provide enormous benefit to families struggling with Alzheimer's, at both a spiritual and a practical level. Beyond the engagement of persons with Alzheimer's in religious activities, volunteers from religious communities can provide practical and emotional support. Volunteers have been successfully trained to lead support groups—for caregivers and for those in the early stage of Alzheimer's who can participate at their own level—that offer the opportunity not only to share good and bad stories but also to share knowledge and skills for caregiving. Volunteers have also been trained to provide in-home respite care and to lead more complicated psychoeducational groups. Such programs could be extended and made more widely available. The parish nurse concept—sporadically in place—could also be extended, engaging these professionals in training and providing consultation to the cadres of volunteers engaged in Alzheimer's support in communities.[13]

Spiritual Dimensions of Caregiving

Family caregiving is a complex and sustained enterprise that almost always exacts a price.[14] Just as religious communities can find ways to minister to persons with Alzheimer's, they can find ways to minister to their caregivers. In some sense, ministry to one necessitates ministry to the other—the level of participation afforded to the person with Alzheimer's may determine the level of participation with which the caregiver can engage. In engaging in caregiver ministry, however, it is useful to understand that caregiving is heterogeneous and nuanced; caregivers act from a variety of possible motives, they encounter a variety of experiences, and they take on a variety of roles.

Ministry. Family caregiving can be construed as ministry: the person with Alzheimer's is multiply vulnerable; over time he or she becomes helpless and often shunned. These persons cannot speak their own needs, defend themselves, or even speak their own name. Caregivers provide care for whole persons, meet their needs, protect them from the hurts that others might do intentionally or unintentionally, assert their personhood, and guide them through the frightening universe.

Fidelity. The most common context of caregiving is that of constancy or fidelity: the added care and commitment that occurs as an integral part of an existing relationship. This is freely given and freely embraced caregiving. While it taxes the caregiver and entails as many challenges as any other form of caregiving, those who take on this role out of a sense of continued love appear to experience less distress than other caregivers.[15]

Instrumentality. For most, caregiving occurs along with other contexts and entails other consequences. Some cast it as obligation ("If not me, who?). At its best, this is a form of caritas, though it is often reluctantly or begrudgingly—and imperfectly—performed. We have, for example, seen persons long separated or divorced reunite so that the well person could care for the person with Alzheimer's; these are not happy arrangements, but they are caring ones. We have also seen children keep a parent at home in the community, not only out of a sense of obligation but also to preserve their inheritance. Such obligational caregiving can be kind and effective, but it can also be the source of sustained elder abuse.

Isolation. Alzheimer's family caregivers commonly speak of abandonment. Other family members deny the problem or seek to avoid becoming as involved as the primary caregiver. Friendship connections evaporate as the capacities of the person with Alzheimer's and the energies of the caregiver wane. Primary healthcare providers, seldom expert in dementing diseases and without clear remedies to offer, become therapeutic nihilists ("It's dementia; there's nothing we can do"). Community organizations—including religious organizations—have no well-charted place for persons with Alzheimer's and their caregivers.

Trials, gifts, and beyond. Religious or spiritual constructions may also come into play for caregivers. For some, life is a trial, and challenges are opportunities to demonstrate faith. Being asked to care for a person with Alzheimer's is a kind of gift, a sign of favor to be accepted and embraced as a sign of a deity's love and a chance to demonstrate the power of a life of faith. In some traditions, a notion of silent suffering is held out, particularly to women, as a model of behavior in the face of adversity; one's lot must be accepted, without complaint. For some, caregiving may be perceived as an opportunity to win a greater reward in the afterlife. For others, the burden of caregiving may precipitate a crisis in which the caregiver rejects either a deity or the broader transcendental possibilities offered by a particular faith tradition; alternatively, a more profound reaction of despair is possible.

These varieties of the caregiving experience offer, individually and in their permutations, avenues for ministry to caregivers. The caregiver can be viewed as one on a journey who needs sustenance and guidance. Only when religious institutions and faith communities recognize and embrace the profound challenges of Alzheimer's and the varieties of Alzheimer's caregiving will they be able to provide adequate and appropriate responses to them.

We are especially grateful to Grant Glowiak for his review of early drafts of the chapter and for his suggestions in the areas of liturgical participation by persons with dementia and ways of understanding spiritual dimensions of caregiving. Mr. Glowiak's perspective as a student preparing for the ministry and as a caregiver for his own father were invaluable contributions to the chapter.

Notes

1. Alzheimer's Association, *2013 Alzheimer's Disease Facts and Figures, Alzheimer's & Dementia* 3, no. 2 (2013), http://www.alz.org/downloads/facts_figures_2013.pdf.

2. L. E. Hebert, P. A. Scherr, J. L. Bienas, D. A. Bennett, and D. A. Evans, "Alzheimer Disease in the US Population: Prevalence Estimates Using the 2000 Census" *Archives of Neurology* 60(2003): 1119–1122.

3. G. M. McKhann, D. S. Knopman, H. Chertkow, B. T. Hyman, C. R. Jack Jr., C. H. Kawas, W. E. Klunk, et al., "The Diagnosis of Dementia due to Alzheimer's Disease: Recommendations from the National Institute on Aging-Alzheimer's Association Workgroups on Diagnostic Guidelines for Alzheimer's disease," *Alzheimer's & Dementia* 7, no. 3 (2011): 263–269.

4. M. Pinquart and S. Sorensen, "Correlates of Physical Health of Informal Caregivers: A Meta-Analysis, *Journals of Gerontology Series B: Psychological Sciences and Social Sciences* 62, no. 2 (2007): P126–137; R. Schulz and P. R. Sherwood, "Physical and Mental Health Effects of Family Caregiving, *American Journal of Nursing* 108, no. 9 Suppl (2008): 23–27.

5. C. R. Jack Jr., M. S. Albert, D. S. Knopman, G. M. McKhann, R. A. Sperling, M. C. Carrillo, B. Thies, and C. H. Phelps, "Introduction to the Recommendations from the National Institute on Aging-Alzheimer's Association Workgroups on Diagnostic Guidelines for Alzheimer's Disease," *Alzheimer's & Dementia* 7, no. 3 (2011): 257–262.

6. D. Algase, C. Beck, A. Kolanowski, A. Whal, S. Berent, K. Richards, and E. Beattie, "Need-Driven Dementia-Compromised Behavior: An Alternative View of Disruptive Behavior," *American Journal of Alzheimer's Disease & Other Dementias* 11, no. 6 (November 1996): 10–19.

7. L. Teri, L. E. Gibbons, S. M. McCurry, R. G. Logsdon, D. M. Buchner, W. E. Barlow, W. A. Kukull et al., "Exercise Plus Behavioral Management in Patients with Alzheimer Disease: A Randomized Controlled Trial," *JAMA* 290, no. 15 (2003): 2015–2022.

8. M. Smith, G. R. Hall, L. Gerdner, and K. C. Buckwalter, "Application of the Progressively Lowered Stress Threshold Model Across the Continuum of Care," *Nursing Clinics of North America* 41, no. 1 (2006): 57–81.

9. W. J. Puentes, "Using an Associational Trends Framework to Understand the Meaning of Obsessive Reminiscence," *Journal of Gerontological Nursing* 34, no. 7 (July 2008): 44–49.

10. M. Neil and P. Barton Wright, "Validation Therapy for Dementia," *Cochrane Database of Systematic Reviews* 3 (2003): CD001394.

11. H. Elliot, "Religion, Spirituality and Dementia: Pastoring to Sufferers of Alzheimer's Disease and Other Associated Forms of Dementia," *Disability and Rehabilitation* 19, no. 10 (1997): 435–441.

12. K. Hepburn, M. Lewis, J. Tornatore, C. W. Sherman, and K. L. Bremer, "The Savvy Caregiver Program: The Demonstrated Effectiveness of a Transportable Dementia Caregiver Psychoeducation Program," *Journal of Gerontological Nursing* 33, no. 3 (March 2007): 30–36.

13. R. Address, "Creating Sacred Scenarios: Opportunities for New Rituals and Sacred Aging," *Journal of Gerontological Social Work* 45, nos. 1–2 (2005): 223–232; D. Everett, "Forget Me Not: The Spiritual Care of People with Alzheimer's Disease," *Journal of Health Care Chaplaincy* 8, nos. 1–2 (1999): 77–88; S. F. Mooney, "A Ministry of Memory: Spiritual Care for the Older Adult with Dementia, *Care*

Management Journal 5, no. 3 (2004): 183–187; S. E. Wilks and M. E. Vonk, "Private Prayer among Alzheimer's Caregivers: Mediating Burden and Resiliency," *Journal of Gerontological Social Work* 50, nos. 3–4 (2008): 113–131.

14. R. Schulz and P. R. Sherwood, "Physical and Mental Health Effects of Family Caregiving," *American Journal of Nursing* 108, no. 9 Suppl (2008): 23–27, quiz 27.

15. M. L. Lewis, K. Hepburn, S. Narayan, and L. N. Kirk, "Relationship Matters in Dementia Caregiving," *American Journal of Alzheimers Disease and Other Dementias* 20, no. 6 (2005): 341–347.

Conclusion

RELIGION'S ROLE AS A SOCIAL DETERMINANT
OF TWENTY-FIRST-CENTURY HEALTH:
PERSPECTIVES FROM THE DISCIPLINES

PAUL ROOT WOLPE, WALTER BURNETT, AND ELLEN IDLER

An Ethics Perspective, *by Paul Root Wolpe*

Early in my career, a colleague and I got a small contract to survey the churches of economically depressed West Philadelphia to determine the role that they played in providing drug treatment, drug counseling, and other substance abuse services to the community. While I do not have access to the exact numbers anymore, I was surprised at the degree to which the religious institutions of the area provided counseling, hosted meetings, provided transportation to treatment centers, and served as a drug treatment, counseling, and social support system, much of it under the radar of the city's "formal" systems. The impact of that informal system on the lives of those in that community with substance abuse challenges was profound.

As this book makes plain, my findings are not unusual. Religion as a conceptual system, religious behavior translated as social action in the world, and religious institutions as social actors all help shape health behaviors and resources in many different ways and often with great influence. Faith communities can be primary initiators of health interventions and promotion, often reaching otherwise hard-to-reach corners of society and having both widespread exposure and unique resources in the communities they serve.[1]

In chapter 21 of this volume, Matthew Bersagel Braley outlines the history of the Christian Medical Commission's program, which shifted away from hospital-based care to a theologically based focus on primary care and influenced the World Health Organization (WHO) in ways that had a global impact. To take another, more localized example, the North Carolina Council of Churches—a statewide ecumenical organization representing eighteen denominations, 6,200 congregations, and 1.5 million individuals— has been engaged in a faith-based health initiative called Partners in Health and Wholeness, which encourages a variety of health behaviors and programs in its clergy and congregants and offers formal recognition of member churches for their health-related efforts.[2] Activities such as these cannot be reduced to "health behaviors." Seeing faith-based intervention as no different than interventions in the secular realm is mistaken, because the mission of Partners in Health and Wholeness, for example, is to "promote health as a practice of faith" in part through "illustrating the spiritual significance of leading healthy lifestyles."[3] Researchers must look closely at religious motivations and framings to fully understand outcomes.

Where does ethics enter this conversation? Considering religion as a social determinant of health raises both theoretical and methodological kinds of ethical questions. We might address the normative question of whether the exclusion of religion from the conceptualization and research focus of the social determinants of health is itself unethical. Or, we might ask more methodological questions about the ethical challenges of including religion as a variable or a focus in research on the social determinants of health. How should we define religion and operationalize definitions so that they are reflective of the lived reality of religion embodied in social institutions, expressed in practice, and shaped in beliefs? What do we include or exclude?

To determine whether there is an ethical mandate to include religion as a social determinant of health, we must first ask what the focus of public health is—how does it identify the subjects of its interest? According to the WHO, health systems include "all the activities whose primary purpose is to promote, restore, or maintain health."[4] Childress and colleagues suggest that "public health systems consist of all the people and actions, including laws, policies, practices, and activities, that have the primary purpose of protecting and improving the health of the public."[5] Such definitions locate the activities of many religious institutions squarely within the area of interest of the public health enterprise and equally recommend much religious activity as healthy behavior. Furthermore, as may seem obvious, "the goal in public health is to improve the health of *communities*."[6] Communities are often self-defined by their religious affiliations or have a religious affiliation as a central feature of community identification.

So, almost by definition, public health as an enterprise has an obligation to acknowledge, incorporate, and evaluate religious community health activity, and research on the social determinants of health must be equally obligated.

The exclusion of religious institutions seems therefore to violate the definitional assumptions of public health as an activity and of the social determinants of health as a research enterprise. If religious institutions, beliefs, and behaviors are themselves important loci of health activity, as the chapters in this book (and my survey of West Philadelphia) seem to make plain, then it is not only prudent and scientifically necessary to include religion in our understanding of determinants of health; the underlying moral justifications of the pursuit of public health itself make it an ethical mandate.

Public health as a social pursuit rests on largely moral claims. Public health shares with clinical medicine certain ethical assumptions—that health is a positive value, that people deserve to have access to means to improve their health, that health professionals have an obligation to promote and support good health behaviors, and so on. As research-driven enterprises, both medicine and public health have also assumed ethical stances on the mandate to perform good research, to be nondiscriminating (in the sense of exclusionary) in scope and application, and to avoid allowing bias to distort scientific theory or methodology.

Public health *ethics* is also a field of its own, with a literature that takes pains to distinguish it from its much larger sibling, medical ethics. Of course, public health practitioners have been confronting unique ethical questions since long before the pursuit was organized into a discipline. In late medieval Europe, the practice of isolating plague victims and incarcerating their contacts as a public health prevention measure—leading to the invention of "medical police" to enforce quarantine regulations and restrictions on movement—was met with strong opposition and debate.[7] While the debates are not new, the emergence of the field of public health ethics has helped define and focus the ethical principles that underlie the enterprise.

While much of public health ethics is concerned with the ethical challenges of designing and implementing public health interventions, the field has also grappled with defining the basic ethical principles upon which public health is based. Public health operates on moral assumptions of fairness, justice, equity, and alleviation of suffering. In their seminal work on public health ethics, Childress and colleagues assert that "public health activities have their grounding in general moral considerations, and . . . public health identifies one major broad benefit that societies and governments ought to pursue."[8] After enumerating many of the relevant general moral considerations, they conclude that a number of them, such as benefiting others, preventing and removing harm, and maximizing the balance of benefits over harms and other costs (ensuring utility), provide a prima facie justification for public health activity.

Such ethical justifications are necessary because the work of public health involves social manipulations to change health behaviors and outcomes and is, therefore, to greater or lesser degrees, an imposition on liberty. Public health interventions involve a kind of ethical calculus: weighing individual autonomy versus public good; balancing the severity of the harm, the likelihood of occurrence without intervention, and the effectiveness of the intervention; and determining the level of coerciveness of the intervention, from health education to behavioral incentives to mandatory actions or prohibitions. Such impositions on the public, even if putatively for their benefit, must be based upon and answerable to defensible ethical presumptions.

As a medical sociologist who labors largely in the world of bioethics, I find the ethical mandate to include so fundamental a part of social life in research on the social determinants of health theoretically and methodologically plain. The assertion is only the beginning of the work of public health ethics, only the foundation for the construction of the ethical underpinnings of research on the social determinants of health. Religious institutions can be instrumental there as well, standing as they do as both sources and arbiters of public moral conversation. Still, once established, the ethical mandate stands as a beacon and touchstone for the hard work of both public health research and public health planning and intervention.

A Health Policy Perspective, *by Walter Burnett*

When most people think of health policy, they assume that the decisions affecting health emanate from a legislative process at one level of government or another. The Affordable Care Act of 2010 serves as a typical example. Health policy decisions, however, also come from religious institutions. Consider the effort of the Patriarch of the Georgian Orthodox Church to address a decreasing birth rate that was contributing to the aging of the population of the former Soviet Republic; Patriarch Ilia II offered to become the godfather of all babies born into the church from families that already had two or more children. He began the mass baptisms in 2008, and by 2010 the nation's birth rate was 20 percent higher than it had been in 2005; many new parents said the Patriarch's offer was instrumental in their decision to have more children.[9]

The essence of religion is the age-old and ongoing quest for the meaning and purpose of life and the institutions in which that quest is centered. With these teleological and institutional orientations, both individuals and communities develop and institutionalize their values through public policy. Faith traditions and institutional religion often play a key role in both the formulation and implementation of policy. As religion becomes recognized as an increasingly important factor in public health[10] decision-making, communities[11] will tend to adopt policies that are more consistent with the values of their members. Our focus here is on what we might expect to see over the coming decade in the relationship between religion and public health from the perspective of health policy.

The observations presented here are predicated on the argument of the earlier chapters of this book: Religion is and should increasingly be taken into account as a social determinant of health. It is also predicated on the WHO definition of health: "Health is a state of complete physical, mental and social well-being and not merely the absence of disease or infirmity."[12] This idea of health can be conceptualized from two perspectives: a focus on the health of an individual or a focus on the health of a population. Here we are looking at the policy implications from the population-based perspective. The paradigm change is that religion is added to the social determinant themes. The following speculations relating to the policy-relevant intersection of religion and public health are based on the assumption that a significant number of people around the world will continue to be religious for the next decade, as measured by religious practice and a belief in God. While changes in institutional affiliation beyond the coming decade may shift, faith traditions may be expected to continue to be basic to health-related decision making. As public health and health services policy development increasingly takes into account religion and faith tradition as a social determinant, we can reasonably expect see three trends develop.

An increased awareness of religion's role in healthcare decision-making and in promoting healthy behaviors. As health literacy increases and health professionals continue to expand the involvement of individuals in shared decision-making, the value systems expressed in religious behavior and commitment will bring religion into the mainstream of thinking for the development and implementation of public health interventions. Religious institutions have developed health-related programs that focus on the shared interests of subsets of their members. These affinity groups are characteristic of both large and small churches, temples, and mosques, regardless of theological orientation, and they will continue to expand in several forms. Some will focus on health behaviors, such as weight control. Others will take the form of health advocacy groups, working for such health infrastructures as bike lanes, greenways, or women's health facilities. Still others may take the form of outreach groups, for instance, serving as clinic volunteers.

Facilitation of the search for common cause for health policy interventions. As the role of religion and faith-based decision-making is taken into account as a social determinant of health, the tensions that currently exist between many of the doctrines of institutional religious organizations and evidence-based and population-based public health organizations may become less problematic. The July 2013 comments of Pope Francis on the role of women in the church and acceptance of gay individuals as persons is an example of an attempt to find common cause that has the potential of moving forward public policy discussions dealing with health disparities. The Moral Monday protests in North Carolina beginning in the summer of 2013, organized by clergy along with other nonreligious groups to protest state cuts to the social safety net and the state legislature's failure to expand Medicaid under the Affordable Care Act, are another example of an attempt to find common cause and bring religious values into health policy decisions. A better understanding of the relationship between health determinants and public health interventions will facilitate the search for public policy common cause.

Much of the impetus to common cause will be driven by the search for interventions to reduce health disparities among population groups. There are several areas where the search for common cause may lead to constructive and agreed-upon interventions. Many of these interventions will be developed at the state rather than the federal level. These include but are not limited to end-of-life care, maternal and child health, gene therapies, access to electronic health records, medication adherence, and reproductive health.

An increase in the sophistication of health policy and health services research. The twenty-first century presents a number of challenges to health policy and health services research. Much of the current research is predicated on the use of large secondary databases built on survey research or insurance claim data. With the development of electronic health records and their use in large healthcare delivery organizations, a new set of possibilities is opening for the establishment of population-based research protocols that bring together clinical and administrative data.[13] As the understanding of religion as a social determinant becomes more widely accepted, the inclusion of data about religious affiliation or beliefs in electronic health records will offer an opportunity to understand decision-making and adherence issues among populations experiencing health disparities. This will bring religion as a social determinant into the formulation of evidence-based health policy.

A yet unexplored area for increasing the understanding of the role of religion in disparate population groups is the use of the inferences that can be developed using "big data," gathered through digital social networks and Internet search engines. Interesting and promising models in health have been developed for predicting flu epidemics using big data.[14] The data-mining technologies and predictive models that are being developed offer great potential for understanding the health determinants of populations. How these will incorporate religion remains to be seen, but network models that overlook ties based on religious affiliation will risk ignoring an important sector of social connections. Furthermore, the lessons learned from these models may serve as a basis for the incorporation of a more comprehensive behavioral economics into public health policy-based interventions.[15] As the role of religion in determining the health of populations is better understood, it is reasonable to expect that policy proposals that focus on reducing health disparities and increasing the health status of the population in general will include and acknowledge the role of religion.

Understanding the social determinants of health has added significantly to the evidence-based development of health policy interventions at both the state and federal levels of government. The addition of religion as a social determinant offers the possibility of developing even more effective interventions to reduce health disparities and increase positive health status.

Conclusion, by Ellen Idler

Where is religion going in the twenty-first century? Where is public health going? Are the two on a collision course, or will they open up new pathways for each other? In Part V of this book, we explored the role of religion in three epidemics of the beginning of this new century, and we saw the institutions of public health and religion intersecting in complex and contradictory ways. Even in the context of the same public health threat, the response of different religious communities has been and continues to be diverse and contradictory, aligned with public health interests in some times and places and opposed in others. This should remind us again of the dangers of generalizing about *religion*, as if it were one thing, when it is many things. Not only are there many religions, defining their own interests and values with respect to health, but those interests and values are themselves evolving in the context of ongoing public health crises to which they respond in one way or another.

The simple argument of this book is that we must end the exclusion of the essential sector of religion from the paradigm of social health determinants if fully effective challenges to the world's current and future public health challenges are to be found. The social determinants of health paradigm is now the dominant lens through which research and intervention in public health is viewed. Thomas Frieden, Director of the Centers for Disease Control and Prevention, has described a "health impact pyramid" that organizes the continuum of public health interventions from those that have the greatest impact at the lowest cost to those that have the least impact at the greatest cost.[16] He places socioeconomic factors—the "usual suspects" of social determinants—at the broad base of his pyramid of public health intervention to signify that public health interventions to reduce poverty and improve nutrition, sanitation, and housing have the greatest potential to improve population health.

Moving up the pyramid, the next most effective public health intervention, according to Frieden, is "changing the context to make individuals' default decisions healthy," by which he means societal efforts to be sure that the water, food, and air are clean and safe. Moving up another level, where the impact again narrows, he places "long-lasting protective interventions," one-time or infrequent preventive actions delivered to individuals, such as immunizations or circumcision. Narrowing the impact once again, the next level is for "clinical interventions" for people who already have disease diagnoses, to prevent the condition from getting worse; these would include treatment for HIV or tuberculosis or methadone programs for drug addiction. Finally, at the top of the pyramid are the most individualized and expensive interventions of "counseling and education," for individual behavior change in diet, exercise, or smoking. Like the report from the Commission on the Social Determinants of Health discussed in chapter 1, Frieden's health impact pyramid does not mention religious practices or religious institutions as sites for public health interventions or agents for change in other social determinants.

In this book we have described religions around the world acting as social determinants of health, alongside the political, economic, and social structures from which the social determinants paradigm is built. Religious practices and institutions play a role across the spectrum of interventions categorized in Frieden's pyramid. In an interdisciplinary graduate seminar on religion and public health taught at Emory University, students (from public health, theology, religious studies, sociology, and anthropology) were asked to locate research papers that they had read during the semester at some level on Frieden's pyramid. They did this easily, quickly covering the pyramid at every point with examples of effective public health interventions supported by religious practices and institutions. They named Shri Kshetra Dharmasthala anti-alcoholism camps (described in chapter 22) as an example of "counseling and education," faith-based nongovernmental organizations as sources of "clinical intervention" for HIV treatment (chapter 24), Jewish and Muslim circumcision as examples of "long-lasting protective interventions" (chapter 18), Mormon Utah or Israeli *kibbutzim* as "contexts that make individuals' default decisions healthy" (chapter 18), and Heifer International's work in taking action on "socioeconomic factors" by reducing poverty and hunger (chapter 22). It was clear that religion's influence on public health and public health interventions was pervasive.

Frieden's pyramid calls attention to both the upstream and downstream factors in public health. Some determinants of public health, those referred to as downstream, have their point of impact after disease processes are already under way; the goal at this point is to stop the progression of the disease or reduce the associated disability. Religions play a role here, as the students demonstrated. But current thinking in public health and the official position of the WHO are that it is the background, upstream factors that have by far the most influence on population health—these are the social determinants of health that influence every moment of the life course, beginning even before birth. Religion is present in most societies both downstream and upstream and should be considered alongside its social, political, and economic counterparts if we are to have a complete framework of the social determinants of health.

In this work, with the insights of authors from many perspectives, we have seen where, when, and how religions have acted as social determinants of health in their communities. Beginning in Part I with practices performed by the laity of the world's religions, we saw the potential for widespread, direct health effects on billions of people who perform ritual practices relating to diet, exercise, clothing, and other central aspects of life every day. In Part II we saw the roles played by well-established religious institutions and their clergy leadership in the dissemination of health information and the historical development of modern Western public health institutions. In Part III we reviewed the many ways in which religions influence the health of individuals and communities, beginning with fertility, pregnancy, and birth, and extending through the life course to old age and death. In Part IV we saw the effect of missionary medicine, religiously inspired innovative institutions on global health, and the role of local religious health assets. In Part V we saw the complicated role of religions in three ongoing epidemics.

Throughout, it is clear that religions not only affect the lives and health of the religious; to the extent that they help to curb infectious outbreaks with vaccination programs or work to pass laws that clean the air, they improve conditions for all members of the local community. A male child who has been ritually circumcised will have a reduced risk of HIV infection throughout his life and will put his female sexual partners at lower risk of cervical cancer, even if he does not observe the religious traditions of his parents. We also saw that the effect of religion can be negative. The Comstock laws restricted birth control information and access to contraception not only for conservative Christians like Comstock, but for everyone who used the US Postal Service. As a social determinant, for good or ill, religion has widespread and persistent effects well beyond the borders of its own institutions.

Religion also belongs among the social determinants of health because it is related to the other social determinants in complex ways. The social determinants perspective in the WHO Commission report drew attention to social inequality as the primary source of poor health around the world. Its formulation was at its core an ethical one. Social inequality hurts; it hurts individuals and societies as a whole, even those who sit on top of the hierarchy. Religions around the world speak to this inequality with a central, shared message of compassion and concern for the poor and with structures that deliver care. They focus our attention upstream, to what matters most to people.

There are times and places when religious values and ultimate concerns are at odds with the interests of public health, but there are also many times when their core values are shared. We see religions and public health as having aligned interests—frequently—when the good of the group is seen as outweighing the interests of single individuals, and where an ethic of reducing harm and promoting care is paramount. Religions' role in health is upstream and downstream and in between, but religions have a singular capacity to refocus our attention upstream. By directing attention to shared values and common purposes and lending their social capital, religions can help to create the conditions for social change that are critical to altering conditions of inequality and improving public health.

Notes

1. Marci Kramish Campbell, Marlyn Allicock Hudson, Ken Resnicow, Natasha Blakeney, Amy Paxton, and Monica Baskin, "Church-Based Health Promotion Interventions: Evidence and Lessons Learned," *Annual Review of Public Health* 28 (2007): 213–234.
2. Annie Hardison-Moody and Willona M. Stallings, "Faith Communities as Health Partners: Examples from the Field," *North Carolina Medical Journal* 73, no. 5 (2011): 387–388.
3. Hardison-Moody and Stallings, "Faith Communities as Health Partners," 387.
4. World Health Organization, *World Health Report 2000—Health Systems: Improving Performance* (Geneva: World Health Organization, 2000), 5.
5. James F. Childress, Ruth R. Faden, Ruth D. Gaare, Lawrence O. Gostin, Jeffrey Kahn, Richard J. Bonnie, Nancy E. Kass et al., "Public Health Ethics: Mapping the Terrain," *Journal of Law, Medicine & Ethics* 30, no. 2 (2002): 170.
6. Nancy E. Kass, "Public Health Ethics from Foundations and Frameworks to Justice and Global Public Health," *Journal of Law, Medicine & Ethics* 32, no. 2 (2004): 232–242; emphasis in original.
7. Paul Slack, "Responses to Plague in Early Modern Europe: the Implications of Public Health," *Social Research* 55 no. 3 (1988): 433–453.
8. J. F. Childress, R. R. Faden, R. D. Gaare, L. O. Gostin, J. Kahn, R. J. Bonnie et al., "Public Health Ethics: Mapping the Terrain," *Journal of Law, Medicine & Ethics* 30, no. 2 (2002): 171.
9. Misha Dzhindzhikhashvili, "Georgia's Patriarch Baptizes 400 Babies," Associated Press, May 7, 2012.
10. Here the term "public health" is used in the context of the health of a population as opposed to health services provided by a governmental agency. In this context, populations are not constrained to geographical divisions. Rather the term "population" is used to refer to any group that shares a common characteristic; examples include ethnic groups, employees, age groups, income cohorts, and congregations. Comparison of groups serves as the basic method for uncovering disparities in health status.
11. Communities may be thought of as functioning at multiple levels of government, that is, municipal, state, and federal.
12. World Health Organization, "WHO Definition of Health," citing the Preamble to the Constitution of the World Health Organization as adopted by the International Health Conference, New York, 19–22 June, 1946; signed on 22 July 1946 by the representatives of 61 States (Official Records of the World Health Organization, no. 2, p. 100) and entered into force on 7 April 1948, http://www.who.int/about/definition/en/print.html.
13. The Veterans Administration and Kaiser-Permanente are the most often cited examples.
14. The potential uses and challenges of big data are discussed in Victor Mayer-Schonberger and Kenneth Niel Cukier, *Big Data: A Revolution That Will Transform How We Live, Work, and Think* (New York: Houghton Mifflin Harcourt, 2013).

15. D. King, F. Greaves, I. Vlaev, and A. Darzi, "Approaches Based on Behavioral Economics Could Help Nudge Patients and Providers toward Lower Health Spending Growth," *Health Affairs* 32, no. 4 (April 2013): 661–667.
16. Thomas Frieden, "A Framework for Public Health Action: The Health Impact Pyramid" *American Journal of Public Health* 100 (2010): 590–595.

CONTRIBUTORS

Abdullahi An-Na'im, LLB, PhD. Charles Howard Candler Professor of Law, School of Law, Emory University, Atlanta, Georgia.

John Blevins, ThD. Associate Research Professor of Global Health, Rollins School of Public Health, Emory University, Atlanta, Georgia.

Matthew Bersagel Braley, PhD. Assistant Professor of Religious Studies and Philosophy, Viterbo University, La Crosse, Wisconsin.

Peter J. Brown, PhD. Professor of Anthropology, Emory University, Atlanta, Georgia.

Walter Burnett, PhD. Professor of Health Policy and Management, Rollins School of Public Health, Emory University, Atlanta, Georgia.

James R. Cochrane, PhD. Professor of Religious Studies Emeritus, University of Cape Town, Cape Town, South Africa.

James W. Curran, MD, MPH. Dean and Professor of Epidemiology, Rollins School of Public Health, Emory University, Atlanta, Georgia.

Safiya George Dalmida, PhD. Assistant Professor, Nell Hodgson Woodruff School of Nursing, Emory University, Atlanta, Georgia.

L. Wesley de Souza, PhD. Arthur J. Moore Associate Professor in the Practice of Evangelism, Candler School of Theology, Emory University, Atlanta, Georgia.

Laura M. Gaydos, PhD. Assistant Professor of Health Policy and Management, Rollins School of Public Health, Emory University, Atlanta, Georgia.

George H. Grant, PhD. Clinical Assistant Professor, Nell Hodgson Woodruff School of Nursing, Emory University, Atlanta, Georgia.

Gary R. Gunderson, DDiv, MDiv. Vice President, Division of Faith and Health Ministries, Wake Forest Baptist Health, Winston-Salem, North Carolina.

Kenneth Hepburn, PhD. Professor, Nell Hodgson Woodruff School of Nursing, Emory University, Atlanta, Georgia.

Carol Hogue, PhD, MPH. Jules and Uldeen Terry Professor of Maternal and Child Health and Professor of Epidemiology, Rollins School of Public Health, Emory University, Atlanta, Georgia.

Lynn Hogue, PhD. Professor of Law Emeritus, Georgia State University, Atlanta, Georgia.

Ellen Idler, PhD. Samuel Candler Dobbs Professor of Sociology, and Director, Religion and Public Health Collaborative, Emory University, Atlanta, Georgia.

Theodore M. Johnson II, MD, MPH. Paul W. Seavey Chair in Medicine and Professor of Medicine, School of Medicine, Emory University, Atlanta, Georgia.

Mimi Kiser, DMin, MPH. Assistant Research Professor of Global Health, Rollins School of Public Health, Emory University, Atlanta, Georgia.

Emmanuel Yartekwei Amugi Lartey, PhD. L. Bevel Jones III Professor of Pastoral Theology, Care, and Counseling, Candler School of Theology, Emory University, Atlanta, Georgia.

Bhagirath Majmudar, MD. Professor of Pathology and Associate professor of Obstetrics and Gynecology, School of Medicine, Emory University, Atlanta, Georgia.

Deborah McFarland, PhD, MPH. Associate Professor of Global Health, Rollins School of Public Health, Emory University, Atlanta, Georgia.

Jose Montenegro, MDiv. Chaplain, Emory Center for Pastoral Services, Emory University, Atlanta, Georgia.

Geshe Lobsang Tenzin Negi, PhD. Senior Lecturer in Religion and Director, Emory-Tibet Partnership, Emory University, Atlanta, Georgia.

Brendan Ozawa-de Silva, PhD. Associate Professor of Psychology, Life University, Marietta, Georgia.

Chikako Ozawa-de Silva, PhD. Associate Professor of Anthropology, Emory University, Atlanta, Georgia.

Patricia Z. Page, MS, CGC. Director, Genetic Counseling Services, School of Medicine, Emory University, Atlanta, Georgia.

Laurie Patton, PhD. Dean of the Faculty of Arts and Sciences, Duke University, Durham, North Carolina.

Eric Reinders, PhD. Associate Professor of Religion, Emory University, Atlanta, Georgia.

Don E. Saliers, PhD. William R. Cannon Distinguished Professor of Theology Emeritus, Candler School of Theology, Emory University, Atlanta, Georgia.

Scott Santibañez, MD, MPHTM, MA. Associate Director for Science, Division of Preparedness and Emerging Infection, Centers for Disease Control and Prevention, Atlanta, Georgia.

Karen D. Scheib, PhD. Associate Professor of Pastoral Care and Pastoral Theology, Candler School of Theology, Emory University, Atlanta, Georgia.

Don Seeman, PhD. Associate Professor of Religion, Emory University, Atlanta, Georgia.

Phillip M. Thompson, PhD. Executive Director, Aquinas Center of Theology, Emory University, Atlanta, Georgia.

Sandra Thurman, MA. Director, Interfaith Health Program and the Joseph Blount Center for Health and Human Rights, Rollins School of Public Health, Emory University, Atlanta, Georgia.

Paul Root Wolpe, PhD. Asa Griggs Candler Professor of Bioethics and Director, Center for Ethics, Emory University, Atlanta, Georgia.

Kathryn M. Yount, PhD. Asa Griggs Candler Chair of Global Health, Rollins School of Public Health, Emory University, Atlanta, Georgia.

INDEX

African Christian Health Associations, 350

African Religious Health Assets Programme (ARHAP): creation of, 270; healthworlds concept and, 271, 361; HIV/AIDS epidemic and, 344–345; leadership structure at, 347; religious health assets (RHAs) documentation by, 271, 281, 345, 347, 350–351, 353–361; village mapping project of, 271; World Health Organization (WHO) and, 271, 344–346, 348, 351, 353–354, 356

aggrey (Krobo beads), 95

Ahsanullah, Khan Bahadur, 329–332, 337

AIDS. *See* HIV/AIDS

air pollution, 1–2, 113

akori (Krobo beads), 95

Alameda County Study, 4, 231

alcohol: abuse of, 13, 16, 145, 327; adolescents' use of, 215–217, 219; Nevada-Utah comparison regarding, 204; pauperism and, 137–138; religious group membership and, 5, 216–217, 231–232; religious prohibitions against, 51–52, 176, 231; religious service attendance rates and, 212, 232; temperance movement and, 145–146, 157; treatment programs for alcoholism and, 327–328, 338–339, 416; Wesley on, 125

Alcorta, Candace, 220

All Saints Episcopal Church (Atlanta, Georgia), 371

Alma-Ata Declaration on Primary Health Care (1978): criticisms of, 313; limited impact of, 314, 345–346; principles articulated in, 270, 299, 311–314, 349

Alzheimer's Disease. *See also* dementia: caregivers and, 396, 398–405; compassion for sufferers of, 401, 403–405; counseling and, 402–403; isolation issues and, 405; music and, 398, 400; number of people who suffer from, 396; person-centered care and, 398–399; personhood and, 397–402,

404; prayer and, 400; religious institutions and, xvi, 365–366, 397, 400–404; religious participation and, 239, 399–402; symptoms of, 396–398; treatment for, 366

Alzheimer's Resources of Alaska, 402

"Amazing Grace," 65–66

American Baptist Church, 182, 189

American Indians, 216

American Public Health Association, 383

American Tract Society, 110, 139–140

The Amish: cancer rates among, 228; contraception and, 183; genetic disorders among, 6–7; standardized mortality ratios among, 222–223, 237

Ammerman, Nancy, 16, 257

amniocentesis, 193

Anabaptism, 324

anatta (Buddhist doctrine of no self), 15

And the Band Played On (Shilts), 370, 377

Anglican Church: contraception and, 183; Lambeth Conference (1930) and, 183; L'Arche communities and, 335; Methodist movement and, 114–115; public health and, 114, 116; Wesley and, 109, 113, 115

Appleby, Scott, 154–155

Ark of the Covenant, 333–334

Armstrong, Karen, 15

Arole, Mabelle, 338

Arole, Raj, 338

Ashkenazi Jews, 7

Ash Wednesday, 57–58

Asklepieion, 63

Assemblies of God, 182, 189

Associated Charities, 386

Association of State and Territorial Health Officials, 388

asthma, 1, 123

At-Risk Populations Project (ARPP), 388, 392

authority/respect moral dimension, 259

Avicenna, 184

azl (Islamic term for *coitus interruptus*), 184–185

Bagiella, E., 225
Bahubali, 326
Bailey, Martha J., 169
Baker, Josephine, 187
Banda, Marlon, 286
Bangladesh: Dhaka Ahsania Mission in, 270, 329–332, 337; Ganokendra (social welfare organizations) in, 330–331; health and wealth indicators in, 279; HIV/AIDS in, 330; L'Arche communities in, 335; Muslim-Hindu relations in, 329; prayer frequency in, 281
Ban Ki-Moon, 275
baptism: of adults in Latin American Pentecostalism, 97–101; Georgian Orthodox Church and, 411–412; health research regarding, 101; of infants, 211, 411–412; invocations of Jesus during, 98–100; as means of addressing pain or disease, 97–98, 101, 373; salvation and, 99
Baptists, 18, 182, 189, 218, 391
bar mitzvahs/bat mitzvahs, 214
Barrett, Ron, 385
Bartley, Mel, 207
Bates, Anna Louise, 156–157
Bates, James, 52
Bearman, Peter, 218
Beckwith, Carol, 92–93
Becoming Human (Vanier), 334
Beecher, Henry Ward, 158
Benares (India), 104
Benjamin, Regina, 382
Benjamins, Maureen, 232
Benn, Christoph, 303, 307
Ben-Shlomo, Yoav, 233
"The Beraita of Three Women" *(Talmud),* 185
Berhorst, Caroll, 289
Berkel, J., 222–223
Bernardin, Joseph, 61
Besant, Annie, 168–169
Bhagavadgita, 106
Bhagavatam, 105
Bhajan Mandali (religious meeting), 328

"big data," 414
Bigelow v. Virginia, 165
Bill and Melinda Gates Foundation, 276, 348
Billings, John Shaw, 136
birth control. *See* contraception
birth control pill, 169
Black Report, 10
"Blessed Assurance," 65
bodum (Krobo beads), 95
Bolger v. Young's Drug Products Corporation, 164
Boston (Massachusetts), 187
Botton, Alain de, 236
Boyle, Robert, 116, 123–124
Bradlaugh, Charles, 168
Brazil: health and wealth indicators in, 279; "Jordan River" in, 98–101; National AIDS Program in, 372; Pentecostalism in, 97–101; wealth and religiosity indicators in, 280
breastfeeding: La Leche League and, 270–271, 320–322, 336–337, 339–340; religious service attendance rates and, 212; twentieth-century medicine's discouraging of, 320–321
Briggs, Philothea, 126
brit (Jewish circumcision ritual), 85–87
British Birth Cohort studies, 12, 206
Broad Street Pump (London), 109, 351–352
Brown, Peter, 385
Brückner, Hannah, 218
Bryan, William Jennings, 147–148, 152n37
Buck, Anna, 232
Buconyori, Joy, 338
The Buddha (Siddhartha Gautama), 32
Buddha Maitreya, 32
Buddhas (enlightened beings), 31–33, 35
Buddhism: abortion and, 184, 190, 193; adolescents in monasteries and, 214; *anatta* (doctrine of no self) in, 15; clerical celibacy and, 221; compassion in, 33–35; contraception and, 183–184, 186–187; Dharma (teachings and

Dipo (Kroko women's coming of age ritual), 91–95
disability: among the elderly, 238–239; different religious groups' rates of, 228; L'Arche communities treatment of, 271, 333–334, 337, 340; prenatal screening and, 192–194; religious participation rates and, 239; religious perspectives on, 192–193
Disciples of Christ Church, 371
Diwali, 209
Dor Yeshorim, 194–195, 336, 338
The Doxology, 66
Dupre, M., 226
Durkheim, Emile: on group membership, 5, 7, 230; on suicide, 3–6, 215, 238

Easter, 58–59, 209, 240
Eau Vive, 333, 335
Ecumenical Pharmaceutical Network (EPN), 286
Edwards, Jonathan, 145
egg donation, 196
Egypt: contraception during antiquity in, 180–181; contraception during modern times in, 184; first-person account of veiling in, 44–46; Old Testament and, 15; wealth and religiosity indicators in, 280
Eid al-Fitr, 78, 402
Eighteenth Amendment (U.S. Constitution), 146
Eisenstadt v. Baird, 164–165
Ekstein, Josef, 194–195, 338
Elijah's Promise (New Brunswick, NJ), 336, 338
Elliott, Charles, 312
embodied cognitive logics, 254, 263
Emory University: African Religious Health Assets Programme (ARHAP) and, 346; Engaging Communities in Response to Pandemic Influenza and, 382, 389, 392; graduate students at, 416; Interfaith Health Program (IHP) at, ix, 133, 347–348, 350, 382, 384, 389, 392; mental health research at, 257; Religion and Public Health

Collaborative at, ix; Rollins School of Public Health, 133
endocrine disorders, 229
Eng, P.M., 226
Engaging Communities in Response to Pandemic Influenza, 382, 389, 392
England. *See also* United Kingdom: contraception in, 160; historical decline in mortality in, 282; literacy in, 110; Methodist movement in, 115, 119–120; public health in, xiv, 109–114, 119–128; tract movement in, 138–139
The Enlightenment, 115–116, 300, 302
Episcopal Church: abortion and, 189; clergy in, 221; contraception and, 182; HIV/AIDS epidemic and, 371; household income levels among U.S. members of, 18
Episcopal Church of the Holy Redeemer (Atlanta), 402
An Essay on Regimen, Together with Five Discourses, Medical, Moral, and Philosophical (Cheyne), 122
An Estimate of the Manners of Present Times (Wesley), 127
ethical spirituality, 257–258, 261–264
The Eucharist: Alzheimer's Disease sufferers and, 402; health research regarding, 61; as marker of individual maturation, 214; prayer and, 59–60; weekly celebration of, 57, 59
eudaimonia, 255
eugenics, 147
Europa, Europa (film), 88–89
Evangelical Lutheran Church in America, 182, 189
Evangelical Lutheran Church of Tanzania, 304
Extract from William Cadogan on the Gout (Wesley), 127
Ezekiel 16, 87

fairness/reciprocity moral dimension, 259
Fairview Health Services (Minnesota), 389–391

Galen, 63, 67, 122
Gandhi, Rajiv, 107
Ganges River, 104, 107
Ganokendra (social welfare organizations in Bangladesh), 330–331
Garner, Bruce, 371
Gates, Bill, 276
Genesis: on Abraham's covenant with God, 85; exhortations to fertility in, 195; on food, 50; on Onan, 185; on surrogacy, 196
genetic disorders within specific religious communities, 6–7, 194–195, 336, 338
Georgian Orthodox Church, 411–412
Ghana. See Kroko
The Ghost Map (Johnson), 8, 109
Gillum, Frank, 225
Galvan, Frank, 376
Global Fund to Fight HIV/AIDS, Tuberculosis, and Malaria, 276, 348
global health movement. See also public health: Christian Medical Commission (CMC) and, 310, 312–315; Cold War and, 274; faith-based organizations (FBOs) and, 274, 277–278, 284–286, 290–291; global poverty and, 275, 278–279; health literacy and, xi; HIV/AIDS epidemic and, 274–276; medical missionaries and, 274, 287–290, 301, 304; Millennium Development Goals and, 269, 275, 315, 325; national governments in developing countries and, 285, 287, 304, 306, 308; nongovernmental organizations (NGOs) and, 274, 276–277, 284–286; origins of, 269, 274; pharmaceutical supplies and, 286; religious literacy and, xi, xv–xvi, 106; short-term missions and, 289–290; traditional healers and, 281–284
Global Religious Futures project, 279
The Golden Rule, 15
Good Friday, 58
"The Good Steward" (Wesley), 121
Grace Cathedral (San Francisco, California), 371

Graham, Jesse, 259
Grama Kalyana Yojane (water sanitation program in India), 327
Great Awakening, 145
Greek Orthodox Diocese of America, 182, 189
Green, Edward, 281
Griscom, John: biographical background of, 136; efforts to improve New York City public health by, 135, 140–142, 149; on importance of cleanliness, 135, 141; on pauperism, 111, 136, 141–142, 149; religious worldview of, 136, 143, 145, 150
Griswold v. Connecticut, 163–165
Guatemala, 289
Guide for the Perplexed (Maimonides), 87
Guinness, Arthur, 120–121
Gunderson, Gary, 347

H1N1. See under influenza
Habermas, Jürgen, 350, 354
Hadith (recorded traditions of the Prophet Muhammad), 79–80
haiden (Shinto hall of worship), 71–72
Haidt, Jonathan, 259
The Hajj, 6
Hales, Stephen, 123–124
Hamilton, Margaret, 156
Hamman, R.F., 222, 237
Hansen, Nathan, 375
Harding, Susan, 146, 149
harm/care moral dimension, 259, 261–263
Harper, Malcolm, 325, 327–328
Harris, George, 386
Harris, Sam, 261
Hartley, Robert: American Tract Society and, 139–140; biographical background of, 136; milk studies of, 110, 137–138; New York Association for Improving the Condition of the Poor and, 135–137, 139–140; on pauperism, 111, 136–138; religious worldview of, 138, 143, 145, 150; on the Sabbath, 138
Harvest Moon Festival, 240

"How Great Thou Art," 65
Hsu, H.C., 225
Humanae Vitae (papal encyclical), 181, 183
Hummer, Robert, 226
Hurricane Katrina (2005): destructiveness of, 387; as impetus for public health preparedness reform, 384, 387–388, 391, 393
hygiene, 122, 125, 212, 327
hypertension, 13, 228

ICCO, 285
Idler, Ellen: Emory University and, ix; research on disability rates among the elderly by, 239; research on mortality rates by, 226, 240; research on social determinants of health by, 205
Ilia II (Georgian Orthodox Church patriarch), 411–412
immunizations: Christian Medical Commission (CMC) and, 310; influenza and, 365, 382–384, 387–393; religious communities' roles in, xvi, 6, 365, 382–384, 387–391, 393, 417; religious prohibitions against, 176, 213
income inequality: educational attainment and, 13, 19; premarital pregnancy and, 19; psychological impact of, 16–17; public health outcomes and, 11–12, 14–16, 278–279; religion and, 14, 17–19, 210, 232; in United States, 11, 19, 220
India: health and wealth indicators in, 279; Hindu cremation rites in, 103–107; HIV/AIDS in, 107; infant mortality and health in, 212; L'Arche communities in, 335; water pollution in, 107
infant mortality: family planning's impact on, 168; maternal age's impact on, 168; Nevada-Utah comparison regarding, 204, 212; in nineteenth-century New York City, 110, 137; prenatal care's impact on, 187; in the United States, 278

infertility. *See* fertility, treatment to improve
influenza: African Americans and, 383, 390; community-based organizations' (CBOs) role in combating, 384, 388–389; data projections regarding, 414; epidemiology of, 6; faith-based organizations (FBOs) work in combating, 365, 382–384, 387–391, 393; H1N1 strain of, 382–384, 387–393; immunizations against, 365, 382–384, 387–393; miasma theory of illness and, 124; Spanish influenza epidemic (1918), 384–385
in-group/loyalty moral dimension, 259
An Inquiry into the Effects of Ardent Spirits upon the Human Body and Mind (Rush), 145, 152n32
Institute for Health and Social Justice, 350–351
Institute of Medicine, ix
Interfaith Health Program (IHP, Emory University): African Religious Health Assets Program and, 350; founding of, 133, 347; influenza immunization efforts and, ix, 382, 384, 389, 392; mission of, 348
International Christian AIDS Network, 313
International Covenant on Economic, Social and Cultural Rights, 169
International Religious Health Assets Program, 270. *See also* African Religious Health Assets Programme (ARHAP)
Internet pornography, 218
intrauterine devices (IUDs), 185
Iran, 233, 281
Iraq, 284
Ireland, 120
Ironson, Gail, 375
Islam: abortion and, 190–192; in Africa, 281, 387; attitudes toward disability in, 193; contraception and, 182, 184–185; Eid al-Fitr and, 78, 402; fasting during Ramadan in, 77–80; fertility and, 179,

Islam: abortion and (*continued*)
195; fundamentalism and, 155; Hadith
(recorded traditions of the Prophet
Muhammad) and, 79–80; *hijab*
(headscarf) and veiling in, 44–47, 188;
ijithad (Islamic principle of analysis)
and, 184; *khimars* (waist-length veils)
and, 45; *niya* (principle of intent) and,
79; prayer and, 79–80, 209, 211;
prenatal care and, 188; Prophet
Muhammad and, 79–80, 193; The
Qu'ran and, 79–80, 193; Ramadan
and, 77–80; regulation of personal
behavior and, 5; Sufism and, 79;
surrogacy and, 196; *twhid* (principle of
unity and wholeness of God) in, 79;
zakaat (principle of charity) and,
332
"Islam's Attitude towards Family
Planning," 184–185
Italy, 239

Jains, 326, 338
Jana Jagruthi (anti-alcoholism program in
India), 327–328, 339
Japan: Buddhism in, 74; Christians in,
72–74; group suicides in, 260; health
and wealth indicators in, 279; income
inequality levels in, 11; prayer
frequency in, 281; Shinto shrines in,
71–75; wealth and religiosity
indicators in, 280
Jehovah's Witnesses, 18
Jen (Confucian principle of measuring
feelings), 15
Jenkins, David, 301
Jenner, Edward, 349
Jerusalem, 216
Jesup, Morris, 158 Jesus Christ: baptismal
invocations of, 98–100; compassion
of, 193; on disadvantaged members of
society, 15; Easter celebration of,
58–59; The Eucharist and, 60; healing
ministry of, 298–299; Social Gospel
movement's invocations of,
143–144

Jews. *See also* Judaism: Tay-Sachs
disease among, 22n39, 194–195, 338;
U.S. household income levels
among, 18
jingli (obeisance), 38
Jnana Viakasa program, 327
Johnson, Ifetayo, 382, 384, 391
Johnson, Steven, 8, 109
"Jordan River" (Brazil), 98–101
Judaism: abortion and, 189–190,
192–193, 195, 336; *bar mitzvahs/bat
mitzvahs* and, 214; circumcision and,
85–89, 416; Conservative Judaism,
182, 185, 190; contraception and, 182,
185–187, 197; covenant in, 85–86,
333–334; fundamentalism and, 155;
Hasidic Judaism, 195; Leviticus on
compassion in, 15; masturbation and,
185, 196; Orthodox Judaism, 182, 185,
190, 193, 195–196; prenatal care and,
187; prenatal genetic screening and,
194–195; Reform Judaism, 182, 185,
189; Sabbath in, 209, 240; Seleucid
persecutions and, 88; *shiva* (mourning
ritual) in, 236; surrogacy and, 196

Kagoshima (Japan), 72
kami (spirits or ancestors), 73
karma, 32, 193, 257
Karnataka (India), 326–327
Karpf, Ted, 345–346
Kasl, Stanislav, 239–240
Kawachi, Ichiro, 7
Keeping the Faith, 372
Keister, Lisa, 18–19
Kenya, 285, 338–339
Kerwin, Mary Ann, 320
khimars (waist-length veils), 45
kibbutzim, 336, 416
Kim, Daniel, 7
Kim, Jim, 277
King, Dana, 228–229, 239
King, H., 222
Kingsley, Charles, 349
Kitagawa, Evelyn, 9
klama dance, 94–95

Kleinman, Arthur, 260–261, 267n27
kloyo peemi ("making a Krobo woman"), 91
Knowlton, Charles, 160, 168
Knox, Alexander, 118 Koenig, Harold: research on adolescent health and, 214–215; research on disability rates among the elderly and, 239; research on morbidity rates by, 228–229, 232; research on mortality rates by, 229–230; research on social determinants of health by, 205
Koh, Howard K., 392
koli (Kroko beads), 95
Koplan, J.P., 274
Korman, Edward, 170
Kramer, Michael R., 218
Krause, Neal, 225, 227
Krieger, Nancy, 17
Kroko people (Ghana), 91–95
Kuh, Diana, 220, 233

La Cour, P., 225, 227
La Leche League: Christian Family Movement (CFM) and, 320, 322; expansion of, 336; "like-to-like" ministry and, 339–340; origins of, 270–271, 320–322, 337, 339
Lambarene (Gabon), 288
Lambeth Conference (1930), 183
Lambourne, Robert, 306–307
L'Arche communities: disabled members of, 271, 333–334, 337, 340;"like-to-like" ministry and, 339; religious ideals of, 270, 334–335, 337; skill building emphasis at, 340; Vanier as founder of, 333, 337
Latin American Evangelical Pentecostalism, 97–101
Laungani, Pittu, 104
The Law of Population (Besant), 169
Lawrence v. Texas, 173n41
Laws, Robert, 288
Laws of Manu, 193
Lennon, Viola, 320
Lent, 58

Lesotho, 271, 351, 357–358
A Letter to a Friend Concerning Tea (Wesley), 127
Leviticus, 15, 50, 193
liberation theologies, 289, 300
life course: adolescence's impact on heath over, 217, 219–220; adulthood's impact on health over, 220–233; cyclical religious practices and, xv, 26–27, 208–209; as a framework for public health analysis, 175–178, 205–207, 213, 416–417; old age and, 234–241, 336; one-time rituals and, xiv, 26, 208–209, 211, 214; religious variation over, 207–211
Lindland, E., 288
Litwin, Howard, 226
Livingstone, David, 288
Livingstonia mission station (southern Africa), 287–288
Locke, F.B., 222
Locke, John, 123–124
London (England): air pollution in, 113, 125; Broad Street Pump in, 109, 351–352; cholera outbreak (1854) in, 8, 109–111, 128, 351–352; Wesley's medical clinic in, 113–114, 119–120, 127
Lowell Community Health Center (Lowell, Massachusetts), 389
Lutheran Church: abortion and, 189, 192; contraception and, 182; HIV/AIDS epidemic and, 371; household income among U.S. members of, 18; Lutheran World Federation and, 286, 299; in Tanzania, 304

MacLeod, Arlene Elowe, 46
Madden, Deborah, 117–118, 124
Maddox, Randy, 118–119
Mahler, Halfdan, 312, 314
Maimonides, Moses, 87
Mala (Sanskrit beads), 103
malaria, 275, 282, 312
mammography, 233
Manji, F., 284

marijuana, 212, 216, 219

Marmot, Michael, 8, 10–12

marriage: Krobo religious ceremonies and, 95; religion as a social determinant in, 179, 204; religious attitudes toward, 195, 221

Marshall, Thurgood, 160

Marty, Martin, 154–155

Marx, Karl, 349

Massachusetts, 161–162, 164

masturbation, 157, 185, 196–197

maternal health, 190–192, 275

Matthew, Gospel of, 193

Maundy Thursday, 58

Maurice, F.D., 349

Max-Neef, Manfred, 346

Maya-Kaqchikel population (Guatemala), 289

McBride, Margaret Mary, 191

McCullough, Michael, 205, 228, 255–256

McGilvray, James: on assumptions of Western medicine, 306; Christian Medical Commission (CMC) and, 309, 312; Tübingen I Conference (1964) and, 301–303

McKenna, Jennifer: activism on air pollution of, 1–2, 113–114, 128; congregational leadership of, 8

medical missionaries, 274, 287–290, 301, 303–304

Medicinal Experiments (Boyle), 116

meditation: in Buddhism, 31–36; mental health and, 257–258, 264, 350, 375–376; physical health and, 375–376

Memphis (Tennessee), 386, 389–390

mental health: adolescence and, 214; Cartesian dualism and, 252–253; Cognitively Based Compassion Training (CBCT) and, 257–258, 264; compassion and, 253, 255–261, 263–264; depression and, 10, 16, 36, 254, 257, 375; eudaimonia and, 255; among gay and lesbian population, 260; hedonia and, 255; medicalization of human suffering and, 260–261; meditation and, 257–258, 264, 350,

375–376; moral socialization and, 259–261; negative definition of, 253; physical health and, 252–253; positive psychology and, 253, 255–256, 258, 262, 264; religion as a social determinant in, 7, 176, 251, 253–256, 258–259, 261–263, 283, 376; religious participation and, 254, 376; social rejection and, 260; spirituality and, 253–259, 261–264; traditional healers and, 281; transgender population and, 260

Merriam, Clinton L., 159

Methodist Le Bonheur Healthcare (Memphis, TN), 358–359, 389–390

Methodist movement: care for the poor and, 119–120; discipline regimen in, 116; group meetings within, 115, 128; Wesley and, 109, 114–116, 119–121, 128

Methodists, U.S. household income levels among, 18

Mexico, 216, 232, 279–280

Mexico City, 216

microfinance, 327–328

milk: breastfeeding and, 270–271, 320–322, 336–337, 339–340; Hartley on, 110, 137–138

Millennium Development Goals, 269, 275, 315, 325

Miller, L., 254

Miller v. California, 165–166

"Miracle Mile" (Cumberland Valley, Pennsylvania), 2

Mission Handbook (North American Protestant ministries), 284

Monitoring the Future Study, 216–217

Moral Monday protests (North Carolina, 2013), 413

Moravians, 117

morbidity rates: among different religious groups, 228–229; among the elderly, 238–239; in nineteenth-century New York City, 137

"The More Excellent Way" (Wesley), 125

Morgan, David, 26

Morgan, J. Pierpont, 158

Mormons. *See also* Church of Jesus Christ of Latter-day Saints (LDS): mortality rates among, 206; standardized mortality ratios among, 222–223; U.S. household income levels among, 18

Morrison, Robert S., 128

mortality rates: Fuchs' Utah-Nevada comparison of, 203, 206; gender and, 225–226, 228, 237; in old age, 236–238; private religiousness' impact on, 227–229, 237; relative mortality risk rates and, 225–227; religious groups' different rates of, 205–206, 222–224, 237; religious participation's impact on, 177, 224–232; standardized mortality ratios and, 222–223, 237

The Moviegoer (Percy), 57

Mueller, Paul S., 375

Munaqabat (face-veiled women), 45

music: Alzheimer's Disease and, 398, 400; congregational hymn singing and, 65–67; emotional power of, 63; health research regarding, 67; as means of coping with pain and disease, 66–67; shape-note singing and, 64

Musick, Marc A., 225, 227–228

Musicophilia (Sacks), 63

Muslims: in Bangladesh, 329; diabetes and endocrine disorders among, 229; fertility rates among, 187; intra-group violence among, 284; mammography and, 233; U.S. household income levels among, 18

Nahmanides, 87

Naikan (Japanese principle of reflection), 255

National Academies of Science, ix

National AIDS Program (Brazil), 372

National Congregation Survey, 16

National Episcopal AIDS Coalition, 371

National Influenza Vaccination Week, 382

National Mortality Followback Study, 238

National Study of Youth and Religion, 218

National Survey on Drug Use and Health, 216

Nava Jeevana Samitis, 327

Negi, Geshe Lobsang Tenzin, 257

Nene Kloweki (Krobo Earth Goddess), 92–93

The Netherlands, 285

Nevada: adolescent health indicators and, 214; alcohol use in, 204; cigarette use in, 204; economic conditions in, 206; Fuchs' public health research on, 203–204, 206, 210, 214, 236; mortality rates in, 203, 206, 236

Newell, Kenneth, 313

New Haven (Connecticut), 234, 239–240

New Orleans (Louisiana), 57, 387

New York City: American Tract Society in, 139; early prenatal programs in, 187; infant mortality during nineteenth century in, 110; New York Association for Improving the Condition of the Poor and, 135–137, 139–140; public health problems during nineteenth century in, 134–135, 137–142, 149, 156

New York State, Comstock-style laws in, 161–164

New York v. Ferber, 173n47

Nicene Creed, 59

Niddah 30b (section of The Talmud), 191

Nietzsche, Friedrich, 349

Nigeria, 279–280, 386–387, 392

Nisbet, Paul, 238

niya (principle of intent in Islam), 79

nocebo phenomenon, 284

nongovernmental organizations (NGOs), 274, 276–277, 284–286, 328, 330, 416

Norris, F.H., 391

North American Mission Board, 391

North Carolina Council of Churches, 409

Norway, 212, 224

Nurses for Newborns Foundation (Saint Louis, MO), 389, 392

Nusrat, Ayesha, 46–47

Nussbaum, Martha, 340

Nyumbani Village (organization for children orphaned by HIV/AIDS), 336, 338–339

Obama, Barack, 170, 383
obscenity law in the United States, 158–159, 165–166
O'Coill, C., 284
odds ratios, 222, 225–227
old age: Alzheimer's Disease and dementia in, 239, 396–405; disability in, 238–239; end of life care and, 234–235; isolation during, 234; morbidity rates in, 238–239; mortality rates in, 236–238; private religious belief during, 234; religious participation during, 234–235; religious rituals and, 208; suicide in, 238; timing of death in, 240
Olivier, Jill, 346
Olmsted, Thomas J., 191
omamori (Shinto amulets), 72
Oman, D., 225–226
omikuji (Shinto fortunes), 72
onanism, 185
"On Visiting the Sick" (Wesley), 119
Opoku, Kofi Asare, 91–94
Ordronaux, John, 139–140
Orsi, Robert, 26
Orthodox Church in Cyprus, 195
Orthodox Jews, 182, 185, 190, 193, 195–196
osaisenbako (Shinto offering box), 72
oshōgatsu (Shinto New Year celebration), 72
Østbye, T., 225
Ott, Phillip, 116
Outdooring Ceremony (Krobo religious rite), 94–95
Outhwaite, William, 350
Oxfam, 284
Oxford (England), 119

Pace, Thaddeus, 257
pain: baptism as a means of coping with, 97–98; circumcision and, 87; music as a means for coping with, 66
palliative care, 277, 282, 359
Panchamahabhuta (five basic elements of the body in Hinduism), 104

Papua New Guinea, 373
Participatory Inquiry into Religious Health Assets, Networks and Agency (PIRHANA), 356–358
Partners in Health, 350–351
Partners in Health and Wholeness, 409
Passover, 240, 402
Pastor Jamil (Santa Cruz, Brazil), 100–101
Patch, Denise, 338
Patterson, Gillian, 309
"Paul Farmer Made Me Do It!" (study of short-term medical missions), 290
Paul VI (pope), 181
pauperism: alcohol and, 137–138; Griscom on, 111, 136, 141–142, 149; Hartley on, 111, 136–138; moral interpretations of, 136, 142, 149–150; Social Gospel movement's emphasis on combating, 136–137, 139, 141–142, 149; socioeconomic interpretation of, 142–143, 149; tract societies' publications on, 139
Peel, Jesse, 373
Pennsylvania Department of Environmental Protection, 2
Penrose-St. Francis Mission Outreach (Colorado Springs, Colorado), 389
Pentecostalism in Brazil, 97–101
Percy, Walker, 57
Perel, Solomon "Solek," 88–89
personhood: abortion and, 191, 194; Alzheimer's Disease and, 397–402, 404
Pew Foundation, 279–280
Philadelphia (Pennsylvania), 372, 408, 410
Philippe, Thomas, 333–335
Phillips, David, 222, 240
Pickett, Kate, 278–279
Pietism, 324
Pius XI (pope), 339
Place, Francis, 160
Plan B One-Step, 170
Plan International, 284
Planned Parenthood of Southeastern Pennsylvania v. Casey, 163, 167

Plato, 63
Plevak, David J., 375
Pol, Muktabai, 340
polio, 387, 392
positive psychology, 253, 255–256, 258,
  262, 264
Postal Clause (U.S. Constitution), 159
Post Office Act of 1872 (anti-obscenity
  statute), 158–159
Powell, Lynda, 205, 228–229
pox outbreak (1490s), 385
Pragathi Nidhi (Indian term for
  microfinance), 328
"Praise God from Whom All Blessings
  Flow," 66
prayer: Alzheimer's Disease and, 400; in
  Buddhism, 31; circumcision and, 87;
  The Eucharist and, 59–60; healing
  and, xii, 67, 350, 375–376;
  international data on, 281; in Islam,
  79–80, 209, 211; mental health and,
  254; religious rituals and, 211
preconception genetic carrier screening,
  194–195
pre-implantation genetic diagnosis (PGD),
  194
prenatal care, 187–188
prenatal screening and diagnosis, 192–195
Presbyterian Church: abortion and, 189,
  192; contraception and, 182;
  household income levels among U.S.
  members of, 18
Presbyterian Church (USA), 16
Presidents' Emergency Plan for AIDS
  Relief (PEPFAR), 276–278, 344
Presidents' Malaria Initiative, 276
Price, George, 143
Primitive Physick (Wesley), 109–110,
  113–114, 117, 120, 122–123,
  125–128, 271
privacy doctrine, 164–165
Prohibition Era (United States), 146
Project FAITH, 372
Prophet Muhammad, 79–80, 179, 193
Protestantism. *See also specific*
  denominations: abortion and, 191;
  colonial-era missionary activity and,

287; congregational hymn singing in,
  65–67; contraception and, 186–187,
  218; fundamentalism and, 147–149,
  154–157, 186–187; individual
  salvation emphasis in, 144–145, 147;
  Social Gospel movement and, xiv, 110,
  134–144, 148–149; suicide and, 238;
  temperance movement in the United
  States and, 145–146; tract societies
  and, 110
Provisional Integration Team, 347
Psalm 91, 100–101
Psalms, 63
puberty: beginning of Ramadan fasting
  during, 77–78; impact on an
  individual's health over the life course
  of, 207–208; religious rites marking,
  91–95, 208, 214
public health. *See also* global health
  movement; mental health; reproductive
  health: Comstock Law's overall impact
  on, 169, 171; definition of, 3; ethics
  and, 410–411; Griscom on the origins
  of, 135; Hartley's research on milk as
  a disease vector and, 137–138; in
  nineteenth-century New York City,
  134–135, 137–142, 149, 156;
  Protestant fundamentalism and, 149;
  religion as social determinant of,
  ix–xvi, 3–7, 9, 13–14, 16–17, 19–20,
  25–26, 110, 154, 156–157, 170–171,
  175–188, 191–197, 203–205,
  209–210, 212–217, 222–233, 251,
  253–256, 258–259, 261–263,
  271–273, 282–284, 360–361,
  375–377, 384, 386–387, 389–393,
  408–410, 412–418; religious
  organizations' role in promoting, 2–3,
  109, 113–119, 121–122, 128–129,
  133–144, 148–150, 180, 270,
  277–278, 288, 319–341, 344–361,
  365–367, 371–373, 382–393,
  408–410, 416–417; Social Gospel
  movement and, xiv, 110, 134–144,
  148–149; spiritual aspects of wellness
  and, 106–107
Public Health Service Act of 1970, 167

Sabbath: Hartley on the importance of preserving, 138; in Judaism, 209, 240; Seventh-day Adventist (SDA) Church and, 49, 52

Sacks, Oliver, 63

sacred harp singing, 64

"Sahar" (pseudonym), 45–46

Saint Christopher's Hospice (London), 337

Saint Joseph's Hospital and Medical Center (Phoenix, Arizona), 191–192

Saint Mary's Cathedral (Memphis, Tennessee), 386

Saint Paul, 138

Saint Vincent's Hospital (New York City), 371

salvation: baptism and, 99; L'Arche communities focus on, 335; Seventh-day Adventist Church emphasis on, 52; Social Gospel movement and questions of, 143–144; Tübingen I Conference (1964) on, 300–303, 305, 307–309; Wesley on, 115, 118–119, 121

Sampoorna Suraksha, 327

San Francisco (California), 371

Sanger, Margaret, 163, 168

Sanger case, 163

Sangha (spiritual community in Buddhism), 31, 33–35

The Sanitary Conditions of the Laboring Population of New York (Griscom), 140–142

sanitation: Dhaka Ahsania Mission's efforts to improve, 330, 332, 337; mass gatherings' impact on, 6; public health and, 3, 278, 282, 327; Shri Kshetra Dharmasthala Rural Development Programme (SKDRDP) and, 327, 338

sannyasi (Hindu recognition of asceticism), 234

sanskaras (Hindu sacraments), 103

Santa Cruz (Brazil), 97–101

Santa Cruz (documentary film), 97

Satcher, David, 8

Sati (tradition of funeral burning of widows in Hinduism), 105

Saunders, Cicely, 235, 337

Save the Children, 284

Schad v. Mount Ephraim, 166

Schnall, Eliezer, 225, 227–228, 232

Schoenbach, V. J., 226

Schuylkill County VISION, 389

Schweitzer, Albert, 288–289

scientism, 350

Scopes Monkey Trial (1925), 147–148, 152n37

secondary prevention, 282, 372

Second Ebenezer Baptist Church (Detroit, Michigan), 382

Second Presbyterian Church (Carlisle, Pennsylvania), 1, 4, 16

"secular spirituality" (Dalai Lama), 256, 258

selective primary health care (SPHC), 312–313

Sen, Amartya, 8, 340

"sensible regimen" (Wesley), 113, 121–126

Senturias, Erlinda, 303, 307

Service Availability and Readiness Assessment tool (SARA), 353, 355, 357

Seux, Philippe, 333–334

Seventh-day Adventist (SDA) Church: abortion and, 189; contraception and, 182; health research regarding, 53; Hispanic members of, 49; infant health in, 212; in Norway, 212, 224; physical health emphasis in, 49; prohibition against alcohol in, 51–52; regulation of personal behavior and, 5; Sabbath and, 49, 52; salvation emphasis in, 52; standard mortality ratios among, 222–224; vegetarianism in, 49–53

Seventh Day Adventists, morbidity rates among, 228

sex. *See also* contraception; family planning; fertility; reproductive health: during adolescence, 215, 218–219; Comstock's fears regarding, 157–158, 160; HIV/AIDS and, 370, 376; obscenity and, 165–166; oral sex, 218; Ramadan abstentions from, 77, 79; religion and, 181, 204, 218–219

Society for the Prevention of Pauperism, 136

"Sometimes I Feel Like a Motherless Child," 66

South Africa, 373

Southern Baptist Church, 182, 189, 218

Southern Baptist Convention, 391

Spanish influenza epidemic (1918), 384–385

sperm donation, 196

spirituality: among HIV/AIDS victims, 374–376; ethical spirituality and, 257–258, 261–264; mental health and, 253–259, 261–264; "secular spirituality" (Dalai Lama) and, 256, 258

standardized mortality ratios (SMRs), 222–223, 237

Stanley v. Georgia, 165, 173n47

"Statement on the Christian Concept of the Healing Ministry of the Church," 299–300

Steele, Richard, 125

Stenberg v. Carhart, 163

sterilization, 183–184, 186

Stokols, Daniel, 346

Strawbridge, W.J., 231–232

stroke, 366

Stuetzle, Rick, 375

Subramanian, S.V., 7

subsidiarity, 271, 307, 311, 339

Sufism, 79

suicide: among adolescents, 214–215; among the elderly, 238; *anomie* and, 5; Durkheim on, 3–6, 215, 238; in Japan, 260; religiosity and, 214–215, 238, 375; social determinants and, 4, 10, 215, 238

Sunni Muslims, 284

surrogacy, 196

Taiji (T'ai-chi): balance in, 39–41; compared to *vipassana,* 40; compared to yoga, 39, 41; *Daodejing (Tao Te Ching)* on, 41; health research regarding, 42; *jingli* (obeisance) and, 38; martial arts roots of, 40–41; push hands exercise in, 41; *qi (ch'i)* and, 39–40; Twenty-Four Form maneuvers in, 39–40; Yang-style series in, 39

The Talmud, 90n1, 185, 191

Tanzania, 280, 285, 304

Taoism: contraception and, 183; Taiji (T'ai-chi) and, 38–41

Tarakeshwar, Nalini, 375

Tay-Sachs disease, 22n39, 194–195, 338

Teinonen, Timo, 225

Tekpete stone, 92–94

temizuya (Shinto shrine font), 71

temperance movement, 145–146

Temple, William, 349

thalassemia, 195

Thoresen, Carl, 228

Three Precious and Sublime Jewels of Buddhism, 31, 33–35

timing of death, 240

Title X (Public Health Service Act in 1970), 167

tobacco. *See* cigarettes

Tomatis, Alfred, 64–65

Tompson, Marian, 320

Tontonoz, Matthew, 147

torii (Shinto shrine archway), 71

toshikomori (welcoming new year's spirits in Shintoism), 73

traditional healers in Africa, 281–284

transgender population, 260

Trinidad, 216

Trosly-Breuil (France), 333–335, 337

tuberculosis (TB), 124, 275, 386, 415

Tübingen I Conference (1964): on Christian medical missions, 299–305, 307; on salvation and health, 300–303, 305, 307–309; Statement on the Christian Concept of the Healing Ministry of the Church and, 299–300

Tübingen II Conference (1967): on assumptions of Western medicine and, 306–308; on Christian medical missions, 305–307; on health care access issues, 305; on holistic health, 307–308

Tutu, Desmond, 298–299, 315

117; on importance of fresh air, 123–125; London medical clinic for the poor of, 113–114, 119–120, 127; medical care for the poor and, 118–120; medical training of, 116–117; Methodist movement and, 109, 114–116, 119–121, 128; on personal cleanliness, 125, 128; "practical holiness" emphasis of, 115; "sensible regimen" and preventive health care emphasis of, 113, 121–126; on sleep, 125–126

West, Dan, 323–324, 337

"What Is Man?" (Wesley), 124

White, Ellen, 52

White, Helen G., 50–52

White, Mary, 320

Whitehall Studies, 10

Whitehead, Henry, 8, 109–111, 128, 351–352

White House Office of Faith-Based and Neighborhood Partnership, 383–384

Who Shall Live? (Fuchs), 203–204, 206, 210, 214, 236

Wilkinson, Richard, 11, 14, 16, 278–279

Williams, George, 337

Willoughby, Brian, 255–256

Winslow, Charles-Edward Amory, 3

Women's Health Initiative Study, 225, 227, 232

Woodhull, Victoria, 158–159

The Woodhull and Claflin Weekly, 158

World Bank, 276, 278

World Council of Churches (WCC): Christian Medical Commission (CMC) and, xv, 269–270, 298–299, 309–310, 313, 345; Committee for Specialized Assistance to Social Projects, 305; Division of Inter-Church Aid, Refugee, and World Service, 309–310; Division of World Mission and Evangelism in, 299, 309

World Health Organization (WHO): African Religious Health Assets Programme (ARHAP) and, 271, 344–346, 348, 351, 353–354, 356; Alma-Ata Declaration on Primary Health Care and, 270, 299, 311–314, 345, 349; Christian Medical Commission and, xv, 269, 298–299, 312, 314, 345, 409; Commission on the Social Determinants of Health (CSDH) and, x, 8–9, 12, 20, 205, 415; definition of health by, 348, 412; definition of health systems by, 409; global health movement and, 274; *Health by the People* report and, 345; HealthMapper GIS database and, 353, 355, 357; primary health care emphasis and, 314; religion as a complicating factor for, 344–345, 350; Service Availability and Readiness Assessment tool (SARA) and, 353, 355, 357; Tutu's plenary remarks to (2008), 298–299, 315; WHO Action Programme on Essential Drugs and, 313; WHO Guidelines for Primary Health Care (1974) and, 299; World Health Assembly (governing body of WHO), 298, 311, 315

World Vision, 285

Wynder, Ernest L., 228

Yeager, D.M., 225, 227

Yebamoth 69b (section of *The Talmud*), 191

yellow fever, 135, 282, 386

yoga, 39, 41, 263–264

Yom Kippur, 240

Young Christian Workers, 322

Young Men's Christian Association (YMCA), 157–159, 336–337

Your Blessed Health, 372

Youth with a Mission, 289

Zahniser, A. H. Mathias, 99, 101

zakaat (Islamic principle of charity), 332

Zambia, 271, 288, 351, 357

Zimbabwe Demographic and Health Survey, 219